Veterinary Clinical Pathology and Laboratory Diagnosis

NIPA® GENX ELECTRONIC RESOURCES & SOLUTIONS P. LTD.
New Delhi-110 034

Veterinary Clinical Pathology and Laboratory Diagnosis

R.S. Chauhan M.V.Sc., Ph.D. (Path.), FNAVS, FSIIP, FIAVP, PDCR, OCTT, ACPPM, MBA
(Ex- Advisor WHO, Ex- Director IVRI, Ex-JD-CADRAD, Ex-Director IBT
Ex- National Fellow ICAR)
Member Animal Welfare Board of India (Govt. of India)
Member, CCSEA (Govt of India)
Chairman, SAC, NARFBR (ICMR)
Professor, Department of Veterinary Pathology
GB Pant University of Agriculture & Technology
Pantnagar - 263 145, Uttarakhand, India

Desh Deepak Singh M.V.Sc., Ph.D.
Professor & Head
Department of Veterinary Pathology
Uttar Pradesh Pandit Deen Dayal Upadhyay Pashu Chikitsha Vigyan Vishwavidyalaya
Evam Go Anusandhan Sansthan (DUVASU)
Mathura-281001, Uttar Pradesh, India

NIPA® GENX ELECTRONIC RESOURCES & SOLUTIONS P. LTD.
New Delhi-110 034

NIPA. GENX ELECTRONIC
RESOURCES & SOLUTIONS P. LTD.

101,103, Vikas Surya Plaza, CU Block
L.S.C.Market, Pitam Pura, New Delhi-110 034
Ph. +91 11 27341616, 27341717, 27341718
E-mail: newindiapublishingagency@gmail.com
www: www.nipabooks.com

For customer assistance, please contact
Phone: + 91-11-27 34 17 17
Fax: + 91-11-27 34 16 16
E-Mail: feedbacks@nipabooks.com

Print ISBN: 978-93-58872-90-3

ebook ISBN: 978-93-58879-88-9

Composed and Designed by NIPA®.

Preface

The need of a suitable literature for students of Veterinary Sciences on disease investigation was felt since long. Many times it has been observed that Clinical Pathology and Laboratory Diagnosis requirements for disease investigation are required to be at one place so that the Veterinarians and disease investigation experts find it useful for their routine disease investigation work. The need of rapid and specific diagnostic tool(s) for detecting a wide variety of viral, bacterial, fungal, toxic, metabolic and parasitic diseases of animals has always been an area of considerable importance for clinicians. Many infectious diseases are diagnosed by isolating, growing and identifying the infectious agent from clinical specimens. These methods demand well equipped and well-staffed Pathological laboratories. Days to weeks are sometimes spent in arriving at an unambiguous diagnosis which lead into failure to meet the need for an early management of the disease by the clinician. Although isolation and identification of the micro-organism provides incontrovertible diagnosis and the disease but the rate of success is limited. Alternatively, methods detecting seroconversions to particular micro-organisms can be of great diagnostic importance. Laboratory based diagnosis of majority of infectious disease involve seroconversion has largely been depended on the assays using antigen-antibody reactions. Amongst the various immunodiagnostics tools enzyme immunoassay becomes increasingly popular for the detection of humoral immune response (seroconversion) or microbial antigens for the purpose of diagnosis. Besides, regulatory and safety requirements are given in this book for the first time in this book for Veterinary disease investigation. The field veterinarians will also find it useful in their day to day routine work of diagnosing the diseases, identification of the causative agents and thereby suggesting the effective therapeutic and preventive measure to contain the livestock and poultry diseases. The animals cannot speak their illness, it is the veterinarians who may apply his/her mind to identify the disease and its cause mainly based on the characteristic symptoms and macroscopic or microscopic lesions which are exhaustively presented in this book along with illustrations. More emphasis is given on rapid diagnosis of diseases on the basis of history, clinical manifestations, post mortem lesions based on my experiences of more than 40 years as disease investigation expert.

In a work of this magnitude, it is natural for the authors of a book to solicit help and cooperation from others. The most overwhelming enthusiasm, good will, love and affection have generously come from my students for which we shall remain always indebted to them. Lastly, in spite of our best efforts at perfection, element of human error is still likely to creep in which the readers are welcome to point out since that would help us in improving the text further.

R.S. Chauhan
D.D. Singh

Contents

1

Examination of Blood

- General considerations
- Collection of blood
- Storage
- Examination of blood
    - Coagulation time
    - Bleeding time
    - Determination of movement of parasites under wet film
    - Total erythrocyte count
    - Total leucocyte count
    - Differential leucocyte count
    - Hemoglobin
    - Erythrocyte sedimentation rate
    - Hematocrit value
    - Mean corpuscular volume
    - Mean corpuscular hemoglobin
    - Mean corpuscular hemoglobin concentration
    - Erythrocyte fragility test

General Considerations

Blood is red, slightly alkaline fluid and contains erythrocytes, leucocytes and platelets suspended in plasma. The amount of blood in the body of animals is given in Table 1.1. Blood travels in blood vessels, i.e. arteries, veins and capillaries through the pumping action of heart. The main functions of blood are:

1. It serves as a carrier of nutrients from the digestive tract to various tissues of the body.
2. It transports oxygen from lungs to tissues and carbon dioxide from tissues to lungs
3. It carries hormones from endocrine glands.
4. It maintains water balance in body.
5. It carries waste products to the kidneys for filtration.
6. It maintains temperature of body.
7. It plays an active role in defense of body.
8. It maintains the pH of body tissues.

Blood constitutes the cells and plasma; the cells are erythrocytes, leucocytes and platelets. Plasma contains fibrinogen, globulins and albumin. Besides, the plasma contains certain non-proteinous substances like amino acids, urea, glucose, fat, sodium, potassium, calcium, magnesium and phosphorus. The coagulated blood releases serum which is like plasma but it does not have fibrinogen.

Collection of Blood

The blood is collected from animals through puncture of vein using syringe and needle. In laboratory animals or poultry, however, it is collected directly from the heart. The sites of blood collection in different animal species are as under:

1.	Cattle and buffaloes	Jugular vein, ear vein
2.	Horse	Jugular vein
3.	Camel	Jugular vein
4.	Sheep	Jugular vein
5.	Goat	Jugular vein
6.	Pig	Ear vein, anterior vena cava
7.	Dog	Cephalic vein
		Recurrent tarsal vein.
8.	Poultry	Wing vein, Heart

Table 1.1: Amount of blood and specific gravity

Sr.No.	Species	Quantity of blood	Specific gravity
1	Cattle	7.71% of body wt.	1.060
2	Horse	6.60 % of body wt.	1.060
3	Pig	4.06 % of body wt.	1.060
4	Sheep	8.01 % of body wt.	1.050 -1.058
5	Goat	8.01 % of body wt.	1.050 -1.058
6	Dog	5.5- 9.1% of body wt.	1.050

Jugular Vein

The jugular vein is situated in the jugular groove, over the trachea and carotid artery on both sides of the neck. Before collection of blood, the hairs of the area are removed with the help of scissors and the area is shaved with razer. The antiseptics like spirit is applied over the area of vein puncture and the animal is properly restrained. The vein is raised by applying pressure at ventral point of puncture. The vein can be felt by finger tapping. Blood is collected by using a 16 gauge needle in large animals and 18 gauge needle in small animals. The needle is inserted in the vein by force in an angle; blood can be collected directly in the collection tube or by applying syringe over needle to suck the blood (Fig.1.1). After collection of blood, the pressure is released and needle is removed. Apply antiseptics at the site of vein puncture. In casted animals, the neck should be turned upwards as it helps in distention of vein for puncture.

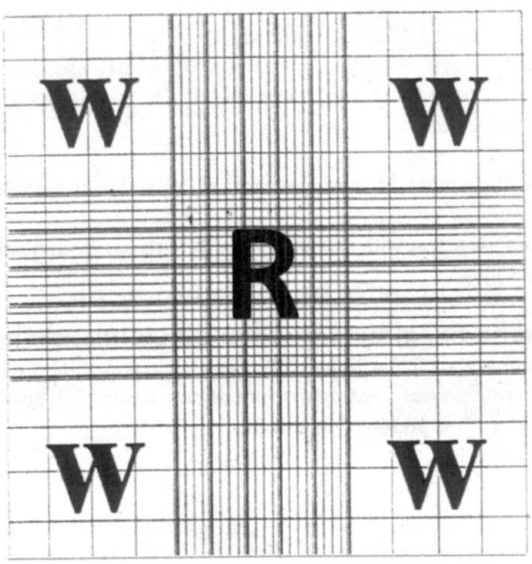

Fig. 1.1: Neubauer's chamber (W=Counting area for leucocytes; R= Counting area for erythrocytes)

Ear Vein

Small amounts of blood (1-2 ml) can be collected from ear vein. The area should be cleaned and shaved properly at the dorsal side of the ear. Antiseptics should be applied over the area. The vein is raised by applying pressure of thumb and index finger of left hand and blood is collected using a 20 or 22-gauge needle with syringe. After collection of blood, the pressure is released and the vein puncture site is rubbed with cotton dipped in spirit.

Anterior Venacava

The blood is collected from pigs through anterior vena cava. For this purpose the pig is placed on its back with extended neck and forelegs stretched backward against the chest. The area is shaved and antiseptic is applied to disinfect the skin. A 10-12 cm long needle of 18 gauge with syringe is inserted on a line between cariniform cartilage and base of ear about 4-5 cm anterior to the apex of cariniform cartilage. The needle is directed downwards and backwards between the first ribs and pushed till the blood appears in syringe. Collect the blood and remove syringe and needle and apply antiseptic over the area of puncture.

Cephalic Vein

The cephalic vein is situated in the anterior surface of the forelegs, from where hairs should be removed and the area is shaved. For proper disinfection, 70% alcohol spirit is applied over the area. Use a torniquet around the elbow to raise the vein. Vein is felt by finger tip and a needle of 20-22 gauge is inserted along with syringe. The needle should be in the right side of the vein and a clik like sound appears when the needle penetrates the vein. Collect blood in desired quantity and remove the torniquet, needle and syringe. Apply antiseptic at the site of puncture.

Recurrent Tarsal Vein

This vein is situated on the lateral side of the hock joint where it takes a round. The pressure should be applied over the stifle joint. The area must be cleaned, shaved and properly disinfected. The blood is collected with a 20 gauge needle with syringe. After collection of blood, pressure is released and needle is removed. The antiseptics are applied over the vein puncture area.

Poultry

In poultry, small amount of blood (1-2 ml) can be collected from wing vein. However, if more blood is required, it should be collected directly from the heart. The wings are extended and the area should be cleaned. Feather or fluffs are removed from the site and then the vein is raised by applying pressure at the root of wing. The needle (20 gauge) is inserted in the vein and blood is collected slowly. Remove the pressure, before withdrawal of needle and apply proper disinfectant at vein puncture site.

For the heart puncture, the bird is placed on its back with extended neck and wings against the chest. The needle (20 gauge) along with syringe is applied from dorsal side in the groove of neck and the needle is directed forward in slightly raised position. When it punctures the heart, blood comes out in the syringe. Collect the desired quantity of blood and remove the needle. Apply proper disinfectant on the area of needle puncture.

Some scientists have used the jugular vein for collection of blood in birds. The neck is cleaned and fluffs are removed and the area is properly disinfected. The head of the bird is held at its base between fore and middle fingers and then with the help of the thumb the jugular vein is so placed that it rests on the ridge or the solid background of cervical vertebrae. The needle is inserted into the vein and collect the blood in syringe. After collection of blood, remove the needle and syringe and apply disinfectant at the site of vein puncture.

After the collection of blood from animal, the needle is removed from syringe and the blood is slowly transferred to the collection tube in order to avoid the breakage of erythrocytes and formation of hemolysis.

Storage

The blood has tendency to clot outside the body. To store the blood sample for analysis, it is necessary to mix a proper anticoagulant which prevents coagulation of blood. A number of anticoagulants are used in hematological studies. It should be mixed slowly and gently to avoid hemolysis. The collection vials should be shaked by rotating in between the palms for proper mixing of the anticoagulant. Vigorous shaking should be avoided as it may lead to hemolysis and production of foam.

It is always advisable to start the examination of blood soon after its collection. But if delay is expected, the blood samples must be kept in refrigerator at 40C for 24 hours without much alterations. The refrigerated blood samples should be taken out at least 30 min before the start of examination and the sample should be mixed properly by gently shaking it. The routinely used anticoagulants and their dose are described in Table 1.2

Table 1.2: Anticoagulants

Sr.No.	Anticoagulants	Dose per 10 ml blood
1	Lithium oxalate	10-15 mg
2	Potassium oxalate	20 mg
3	Sodium oxalate	20 mg
4	Sodium fluoride	40 mg
5	Lithium citrate	30 mg
6	Sodium citrate	60 mg
7	Heparin	Few drops of 1% solution
8	EDTA	20 mg
9	Ammonium oxalate	1.2%
	Potassium oxalate	0.8% in -1 ml

Examination of Blood

Coagulation Time

To determine the coagulation time, fresh blood should be used immediately after its collection and without addition of any anticoagulant. The coagulation time is determined by one of the following methods.

1. *Capillary tube method:* In this method the microhematocrit capillaries having 0.5 to 1 mm diameter and 8-10 cm length can be used. The blood is directly taken from the puncture of ear vein/wing vein into the capillary, in which the blood is filled by capillary action. The time should be noted when blood comes out from vein. Keep the capillaries at room temperature and break the capillaries at an interval of 30 sec until the strands of fibrin are seen across the gap between ends of tube. The coagulation time is the time interval between appearance of blood from vein and appearance of fibrin strand in capillary break ends.

2. *Lee-white method:* The blood is collected by sterile syringe and needle. The time should be recorded at the first appearance of blood in syringe. Air should not be allowed to enter with blood, which may affect the coagulation time. The needle is removed from syringe and 1 ml of blood is kept in each of three tubes (8 mm diameter, 7.5 cm length) Prior to placing the blood in tubes, the tubes are thoroughly cleaned and siliconized or rinsed with normal saline solution and maintained in water bath at 37°C. These tubes are tilted at 30 sec interval and the record time of coagulation of blood in all three tubes to calculate the average clotting time. Complete clotting can be observed by inverting the tube without spilling its contents.

Normal coagulation time in different species of animal is given in Table 1.3.

Table 1.3: Normal coagulation time in different species of animals

Sr.No.	Species	Time in min Lee-white method	Time in min Capillary method
1	Cattle & Buffaloes	4-15	3-15
2	Sheep	4-8	1-6
3	Goat	-	2.5-4.5
4	Horse	4-15	3-15
5	Pig	6.2	4
6	Dog	6-7.5	4

3. *Slide method:* In this method two drops of fresh blood are taken on a clean, dry glass slide and with the help of a pin, the presence of fibrin strands is checked after every 30 sec. Time gap between blood appearance in syringe and appearance of fibrin strand on slide is the coagulation time.
4. *Glass bead method:* In a watch glass containing glass beads, take 2-3 drops of fresh blood collected from animal and move the watch glass to see the movements of glass beads. The movements of glass beads stop indicating the coagulation; note the time. The time of coagulation is difference between the first appearance of blood in syringe and restriction of the movement of glass beads.

The coagulation time increases in following blood disorders:

a. Hemophilia
b. Idiopathic thrombocytopenic purpura
c. Infectious canine hepatitis
d. Warferrin poisoning.

Bleeding Time

The skin of animal is cleaned and antiseptic is applied, and the area dried. Make a deep puncture with blade. The time should be noted when blood first appears. The drop of blood is carefully removed after a gap of 30 sec without touching the skin. When blood stops and there is no drop of blood then the time should be noted. The time interval between these two is the bleeding time. Normally it varies from 1 to 5 min in all domestic animals.

Determination of Movements of Parasites Under Wet Film

The wet film of blood is examined for the demonstration of movements of microfilaria or trypanosomes. For this a drop of fresh or anticoagulant added blood is placed over a clean and dry slide. It is covered with a cover slip and examined under microscope. The parasites are seen moving in between the erythrocytes. The trypanosomes are recognized by their swirling movements. These parasites can also be demonstrated by lysis of blood using saponin. In this method, 2 ml of blood and 2 ml of 2% saponin is mixed and centrifuged. The erythrocytes get hemolysed and the parasites are settled down in sediment. Examine a drop of sediment under microscope for the movements of parasites. In an another method, the hematocrit capillary is filled with blood and sealed at one end with plasticin/clay. It is centrifuged at 1000 rpm for 5 min and cut at cell fluid interphase. Make a wet film from plasma just over the buffy coat for demonstration of the movements of parasites.

Total Erythrocyte Count

The erythrocytes constitute 32% of the total amount of blood. Under microscope their shape is recognized as biconcave, circular disc and they do not possess nucleus, However, the erythrocytes of birds are nucleated. In camels, its shape is oval and outline is convex. The erythrocytes are soft, flexible and have elastic envelops containing hemoglobin.

Total erythrocyte count is determined by using hemocytometer. First of all, one should clean the Neubauer's counting chamber and put the coverslip on the area demarcated for counting, i.e. ruled area. Using the RBC diluting pipette suck the fresh or anticoagulant added blood up to 0.5 mark and fill the pipette with RBC diluting fluid up to 101 mark and hold the pipette in horizontal position quickly. Remove the rubber tubing from the pipette and mix the contents for one minute by rotating the pipette in between the palms keeping the pipette in horizontal position. Discard first few drops from pipette and then place a drop near the edge of the coverslip on the platform of the counting chamber. One should be careful that the space between coverslip and counting chamber is filled properly. If there is overflowing or presence of air bubble is detected, then discard the specimen and repeat the process. Keep the counting chamber for 1-2 min, for settling of the cells and then start counting under high power of the light microscope. Cells are counted in the five medium squares of the central large squares or the 80 tertiary squares. Cells on the top line of squares and the left side are included in count while that of right side and bottom line are excluded from the counting. To get the cells per cumm multiply with 10,000 to the total number of cells counted in 80 tertiary squares (Fig.1.2).

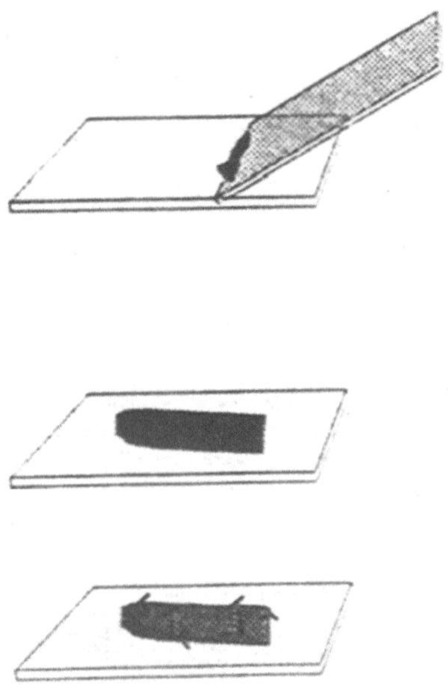

Fig. 1.2: Smear preparation for differential leucocyte count

Precautions

1. Always use clean and dry glass ware in all the processing, including pipette, counting chamber, etc.
2. In case of overfilling of pipette with blood, touch the tip with finger tip to take out the extra blood.
3. Keep one finger on the opening of pipette while removing the rubber tube in order to prevent any loss of fluid or cells.
4. The count of cells should not vary more than 10% among the squares. If it so happens, then discard this and fill the chamber again by repeating the whole process.
5. The RBC diluting pipette should be checked before use. It should have a red bulb which rotates on movement of pipette. If it is fixed, then wash the pipette properly, dry it and use again.

Interpretation

1. Increased total erythrocyte count (erythrocytosis) is reported in following conditions.

Dehydration, hemoconcentration, exercise, occlusion of vein for a longer period, brucellosis, campylobacteriosis, leptospirosis, rinderpest, pasteurellosis, acute poisoning, chronic heart disease, pulmonary fibrosis, shock, vomiting, diarrhoea, hypoxia.

2. Decreased total erythrocytic count (erythropenia) occurs in following conditions:

Anemia, anaplasmosis, babesiosis, leptospirosis, copper, lead and phenothiazine poisoning, equine infectious anemia, defective blood formation, leukemia, hemorrhage, aflatoxicosis, coccidiosis, fasciolosis.

Total Leucocyte Count

1. *Animals:* The total leucocyte count is performed by hemocytometer using a WBC diluting pipette. The blood is sucked in pipette up to 0.5 mark and then WBC diluting fluid, as in case of total erythrocyte count, up to 11 mark. Remove the rubber tubing, keeping the pipette in horizontal position. Mix the contents of pipette by rotating the pipette between the palms and discard the first few drops. Fill the space in between coverslip and counting chamber and wait for 1-2 min for settling of cells. Put the counting chamber under microscope and count the cells in four large corner squares of the ruled area under low power. Calculate the total leucocytes per cumm of blood by multiplying 50 with the count.
2. *Poultry:* For total leucocyte count in poultry, the diluting pipette of erythrocytes is used because of high leucocytic count. Like total erythrocytic count, fill the RBC diluting pipette up to mark 0.5 and fill it with "WBC diluting fluid-poultry" up to mark 101. Remove the rubber tubing and mix the contents, discard a few drops of contents and fill the counting chamber as described earlier. After 1-2 min, count the cells under low power/high power in four corner primary squares of the counting chamber and calculate the number of cells by multiply by 500 to get total leucocyte count per cumm of blood.

Precautions

All necessary precautions should be taken as described in total erythrocyte count.

Interpretation

1. Leucopenia: Leucopenia is the decrease in total leucocyte count and is observed in following conditions:

Canine distemper, infectious canine hepatitis, feline panleukopenia, mucosal disease, hog cholera, swine influenza, chronic intoxication of lead, bismuth, arsenic, mercury, pesticides, prolonged antibiotic therapy, rinderpest, bovine malignant catarrh, extreme debility and loss of resistance, exposure of X-rays, salmonellosis, toxoplasmosis, PPR, brucellosis, chlamydiosis, leishmaniosis, tuberculosis, blue tongue, lymphosarcoma, hepatic cirrhosis, mastitis, copper deficiency, aflatoxicosis, BHV-1 infection, bracken fern poisoning.

2. Leucocytosis: Leucocytosis is the increase in number of leucocytes and is observed in following disease conditions.

Pasteurellosis, leptospirosis, salmonellosis, local infection of *streptococci, staphylococci,* and *corynebacterium*, uremia, diabetes, gout, malignancy, viral infections, rabies, histoplasmosis, tuberculosis, strangles, blood protozoan infections, colibacillosis, chronic enteritis, bovine, immunodeficiency syndrome, acidosis, burn, gangrene, leukemia.

Following are some factors which affect the total leucocytic counts

a.	Age:	TLC high at birth in pups, calves
		TLC low at birth in piglets
b.	Species:	Bovines have more lymphocytic count while canines have more neutrophilic count.
c.	Excitement:	Excitement causes an increase in TLC.
d.	Pregnancy:	During pregnancy total leucocyte count increases.
e.	Estrus:	During estrus TLC increases.
f.	Digestion:	In dogs and pigs after eating food, there is increase in total leucocyte count and neutrophilic count.

Differential Leucocyte Count

For differential leucocyte count, a thin blood smear is prepared on glass slide. A drop of fresh or anticoagulant mixed blood is placed on one corner/end of slide and spread as smear with the help of another slide using its thin edge at an angle of 45^0. Smear should be uniform and thin and it should not have any air bubble (Fig.1.3). Dry the smear in air and mark the identification number in the thick portion of the smear. Thereafter fix the smear in methanol for 5 min and dry in air. Stain the smear with Giemsa stain diluted to 1:10 in distilled water for 30 min. Wash the slides, dry in air and examine under oil immersion of the microscope. Count at least 200 cells by battlement/zigzag method. Cells counted are neutrophils, lymphocytes, eosinophils, monocytes and basophils (Fig.1.4). The cell count is presented in percent.

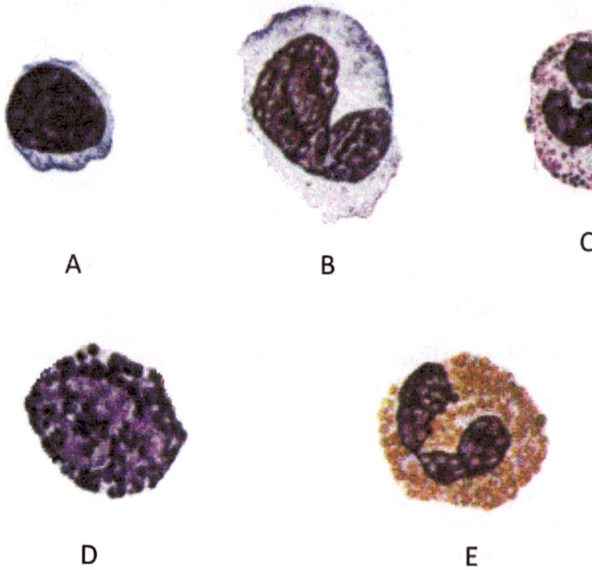

Fig. 1.3: White blood cells (A. Lymphocyte, B. Monocyte, C. Neutrophil, D. Basophil, and E. Eosinophil)

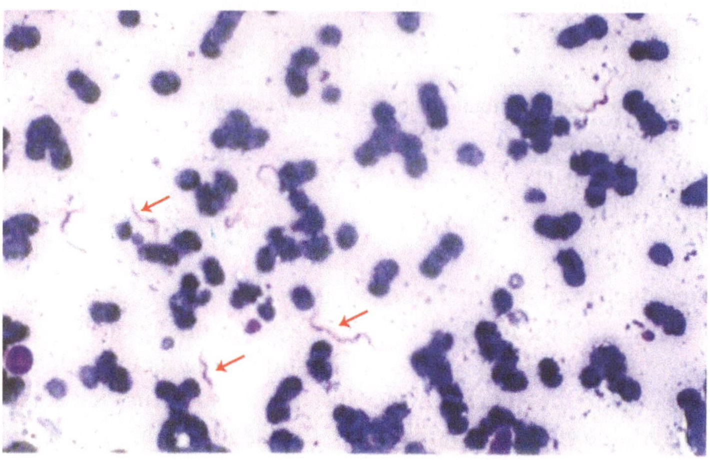

Fig. 1.4: Blood smear examination-Trypanosomes Fig. 1.1. Neubauer's chamber (W=Counting area for leucocytes; R= Counting area for erythrocytes)zz

Interpretation

a. *Lymphocytosis:* Increased number of lymphocytes is observed in viral infections, tuberculosis, brucellosis, hypothyroidism, following vaccination, Leukemia, Adreno-cortico insufficiency etc.

b. *Lymphopenia:* Decrease number of lymphocytes is observed in canine distemper, infectious canine hepatitis, corticosteroid therapy, hypothyroidism, BHV-1 infection, Q-fever, foot and mouth disease, mucosal disease etc.

c. *Neutrophilia:* Increased number of neutrophils is observed in septicemic diseases, uremia, gout, coronary thrombosis, pyogenic infections, acute inflammation, cancer, arthritis, pyometra, post-surgical operation, coronary thrombosis, pregnancy, calf diphtheria, rheumatic fever etc.

d. *Neutrophilia (Shift to left):* Increased number of neutrophils with immature cells is observed in leptospirosis, traumatic reticulopericarditis (TRP), metritis, canine distemper, glanders, endocarditis, synovitis etc.

e. *Neutropenia:* Decrease number of neutrophils is observed in pasteurellosis, bovine viral diarrhoea, infectious canine hepatitis etc.

f. *Eosinophilia:* Increase number of eosinophils is observed in allergy, parasitic infections, skin disease, anaphylactic reactions, convalescence, eosinophilic myositis and granulocytic eosinophilic leukemia.

g. *Basophilia:* Inverse in number of basophils is observed in Pox infections, sinusitis, splenectomy, cirrhosis, Hodgkin's disease, introduction of foreign protein.

h. *Monocytosis:* Increase in number of monocytes is observed in tuberculosis, brucellosis, trypanosomiasis, convalescence, monocytic leukemia, carbon tetrachloride poisoning.

The blood smear, at the time of differential leucocyte count, should also be examined for the presence of intracellular and extracellular blood protozoan parasites like *Trypanosomes* (Fig.1.5), *Theileria, Babesia,* and *Anaplasma.* So care must be taken to examine the erythrocytes also besides leucocytes.

Hemoglobin

It is measured by using Hellige- Sahli hemoglobinometer. Clean and dry the graduated tube of the hemoglobinometer. Take 5 drops of N/10 Hydrochloric acid in tube. Suck the anticoagulant mixed blood in pipette upto 20 marks. Place the pipette in tube containing N/10 HCL and transfer the blood into acid. Suck acid in pipette and leave in tube. Keep the tube for 5 min in dark. Add distilled water in the tube drop-by-drop using dropper, mix with stirring rod and match the colour with standard. Add water till the colour matches with standard. Read the scale on tube; it is the value of hemoglobin gram per 100 ml of blood.

Hyperhemoglobinemia: Increase in hemoglobin is observed in polycythemia, dehydration, leptospirosis, equine influenza, acid indigestion.

Hypohemoglobinemia: Decreased in hemoglobin content is observed in anemia, theileriosis, strangles, anaplasmosis, Degnala disease, fasciolosis.

Erythrocyte Sedimentation Rate

The erythrocyte sedimentation rate (ESR) is measured by using Westergren pipette. Suck the anticoagulant mixed blood in Westergren pipette upto mark 'O' and fix it in stand in vertical position. Leave this for one hour at room temperature. After one hr record the reading on graduated pipette, it is the mm fall of erythrocytes per hour. Care should be taken that there should not be any air bubble in the pipette. Pipette should be filled exactly to 'o' mark. ESR should be performed within one hour of blood collection.

The values of ESR are increased in tuberculosis, carcinoma, nephritis, gout, heavy metal toxicity, rheumatoid arthritis, pleurisy, canine distemper, pyometra., pericarditis, peritonitis, leptospirosis, filariasis, pneumonia, fracture, trypanosomiasis, equine infectious anemia and parasitic diseases.

Decreased erythrocyte sedimentation rate has been recorded in hemolytic jaundice, sickle cell anemia and in brucellosis.

Hematocrit Value

It is also known as packed cell volume. It can be determined by two methods.

1. *Macromethod:* In this method Wintrobe tube is used. With the help of a long needle and syringe, fill the Wintrobe tube with blood up to mark 100. Centrifuge the tubes at 3000 rpm for exactly 30 min. Record the reading of packed cell volume in percent, i.e. mass of erythrocytes settled down in tube.

2. *Micromethod:* In this method microcapillaries of 1.0 mm diameter and 7-8 cm length are used. The capillaries are filled with blood by capillary action from collection vial. Seal one end of capillary with plasticin and centrifuge in microcentrifuge for 5 min. Remove the capillaries and put them on reader scale to calculate hematocrit value.

Increased hematocrit value: Dehydration, ketosis, leptospirosis, rotavirus infection, influenza, rinderpest.

Decreased hematocrit value: Anemia, parasitic infection, muscular dystrophy, gestation, lactation, theileriosis, strangles, anaplasmosis, blue tongue, endocarditis.

Mean Corpuscular Volume (MCV)

MCV is calculated using following formula:

$$MCV\ in\ cubic\ micron\ =\ \frac{PCV \times 10}{RBC\ inmillions\ /\ cumm}$$

Mean Corpuscular Hemoglobin (MCH)

Mean corpuscular hemoglobin is calculated by using following equation:

$$MCH\ in\ micro\ micro\ grams = \frac{Hemoglobin\ gm\ x\ MCH\ in\ micro\ micro\ grams}{RBC\ count\ in\ million\ cumm}$$

Mean Corpuscular Hemoglobin Concentration (MCHC)

MCHC is calculated using following formula:

$$MCHC\ in\ percent = \frac{Hemoglobin\ gm\%x10}{PCV\ \ in\ percent}$$

Erythrocyte Fragility Test

In this test, the fragility of erythrocytes is tested by using distilled water. For this test a series of 16 test tubes (3") are kept in a rack. In tube 1, 0.6 ml of normal saline solution (NSS) and 0.4 ml distilled water is placed in tube 2, 0.58 ml NSS and 0.42 ml distilled water is placed and by decreasing 0.02 ml NSS and increasing 0.02 ml distilled water in each tube, one should keep in 16th tube 0.3 ml NSS and 0.7 ml distilled water. Thereafter, add one drop of freshly collected blood in each tube and place the rack along with all tubes at 37^{0}C for 2 hours. Record the NSS concentration at which the complete hemolysis occurs. Care should be taken to keep a row of tube for control blood sample derived from a normal animal. In complete hemolysis, there will not be any button in bottom. If there is no hemolysis, the RBC will accumulate in the bottom to form a button. This test is very useful in such conditions, where the membranes of erythrocyte become weak resulting into hemolysis. Normal hematological values in domestic animals are given in Table 1.4.

Table 1.4. Normal hematological values in domestic animals

Sr. No.	Species	TEC in million /fl	TLC in Thousand/ pl	PCV%	ESR mm/ 30 min	Hb gm%	MCV Cμ	MCH μmg	MCHC %	Differential leucocyte count				
										Lymphocytes	Neutrophils	Eosinophils	Monocytes	Basophils
1	Cattle	5-8	5.6-9.25	26-42	0	8-14	40-60	11-17	26-34	48-75	15-45	2-15	2-7	0-2
2	Sheep	8-15	5.5-9.2	24-49	0	8-16	23-48	9-12	29-35	40-75	10-50	1-8	1-5	0-3
3	Goat	8-17.5	12.0	20-38	0	8-14	19-37	5-7	30-35	50-70	30-48	3-8	1-4	0-2
4	Horse	7-13	8.2-9.2	32-52	20-40	11-18	34-58	12-18	31-37	15-50	35-75	1-10	2-10	0-3
5	Pig	5-8	11-22	32-50	0-6	10-16	32-50	50-67	30-34	39-60	28-47	1-11	2-10	0-2
6	Dog	6-9	8.2-13.5	37-54	1-6	12-18	60-77	19-25	31-34	12-30	60-75	2-10	3-9	0-1
7	Cat	5-10	8.0-25.0	24-45	1-6	8-15	39-55	13-17	31-34	20-55	35-75	2-10	1-4	0-1
8	Poultry	3-4	29-39	-	-	9-13	-	-	-	76	13	3	6	2

2

Examination of Blood and Serum for Biochemical Attributes

- General considerations
- Blood glucose
- Total serum protein
- Serum albumin
- Serum globulin
- Serum gamma globulin
- Serum calcium
- Serum inorganic phosphorus
- Serum magnesium
- Serum cholesterol
- Serum creatinine
- Serum urea
- Serum chloride
- Serum sodium
- Serum potassium
- Serum Glutamic Oxaloacetic Transaminase
- Serum Glutamic Pyruvic Transaminase
- Serum alkaline phosphatase

General Considerations

Blood chemistry is considered quite sensitive indicator of the diseases of animals. The chemical constituents of blood with other laboratory procedures and history of illness of animals may guide for a final diagnosis and helpful in evaluation of prognosis. In veterinary sciences, the chemical examinations of blood/plasma/serum are not routinely used. However, their significance is unequivocal. The diagnostic significance of some of the important blood chemistry parameters is given in detail for the benefit of readers. Now a days the use of kits for estimation of biochemical attributes is very much in practice in veterinary sciences but the traditional methods have their own significance. Besides, the cost of test becomes very high with the use of kits so these procedures are economical also.

The method for collection of blood and types of anticoagulants are described elsewhere. Most of the biochemical attributes can be determined by using serum; for which the blood should be collected directly in sterile tubes sufficient in quantity to 4-5 ml serum. The serum, after separation from blood clots, is stored at –100C till examination. It should be kept in mind that give the biochemical attributes should be performed from serum as early as possible after its collection.

Blood Glucose

Indications

The blood glucose examination is performed in animals suspected for diabetes mellitus or convulsions, such as in hunting dogs who show fatigue, in sheep and cattle suspected for ketosis and young chicks suspected for hypoglycemia associated with starvation. In animals suspected for pancreatitis, the glucose examination in blood is indicated. In aged animals, it is performed as routine check up.

Procedure

1. In a clean, dry centrifuge tube, take 3.4 ml distilled water and 0.2 ml blood (sodium fluoride used as anticoagulant). Add
2. 0.2 ml/3 N sulfuric acid and mix well.
3. Add 0.2 ml 10% sodium tungstate solution slowly with constant agitation in tube, mix properly and keep the tube on stand for 5 min.
4. Centrifuge the tube at 2000-3000 rpm in a clinical centrifuge and take out the supernatant.
5. Take 4 Wu sugar tubes and mark them as T for test, S_1 and S_2, for standard and B for blank. In tube T place 1 ml of supernatant as produced in step 3. In tubes S_1 and S_2, place 1 ml standard in each containing 0.1 mg/ml and 0.2 mg/ml; these can be prepared by dissolving 10 mg and 20 mg

glucose in 100 ml saturated benzoic acid solutions, respectively. The 0.1 mg/ml and 0.2 mg/ml standard are equivalent to 200 mg/100 ml and 400 mg/100 ml blood glucose level.

6. Add 1 ml distilled water to each tube and mix well. Take 2 ml distilled water in tube 'B'.
7. Add 2 ml alkaline copper sulfate in each tube and mix; place the tubes in boiling water bath for 8 min.
8. Cool the tubes in running tap water for 2-3 min and add 2 ml phosphomolybdic acid solution to each tube, mix properly and place in boiling water bath for 2 min.
9. Cool the tubes in running tap water and keep them on stand for 3-5 min and then dilute to 25 ml mark with distilled water. Apply stopper and mix the contents.
10. Take 3-5 ml from each tube in cuvette and read the absorbance / transmittance at 420 nm wavelength by setting zero with blank and calculate the glucose level in blood by following equation.

$$\frac{\text{Mg glucose ml blood} = \text{Optical density of test}}{\text{Optical density of standard}} \times \text{mg value of standard}$$

Interpretation

Normal values of blood glucose in different animal species are given in Table 2.1

Table 2.1: Blood glucose level in animals

Sr.No.	Species	Blood glucose (mg /100 ml blood)
1.	Bovines	35-55
2.	Sheep	35-60
3.	Goat	45-60
4.	Horse	60-100
5.	Pig	65-95
6.	Dog	55-90
7.	Cat	60-100

The blood glucose level reflects the nutritional, emotional and endocrinal conditions of animal. Increased blood sugar values are called as hyperglycemia which is observed in diabetes mellitus, hyperpituitarism, shock, urinary obstructions, hyperthyroidism, chronic nephritis, burns, increased intracranial pressure, epilepsy, tetany, convulsions, anoxia, stress, excitement, pancreatitis, strychnine poisoning, convulsions, metritis, terminal stage of pregnancy and toxemia. The decreased blood sugar level is known as hypoglycemia and is met in hyperinsulinism, acetonemia, pregnancy toxemia, hepatic insufficiency, starvation, neoplasms of pancreas, hypothyroidism hypopituitarism, severe exertion, Addison's disease, malabsorption, rotavirus infection and reovirus infection.

Total Serum Proteins

Indications

The measurement of total serum protein is not directly indicative of the presence of any disease but indirect correlation with disease process is extremely helpful. The protein examination is indicated in liver diseases, immunosuppression, parasitic diseases, chronic wasting diseases, pregnancy, starvation and edematous swelling of dependent parts of the body. In serum, total proteins, albumin, globulin, albumin and globulin ratio and gamma globulins are measured.

Procedure

1. Take 3 test tubes and place them on a test tube stand. Mark the tubes as 'T' for test, 'S' for standard, and 'B' for blank. Pipette 4.9 ml normal saline solution in tube 'T' and 'S' and 5.0 ml in tube 'B'.
2. Add 0.1 ml test serum in tube 'T' and 0.1 ml standard (4.0% bovine serum albumin in NSS) in tube 'S'.
3. Add 5 ml biuret reagent in all tubes and mix well.
4. Incubate the tubes in water bath at 37 0C for 30 min.
5. Read the absorbance or tansmittance in a spectrophotometer at 454 nm wavelength. Set zero with blank and calculate the total serum protein by using following equation:

$$\text{Total serum protein (gm / 100 ml)} = \frac{\text{OD of test}}{\text{OD of standard}} \times 100$$

Interpretation

A decrease in protein content is known as hypoproteinemia which is observed in maldigestion, malabsorption, starvation, burns, lactation, renal diseases, liver diseases, chronic wasting diseases, proteinuria, pregnancy, parasitic diseases, diarrhoea and dysentry, An increase in total serum protein (hyperproteinemia) is observed in shock, dehydration, neoplasms like lymphosarcoma, and plasmacytoma, aging and infectious diseases.

The normal values of total serum proteins, albumin and globulins are given in Table 2.2.

Table 2.2: Serum proteins in animals

Sr. No.	Species	Total serum protein (gm/100 ml)	Albumin (gm/100 ml)	Globulin (gm/100 ml)		
				Alpha	Beta	Gamma
1.	Bovine	7.56	3.4	0.85	1.08	2.16
2.	Sheep	5.81	2.96	1.10	0.45	1.30
3.	Goat	6.25	3.95	0.42	1.24	0.91
4.	Horse	6.72	2.60	2.63	0.81	0.68
5.	pig	7.40	3.40	1.50	1.10	1.40
6.	Dog	6.1-7.8	3.1-4.0	1.20	1.30	0.80

Serum Albumin

Indications

The albumin is measured in serum in such conditions in which globulin level is to be calculated. The globulin content is calculated by subtracting the albumin values from total serum proteins. The measurement of albumin is indicated in all such situations in which total serum protein is determined.

Procedure

1. Take 6" test tube and pipette 3.0 ml sulfate-sulfite reagent and mix 0.2 ml serum to be tested. Add 3.0 ml ethyl ether and mix thoroughly by shaking the tube 40 times in about 20 seconds. Centrifuge the tube at 2000-3000 rpm in a clinical centrifuge for 5-10 minutes. After centrifugation, suck 2.0 ml clear solution from lower layer by pipette and place in another test tube and mark the tube as 'T' for test.
2. In another tube, take 2.0 ml sulfate-sulfite reagent and mark it as 'B' for blank.
3. In tube 'S', place 2 ml of standard solution prepared in total serum protein estimation as 4% bovine serum albumin.
4. Add 2.0 ml sodium hydroxide (1.5 N NaOH) in each tube and mix.
5. Add 0.8 ml biuret reagent to each tube and mix properly. Keep the tubes for 20 min. Read the absorbance or transmittance against a reagent blank at zero and calculate the albumin contents by following equation:

$$\text{Total serum protein (gm / 100 ml)} = \frac{\text{OD of test}}{\text{OD of standard}} \times 100$$

Interpretation

The increase in serum albumin content is termed as hyperalbuminemia which is observed in shock, hemoconcentration, intestinal obstruction, severe burns, vomitions, diarrhoea, hepatic disorders, chronic skin diseases and acute dehydration. The hypoalbuminemia, decrease in albumin content in serum, is met in starvation, maldigestion, malabsorption, chronic hepatic diseases, prolonged fever, diabetes mellitus, acute nephritis, nephrosis, ascites, malnutrition, burns, candidiasis, chronic gastrointestinal disorders, trauma, leishmaniasis, schistosomiasis, Johne's disease, rotavirus infection, coronavirus infection and parasitic diseases.

Serum Globulin

The globulin content is calculated by subtracting the serum albumin values from total protein values.

Serum globulin = Total serum protein – Serum albumin
(gram / 100 ml)

There are three types of globulin present in serum; alpha, beta and gamma. The level of globulin content increases (Hyperglobulinemia) in bacterial, viral, parasitic infections, dehydration, shock, vomition, diarrhoea, leukemia, infectious hepatitis, endocarditis, hyperlipimia, plasmacytoma and lymphosarcoma. The hypoglobulinemia, decrease in globulin content, is observed in bovine immunodeficiency, infectious bursal disease and in immunosuppression caused by a number of agents. A:G ratio is calculated by dividing the albumin values withcorresponding globulin values. The A:G ratio alters in immunodeficient diseases. It gives an indication about the immunocompetence of the animal. An increase in A:G ratio is indicative of hyperalbuminemia or immunosuppression while decrease in ratio indicats hypoalbuminemia or immunostimulation.

Serum Gamma Globulin

Indications

Serum gamma globulin level is measured in conditions when specific or non-specific immune status of animal is determined. The evaluation of any vaccine or immunomodulator can be done by measuring the level of serum gamma globulins. It is also measured in immunosuppression, immunopathological reactions, including congenital agammaglobulinemia and hypogammaglobulinemia and in determining the prognosis of disease.

Procedure

1. In a test tube take 5.7 ml ammonium sulfate-sodium chloride solution (19.5% ammonium sulfate and 2.03% sodium chloride; pH 6.4). To this overlay 0.3 ml clear serum sample. Mix the contents by gently inverting the tube at least six times and place it on ice baths for 15 min. Centrifuge this at 3000 rpm for 10 min in a clinical centrifuge and discard the supernatant. Repeat the process twice and finally dissolve the contents in 2.0 ml normal saline solution.
2. Add 5.0 ml biuret reagent and keep it for 10 min at room temperature.
3. Make a blank with 2.0 ml normal saline and 5 ml biuret reagent in a tube marked 'B'.
4. Make a standard by taking 2.0 ml of 0.15% bovine serum albumin in a test tube and add 5.0 ml biuret reagent in this tube marked as 'S'.
5. Read the absorbance or transmittance of test and standard against blank set at 'zero' at 555 nm wavelength and calculate the gamma globulin by following equation:

$$\text{Serum gamma globulin (gm/100 ml)} = \frac{\text{OD of test}}{\text{OD of standard}} \times 100$$

Interpretation

Increased values of gamma globulins are observed in immunostimulatory reactions such as after vaccination, administration of immunostimulatory drugs, in hypersensitivity reactions and in infectious diseases. The decrease in serum gamma globulin level is seen in congenital hypogammaglobulinemia, immuno suppression, immunodeficiency diseases and due to environmental pollutants or contaminants.

Serum Calcium

Indications

Serum calcium levels are measured in bone diseases, paralytic diseases or syndrome, convulsions and parathyroid disturbances.

Procedure

1. Take 3 centrifuge tubes and mark them as 'T' for test, 'S' for standard and 'B' for blank. Pipette 2 ml serum in tube 'T', 2 ml standard calcium (5 mg/100 ml) in tube 'S' and 2 ml distilled water in tube 'B'.

2. Add 1 ml chloranilic acid slowly while agitating the tube constantly.
3. Keep the tubes on stand for 30 min and then centrifuge at 2000 rpm for 10 min in a clinical centrifuge; discard the supernatant and collect the precipitate on filter paper.
4. Transfer the precipitate into another tubes by washing with 6-7 ml isopropyl alcohol and resuspend in test tubes.
5. Centrifuge and discard the supernatant; suspend the precipitate in 0.1 ml distilled water.
6. Add 6 ml EDTA solution to each tube, apply stopper and shake vigorously.
7. Read the optical density at 520 nm in spectrophotometer by adjusting zero with blank and calculate the calcium level in serum by following equation:

$$\text{Serum calcium (mg/100 ml)} = \frac{\text{OD of test}}{\text{OD of standard}} \times 100$$

Interpretation

In animals the normal serum calcium levels are given in Table 2.3.

Table 2.3: Serum calcium level in animals

Sr.No.	Species	Serum calcium (mg/100ml)
1.	Bovine	11.08
2.	Sheep	11.40
3.	Goat	10.70
4.	Pig	11.00
5.	Dog	9.80

The increased serum calcium levels are known as hypercalcemia which is observed in hyperproteinemia, hyperthyroidism, polycythemia, bone cancer, myeloma, nephrolithiasis and after administration of vitamin D. The hypocalcemia, decreased serum calcium levels, is met with hypothyroidism, starvation, ketosis, milk fever, eclampsia, osteomalacia, vitamin D deficiency, nephritis pneumonia, theileriosis and rickets.

Serum Inorganic Phosphorus

Indications

The serum inorganic phosphorus is determined along with calcium estimation as the calcium and phosphorus ratio has diagnostic value. The phosphorus level is measured in sera of animals suspected for hemoglobinuria, pica and rheumatism like syndromes.

Procedure

1. Take 3 test tubes and mark them as 'T' for test, 'B' for blank and 'S' for standard. Place 1 ml serum in tube 'T'; 1 ml distilled water in tube 'B'.
2. Add 9 ml trichloroacetic acid to each tube, mix well and place on stand for 5-10 min. Centrifuge the tubes at 2000 rpm in a clinical centrifuge for 10 min and collect 4 ml supernatant from each tube into separate tubes.
3. Add 0.5 ml Elon reducing solution to each tube having supernatant and mix thoroughly.
4. Keep on stand for 30 min and read the optical density in spectrophotometer at 700 nm wavelength, by adjusting zero with blank and calculate the serum phosphorus level by following equation:

$$\text{Serum phoshorus (mg/100 ml)} = \frac{\text{OD of test}}{\text{OD of standard}} \times 100$$

Interpretation

The serum inorganic phosphorus levels in normal healthy animals are given in Table 2.4.

Table 2.4: Serum inorganic phosphorus level in animals

Sr.No.	Species	Serum phosphorus (mg /100 ml)
1.	Bovine	5.56
2.	Sheep	5.21
3.	Horse	3.50
4.	Pig	10.94
5.	Dog	3.0

The increased serum phosphorus levels are known as hyperphosphatemia, which is observed in renal failure, hypoparathyroidism, healing of fractures and hypervitaminosis -D. Hypophosphatemia, decreased serum phosphorus level, is met with inadequate intake, rickets, hyperparathyroidism, heavy parasitism, rheumatism like syndrome, pica, chronic diarrhoea, starvation, chronic hepatitis, epilepsy, bone chewing and hemoglobinuria.

Serum Magnesium

Indications

The serum magnesium is measured in grass tetany, poor growth, formations of bone and skin lesions.

Procedure

1. Take 3 tubes and mark them as 'T' for test, 'S' for standard and 'B' for blank. Place 0.5 ml of serum in tube 'T', 0.5 ml magnesium standard in tube 'S' (4 mEq/l), and 0.5 ml distilled water in tube 'B'.
2. Add 3 ml trichloroacetic acid to each tube and mix well. Allow to stand for 10-15 min on stand; and centrifuge the tubes at 2000 rpm for 10 min.
3. Pipette 2.0 ml clear supernatant from each tube to other tubes and add 0.5 ml polyvinyl alcohol, 2.5 ml titan yellow and 1.0 ml sodium hydroxide in each tube.
4. Place the tubes on stand for 15 min and read the optical density at 540 nm by setting zero with blank and calculate the serum magnesium levels by following equation:

$$\text{Serum magnesium (mg/100 ml)} = \frac{\text{OD of test}}{\text{OD of standard}} \times 100$$

Interpretation

The serum magnesium levels in normal healthy animals are given in table 2.5.

The hypomagnesemia, decreased level of serum magnesium, is met with grass tetany of animals, lactation tetany and wheat pasture poisoning. The increased level of magnesium in serum is called hypermagnesemia which is observed during parturition, chronic infection and in oxalate poisoning.

Table 2.5: Serum magnesium levels in animals

Sr.No.	Species	Serum calcium (mg/100ml)
1.	Bovine	11.08
2.	Sheep	11.40
3.	Goat	10.70
4.	Pig	11.00
5.	Dog	9.80

Serum Cholesterol

Indications

The determination of cholesterol is indicated in liver and thyroid dysfunction. The level of serum cholesterol is influenced by fat rich diet of animal containing saturated fatty acids.

Procedure

1. Take 3 test tubes, mark them as 'T' for test, 'S' for standard and 'B' for blank.
2. Pipette 0.1 ml serum in test tube 'T' and add 0.1 ml distilled water. Take 0.1 ml standard in glacial acetic acid in tube 'S' and add 0.1 ml distilled water in tube 'S'. Take 0.2 ml distilled water tube 'B'.
3. Add 10 ml colour development reagent to each test tube by pipette at the bottom of tube.
4. Leave the tubes for 1 min and read the absorbance or transmittance at 640 nm wave length of spectrophotometer by setting zero with blank and calculate the serum cholesterol by following equation:

$$\text{Serum cholesterol (mg/100 ml)} = \frac{\text{OD of test}}{\text{OD of standard}} \times 100$$

Interpretation

The serum cholesterol level in various species of animals is given in Table 2.6.

Table 2.6: Serum cholesterol level in animals

Sr.No.	Species	Serum cholesterol (mg/100ml)
1.	Bovine	111±08
2.	Sheep	64±12
3.	Goat	80±30
4.	Horse	96.8±2.8
5.	Pig	152-154
6.	Dog	110±28
7.	Cat	93±24

The increased level of serum cholesterol is termed as hypercholesterolemia which has been observed in hypothyroidism, advance nephrosis, stress, chronic glomerulonephritis, cortisone therapy, diabetic acidosis, high fat diet, obstruction of bile duct, leukemia and pregnancy. The decreased serum cholesterol levels are known as hypocholesterolemia which is met with liver diseases, hyperthyroidism, anemia, low fat diet, starvation, acute infections, polycythemia, intestinal obstruction and epilepsy.

Serum Creatinine

Indications

The serum creatinine is measured in kidney diseases especially in uremia in animals. Serum levels of creatinine are not affected by dietary proteins.

The repeated analysis of serum for creatinine is advisable in kidney disorders, as it not only helps in diagnosis but is also useful for assessing the prognosis.

Procedure

1. Take 350 ml flasks and mark them as 'T' for test, 'S' for standard and 'B' for blank, Pipette 16 ml of 2/3 N sulfuric acid in each flask. Add 2 ml serum in flask 'T', and 2 ml standard in 'S'. Add 2 ml of 10% sodium tungstate to each flask, apply stopper and shake vigorously. Filter or centrifuge.

2. Take 5 ml clear fluid in another small flask and take 5 ml distilled water in flask 'B'.

3. Add 2.5 ml alkaline picrate solution to each flask and keep them at room temperature for 15 min.

4. Read the OD at 520 nm wavelength with zero set by blank 'B', within 5 min and calculate the serum creatinine levels as:

$$\text{Serum creatinine (mg/100 ml)} = \frac{\text{OD of test}}{\text{OD of standard}} \times 100$$

Interpretation

The serum creatinine levels of different animal species are given in Table 2.7.

Table 2.7: Serum creatinine levels in animals

Sr.No.	Species	Serum creatinine level (mg/100 ml)
1.	Bovine	1.0-2.07
2.	Sheep	1.2-1.93
3.	Goat	0.9-1.82
4.	Horse	1.2-1.9
5.	Pig	1.0-2.7
6.	Dog	1.0-2.7
7.	Cat	1.0-2.0

The increased level of serum creatinine is observed in severe nephritis, urinary obstruction and severe toxic nephrosis. Serum creatinine level above 5-18 mg /100 ml is an indication of renal impairment and sign of unfavourable prognosis.

Serum Urea

Indications

The determination of urea in blood or serum is indicated in acute or chronic kidney diseases, nephrotoxicity, nephrosis, uremia and in urinary obstruction such as in urolithiasis.

Procedure

1. Take 3 test tubes and mark them as 'T' for test, 'B' for blank and 'S' for standard. Place 2.8 ml distilled water in tube T, and S, and in tube B, pipette 3.2 ml distilled water. Add 0.2 ml serum in tube 'T' and 0.2 ml standard solution in tube 'S'.
2. Add 0.2 ml urease solution to tube T, and S.
3. Mix well and incubate in hot air oven at 50-55°C for about 15 min.
4. Add 0.4 ml barium hydroxide solution to each tube and mix. Add also 0.4 ml zinc sulfate solution to each tube and mix properly and centrifuge at 2000 rpm for 10 min.
5. Take out 2.0 ml clear supernatant from each tube and place it in another tube and add 3.0 ml distilled water.
6. Add a drop of iodine solution to each tube and 5.0 ml of cold Nessler's solution and mix by swirling.
7. Read the OD by setting zero with blank at 480 nm wavelength in a spectrophotometer within 15 min and calculate the serum urea level by following equation:

$$\text{Serum urea (mg/100 ml)} = \frac{\text{OD of test}}{\text{OD of standard}} \times 100$$

Interpretation

The normal serum levels of urea in animals are given in Table 2.8.

The concentration of urea in serum or blood is increased in chronic or acute nephritis, urinary obstruction, metallic poisoning, intestinal obstruction, peritonitis, bleeding, carcinoma of intestines, duodenal ulcers, cirrhosis of liver, leptospirosis and surgical shock.

Table 2.8: Serum urea levels in animals

Sr.No.	Species	Serum urea level (mg/100ml
1.	Bovine	6-27
2.	Sheep	8-20
3.	Goat	13-28
4.	Horse	10-20
5.	Pig	8-24
6.	Dog	10-20
7.	Cat	20-30

The decreased serum urea levels are observed in acute hepatic insufficiency, chronic wasting diseases, nephrosis, pregnancy and amyloidosis.

Serum Chloride

Indications

The serum chloride levels are determined in assessing the electrolyte balance of body and evaluating the regimen of electrolyte therapy.

Procedure

1. Take 3 test tubes and mark them as 'T' for test, 'S' for standard and 'B' for blank. Place 0.2 ml serum in tube 'T' and 0.2 ml standard in 'S'. Add 0.4 ml of 0.3 N barium hydroxide and 1.0 ml distilled water to the tubes, mix thoroughly and keep for 5 min on stand.
2. Add 0.4 ml of 5% zinc sulfate to each tube and mix. Centrifuge the tubes at 2000 rpm for 10 min.
3. Take 0.5 ml supernatant in other tubes and add 4.0 ml of 1.0% nitric acid. Place 4.0 ml of 1% nitric acid and 0.5 ml water in tube 'B'.
4. Add 10-15 mg of mercuric chloranilate to each test tube, mix well and keep it for 5 min. Centrifuge for 5 min and collect the supernatant for determination of OD in spectrophotometer at 540 nm wavelength by setting zero with blank and calculate the chloride level by following equation:

$$\text{Serum chloride (mEq/1000 ml)} = \frac{\text{OD of test}}{\text{OD of standard}} \times 100$$

Interpretation

The normal values of serum chloride levels are given in Table 2.9.

Table 2.9: Serum chloride levels in animals

Sr.No.	Species	Serum chloride levels (mEq/lit)
1.	Bovine	97-111
2.	Sheep	98-109
3.	Goat	118
4.	Horse	98-106
5.	Pig	100-105
6.	Dog	108-111
7.	Cat	117-123

The increased level of chloride in serum is termed as hyperchloremia which is observed in cirrhosis of liver, hypoproteinemia, cardiac decompensation, nephrosis, urinary obstruction, excessive ingestion of salt, dehydration and respiratory alkalosis. The hypochloremia, decreased level of chloride in serum, is met in pneumonia, pulmonary edema, emphysema, pneumothorax, chronic renal diseases, vomiting, diarrhoea, burns, acute infections and shock.

Serum Sodium

Indications

The serum sodium level is measured in order to estimate the electrolyte balance in the body and to assess the electrolyte therapy to animals.

Procedure

1. The serum is diluted as 1:100 with distilled water. For this take 0.1 ml serum in a test tube and add 9.9 ml distilled water.
2. Prepare stock sodium standard by dissolving 5.85 gm of sodium chloride in 1 lit distilled water. The working standards can be prepared by measuring 10 ml, 11 ml, 12 ml, 13 ml, 14 ml and 15 ml in 100 ml volumetric flasks and diluting this upto 100 ml with distilled water. This gives 100, 110, 120, 130, 140 and 150 mEq/lit sodium.
3. Prepare a standard curve by putting the readings of flame photometer and mEq/lit standards on either side of the graph paper. Put the readings of test serum and read the value of sodium from standard curve in mEq/lit.

Interpretation

The normal sodium content of blood in various species of animals is given in Table 2.10.

Table 2.10: Serum sodium levels in animals

Sr.No.	Species	Serum sodium levels (mEq/lit)
1.	Bovine	132-152
2.	Sheep	146-161
3.	Horse	146-152
4.	pig	140-160
5.	Dog	140-154
6.	Cat	150-156

The increased sodium level in serum is termed as hypernatremia which has been observed in dehydration due to diarrhoea, vomiting, and in primary water deficiency in body. Hyponatremia is the decreased serum sodium level and is met with Addision's disease, myxedema and severe burns.

Serum Potassium

Indications

The estimation of serum potassium is performed to assess the electrolyte balance of the body and to evaluate the electrolyte therapy.

Procedure

1. Dilute the serum sample in the ratio of 1:100 by taking 0.1 ml serum in 9.9 ml distilled water in a test tube
2. Prepare stock potassium standard by dissolving 0.746 gm potassium chloride (KCl) in 1 lit distilled water. The working standards are prepared by pipetting 3 ml, 4 ml, 5 ml, 6 ml and 7 ml of stock solution in 100 ml volumetric flasks and diluting the same upto 100 ml with distilled water. These working standards have 3 mEq/lit to 7 mEq/ lit potassium.
3. Read the samples and standards in flame photometer and plot the standard curve by using reading of standards and mEq/lit values on a graph paper. The values of test samples can be read against the standard curve.

Interpretation

The normal values of potassium in serum in various species of animals are given in Table 2.11.

Table 2.11: Serum potassium levels in animals

Sr.No.	Species	Serum potassium levels (mEq/lit)
1.	Bovine	3.9-5.8
2.	Sheep	4.8
3.	Goat	3.6
4.	Horse	*2.7-35*
5.	Pig	4.9-7.1
6.	Dog	3.7-5.8
7.	Cat	4.0-5.8

The increased serum potassium is termed as hyperkalemia and is observed in nephritis, pyothorax, bronchopneumonia, diarrhoea, adrenal cortical insufficiency, uremia, pyometra and in acute infections. Hypokalemia, decreased potassium level in serum, is observed in hypercorticoadrenaline, chronic nephritis, severe acute diarrhoea, hyperinsulinism and over medication of deoxycorticosteriods.

Serum Glutamic Oxaloacetic Transaminase (SGOT) Aspartate Aminotransferase (AST)

Indications

The determination of SGOT is not specific for any organ or tissue. However, its value is determined in liver or muscle diseases or when a widespread damage is suspected in body. It is particularly indicated in muscular degeneration and necrotic conditions.

Procedure

1. A standard curve is prepared by making a series of dilution of sodium pyruvate solution in following manner.

   a. Stock standard solution is prepared by dissolving sodium pyruvate 0.0222 gm in 100 ml phosphate buffer (0.1M, pH 7.5)

   b. Take 6 tubes in a test tube stand and place 0, 0.1, 0.2, 0.3, 0.4 and 0.5 ml stock standard of sodium pyruvate in these tubes. Add 1.0 ml, 0.9 ml, 0.8 ml, 0.7 ml, 0.6 ml and 0.5 ml aspartate-glutamate substrate in the tubes, respectively so that each tube has 1.0 ml content. Add 0.2 ml distilled water in each tube.

   c. Add 1.0 ml of 2, 4-dinitrophenyl-hydrazine reagent in each tube, mix properly and keep for 20 min. Add 10.0 ml of 0.4 N sodium hydroxide and mix vigorously.

   d. After keeping the tubes for 5 min, read the OD in spectrophotometer at 505 nm wavelength and plot the curve. In tubes of sodium pyruate solution, the activity of equivalent SGOT and SGPT is given in Table 2.12.

On the graph paper plot the readings of spectrophotometer against the equivalent SGOT and SGPT values.

Table 2.12: SGOT and SGPT values in standard solution

Tube No.	Sod. pyruvate solution.	Equivalent SGOT (Frankel unit)	Equivalent SGPT (Frankel unit)
1	0 ml	00	00
2	0.1 ml	20	23
3	0.2 ml	55	50
4	0.3 ml	95	83
5	0.4 ml	148	125
6	0.5 ml	216	—

2. Take 0.5 ml asparatate-glutamate substrate in a test tube and add 0.1 ml serum and incubate at 37°C for 60 min.
3. Add 0.5 ml of 2,4- dinitrophenyl hydrazine reagent and mix properly. Keep the tubes at room temperature for 15 min and add 5 ml of 0.4 N sodium hydroxide and mix well. After 20 min, read the OD in spectrophotometer at 505 nm wavelength using water blank.

$$\text{SGOT (unit/100 ml)} = \frac{\text{OD of test}}{\text{OD of standard}} \times 100$$

Interpretation

In normal animals the SGOT values are given in Table 2.13.

Table 2.13: SGOT values in animals

Sr.No.	Species	SGOT (unit/100 ml)
1.	Bovine	43.8
2.	Sheep	56.0
3.	Horse	165.0
4.	Pig	31.1
5.	Dog	22.7
6.	Cat	19.0

Increased levels of serum GOT are observed in association with cell necrosis like, hepatic necrosis, myocardial infarction, muscular necrosis, azoturia, starvation and white muscle disease or stiff lamb disease.

Serum Glutamic Pyruvic Transaminase (SGPT) (Alanine Aminotransferase (ALT))

Indications

The serum glutamic pyruvic transaminase is determined in necrotic liver diseases, poisoning and prolonged antibiotic therapy.

Procedure

1. Take 0.5 ml alpha-ketoglutarate-d-alanine substrate in test tube and add 0.1 ml serum, mix well and incubate for 30 min.
2. Add 0.5 ml 2, 4-dinitrophenylhydrazine reagent and leave the tubes for 20 min at room temperature.
3. Mix 5.0 ml of 0.4 N sodium hydroxide in the tubes.
4. After 15 min, read the OD at 505 nm wavelength against a distilled water blank. Calculate the SGPT values using following equation:

$$\text{Serum GPT (unit/100 ml)} = \frac{\text{OD of test}}{\text{OD of standard}} \times 100$$

Interpretation

The normal serum GPT levels in animals are given in table 2.14.

Table 2.14: Serum GPT levels in animals

Sr.No.	Species	SGOT (unit / 100 ml)
1.	Bovine	19.7
2.	Horse	11.0
3.	Pig	27.3
4.	Dog	21.8
5.	Cat	16.0

The increased level of serum GPT has been recorded in hepatic necrosis in dogs and cats, in which its value reaches even upto 400 units, The increased SGPT levels are also seen in suppurative hepatitis, anemia, arsenic poisoning, hypothyroidism, pyometra, infectious canine hepatitis and hepatic carcinoma.

Serum Alkaline Phosphatase

Indications

Alkaline phosphatase activity of serum is measured in bone abnormalities.

Procedure

1. Prepare a standard curve of the alkaline phosphatase by preparing standard stock solution of p-nitrophenol (0.139 gm/100 ml distilled

water). Working standard is prepared by diluting 0.5 ml of stock standard to 100 ml 0.02 N sodium hydroxide solution. Take 6 test tubes in a stand and place 0.5 ml, 1 ml, 2 ml, 3 ml, 4 ml and 5 ml working standard solution and add 0.02 N sodium hydroxide 5.0 ml, 4.5 ml, 3.5 ml, 2.5 ml, 1.5 ml and 0.5 ml, respectively, so that each tube has 5.5 ml contents. These tubes are having the alkaline phosphatase activity equivalent to 1.0, 2.0, 4.0, 6.0, 8.0 and 10.0 units AP per ml serum, respectively. Read the OD against 0.02 N sodium hydroxide as blank at 410 nm and plot a curve using AP activity and OD on a graph paper.

2. Take test tubes and place 1.0 ml p nitrophenol substrate. Add 0.1 ml serum in tube marked 'T' and in another tube marked 'B', in 0.1 ml distilled water.
3. Add 10 ml of 0.02 N sodium hydroxide to each tube and mix the contents. Read the OD of test samples against a reagent blank at 410 nm wavelength.
4. After recording OD, add 0.1 ml concentrated hydrochloric acid to each tube and mix. Take again OD against reagent blank at same wavelength. For obtaining the correct reading subtract the later reading from earlier reading.
5. Calculate the alkaline phosphatase activity by standard curve.

Interpretation

In normal animals, the alkaline phosphatase activity is given in Table 2.15.

Table 2.15: Serum alkaline phosphatase activity in animals

Sr.No.	Species	Alkaline phosphate activity
1.	Bovine	11.8 KAU
2.	Sheep	14-427 KAU
3.	Horse	6-22 BU
4.	Dog	3-6 BU
5.	Cat	0-7 BU

The alkaline phosphatase activity is increased in rickets, osteomalacia, osteoblastic sarcoma, metastatic carcinoma, obstructive jaundice, infectious hepatitis, hyperparathyroidism, hyperthyroidism, myositis ossificans, pregnancy and multiple myeloma. The decreased levels of alkaline phosphatase activity is observed in severe chronic nephritis, scurvy, hypothyroidism and hypomagnesimic tetany.

Note: All the procedure for enzyme activities in SGOT, SGPT and AP must be carried at 37°C for optimum findings.

3

Examination of Bone Marrow

- General considerations
- Indications
- Limitations
- Techniques of bone marrow examination
- Cell types
- Cellular composition of bone marrow
- Morphology of the cells
- Interpretation of bone marrow examination

General Considerations

Bones are formed by fibrous tissue and phosphates and/or carbonates of lime. In young animals the fibrous tissue is considered to be more than 60 percent and is responsible for toughness of the bones while in older animals the phosphates and carbonates of lime comprise more than 60 per cent of the bones and are responsible for their brittleness. Mainly, the bones are to two types; dense bones and spongy bones. All the bones have a central cavity which contains marrow which is called as bone marrow. The bone marrow is of two types.

1. *Yellow bone marrow*: Yellow bone marrow is composed of mainly fatty tissue or substance and is found in central cavity of long bones. Functionally it is inactive.
2. *Red bone marrow*: Red marrow is found in the tiny spaces of a fine network of bony threads. The red marrow is referred to as bone marrow in routine as it is the only active marrow. The red marrow is engaged in the formation of blood cells and is considered as factory for the blood cells after the birth of animal. In the red marrow three types of blood cells are formed.

a. Erythrocytes

b. Granulocytic leucocytes, lymphocytes and monocytes

c. Thrombocytes.

The main source of lymphocytes and monocytes, however, remians the reticuloendothelial system and lymph nodes. All these cells are derived from a primitive mesenchymal stem cell, hemoblast, which is large with finely granular basophilic cytoplasm, a very large nucleus and several prominent nucleoli. The red marrow is found in the bones of skull, ribs, sternum and flat bones of pelvis of animal. In adult animal, red marrow supplies the cellular components of the blood but under great demand for more cells, the yellow marrow is also replaced by active red marrow. Bone marrow cells are destroyed rapidly after death thus they can be studied only before death through biopsy.

Indications

The bone marrow examination is necessary as indicated under the following conditions.

1. In such diseases of blood abnormality in which the confirmatory diagnosis is not possible from peripheral blood examination.
2. In diseases associated with decreased cellular elements of blood such as leukemia, degenerative anemia and thrombocytopenia.
3. For the confirmatory diagnosis of leukemia and its differentiation from leukemoid reaction.

Limitations

1. A representative sample of bone marrow is difficult because it may contain blood from sinusoids to give a different/false picture.
2. Quantitative analysis of bone marrow is impossible due to inability to make a total cell count.
3. The results of the bone marrow examinations are based on a relative basis.
4. The veterinarian finds it very difficult to differentiate the immature erythrocytes from other nucleated cells.

The bone marrow examination is considered difficult and time consuming. Hence, it is only advisable when without bone marrow examination diagnosis cannot be made.

Techniques of Bone Marrow Examination

The bone marrow examination should be performed by experienced and trained personnel. All cares must be taken in proper examination and interpretation of the findings. The common sites of marrow collections from animals are:

Cattle	Sternum, ribs
Buffaloes	Sternum, ribs
Horse	Sternum, ribs
Sheep	Sternum
Dog	Iliac crest
Cat	Iliac crest, femur.

The bone marrow is collected under aseptic conditions and all precautions must be taken to avoid any contamination of marrow at the time of its collection. For proper aseptic conditions, remove the hairs/wool from the site and shave the area. Apply tincture of iodine and wash the area with 70% alcohol. Local anesthesia is applied over the sternum, the body of the bone with second rib and infiltrate the anesthesia over periosteum of the sternum, when the marrow is to be collected from sternum. Apply 18 gauge short needle with stylet at an angle of 450 and insert till it reaches periosteum of the sternum. Apply pressure to penetrate the bone and remove the stylet and fit a 10 ml syringe over the needle. The bone marrow is now collected/aspirated in the syringe. The smears on clean, dry glass slides are prepared like blood smears and are air dried. Place the Wright's stain over slides to cover the smear for 1 min and add equal amount of PBS or neutral distilled water and mix by blowing till the metallic sheen appears on the slide. The diluted stain is kept over the smear for 2-5 min. Remove the stain and wash the slides in running tap water. Avoid over-washing as it may de-stain the smears. Dry the slides and examine under microscope.

Cell Types

All types of cells that develop in the bone marrow reveal in their morphology as they develop from the primitive cells to the mature cell type. The various cells present in bone marrow are as under:

1. *Stem cells:* The stem cell is an undifferentiated mesenchymal cell.
2. *Granulocytic series:* In this series following cell types are present:
    a. Myeloblast

b. Promyelocyte

c. Myelocyte

d. Metamyelocyte

e. Band cell

f. Segmented granulocyte

3. *Lymphocytic series*: The following cell types are present:

a. Lymphoblast

b. Prolymphocyte

c. Lymphocyte

i. T-lymphocyte

ii. B-lymphocyte

4. *Erythrocytic series*: In erythrocytic series the following cell types are present in bone marrow:

a. Rubriblast

b. Prorubricyte

c. Rubricyte

d. Metarubricyte

e. Reticulocyte

f. Erythrocyte

5. *Thrombocytic series*: In thrombocytic series the following cell types are present in the bone marrow:

a. Megakaryoblast

b. Promegakaryocyte

c. Megakaryocyte

d. Thrombocyte

6. Other cell types present in the bone marrow are as under:

a. Plasma cells

b. Tissue eosinophils

c. Basophils

d. Osteoclasts

e. Osteoblasts.

Table 3.1: Cellular composition of normal bone marrow (%)

Sr. No.	Cell types	Cattle	Sheep	Goat	Horse	Pig	Dog	Cat
1.	Myeloblast	-	0.1-1.1	-	0-1	0.6	0-1	0.3-2
2.	Promyelocyte	0.2-2	0-1.4	0-1	0-1	2.0	—	1-3
3.	Neutrophilic myelocyte	1-5	0.5-4.9	1-4	11-28	6.0	1-8	4-7
4.	Neutrophilic metamyelocyte	1-8	1.5-9.1	6-10	17-30	11.0	8-25	8-20
5.	Neutrophilic band	5-12	2.4-18.2	7-9	7-25	17.0	—	14-30
6.	Mature neutrophils	4-20	1-19.6	7-12	—	21.0	15-30	15-30
7.	Eosinophilic myelocyte	0-2	0.2-5.7	0-1	0-3	--	0-2	0-2
8.	Eosinophilic metamyelocyte	0.5-4.0	0.4-5.0	1-3	1-7	5	0-2	0-1
9.	Eosinophilic band	2-10	0.5-7.1	1-3	0-6	—	0-2	0-1
10.	Eosinophil	—	0.6-9.3	-	—	—	0-4	1-3
11.	Basophil	0-1	0-2	0-1	0-1	0.3	0.5	0-1
12.	Total myeloid	20-55	45-55	30-40	55-65	—	45-60	50-70
13.	Lymphocyte	5-18	1-11	5-9	2-20	-	1-5	2-10
14.	Monocyte	0-0.5	0-4.3	0-1	0-2	—	0-5	0-2
15.	Plasma cells	0-3	0-1	0-1	0-2	—	0-3	0-1
16.	Rubriblast	0-1	1-7.2	-	0-1	0.5	0-2	0-2
17.	Prorubriblast	0.5-2.0	-	1-2	0-5	3.5	1-4	1-8
18.	Rubricyte	15-30	11-37.7	27-35	2-13	24	10-25	10-30
19.	Metarubricyte	10-35	13-39.9	18-30	4-30	9.1	8-25	-
20.	Total erythroid	30-60	40-50	50-60	25-35	—	30-45	20-45
21.	ME ratio	0.7:1	1.59:1 to 2.35:1	0.69:1.0	1.6:1	1.7:1	1.2:1	1.6:1

Cellular Composition of Bone Marrow

The cell counts are made by examination of stained smears and about 500-1000 cells per smear must be counted in order to arrive at a fairly good differential count. The counting and identification of cell types is very difficult.

There are no universal data of the normal animals as it has to be established in each laboratory doing bone marrow examination. However, for the benefit of readers and to give an idea about the differential cell count of bone marrow a generally accepted and described data is given in Table 3.1.

Morphology of the Cells

1. *Stem cells:* The stem cells have a large round nucleus with fine chromatin, which takes a reddish colour. The fine nucleoli is present. Cytoplasm takes blue colour and shows a foamy appearance. The size of the cell is comparatively large. The margins of stem cells are torn and may have projections. If the stem cells are present with large number of lymphocytes, they are called lymphoblast and when they are with erythrocytes, and known as rubriblast.

2. *Myeloblast:* In myeloblast cells, cytoplasmic granules are absent. The cytoplasm is basophilic and nucleus has fine chromatin structure alongwith nucleoli. These cells are increased in number with other cell types of granulocytic series, and are termed as myeloblast.

3. *Promyelocyte:* Promyelocytes have more dense nucleus and darkly stained azurophilic cytoplasmic granules which are non-specific. The nucleoli are visible but in less number. Cytoplasm takes blue stain and increases in size in comparison to nucleus and thus the nucleus cytoplasm ratio is altered.

4. *Myelocyte:* The nucleus of myelocyte is round or oval and it has coarse chromatin. Cytoplasm takes faint greyish pink colour and has specific cytoplasmic granules. On the basis of granules, these cells can be identified as neutrophilic, eosinophilic or basophilic.

   a. *Neutrophilic myelocyte:* These cells do not have definitive granules but their cytoplasm has granular appearance.

   b. *Eosinophilic myelocyte:* In dogs, the granules of eosinophilic myelocyte stain lightly and vary in size while in cat these are rod shaped and greyish orange in colour. In cow, small, round granules are present which stains red. In sheep, eosinophilic myelocyte has ovoid shaped red granules while in horse the granules are large and dull red to orange in colour. In pig's eosinophilic myelocyte the granules are orange to light red in colour and ovoid in shape.

   c. *Basophilic myelocyte:* In basophilic myelocyte, the granules are distinctly present and may hide the nucleus. These take dark blue to black stain and vary in size.

5. *Metamyelocyte:* The metamyelocyte resembles with myelocyte but their nucleus becomes kidney or bean shaped. The nuclear chromatin becomes more coarse and granules are present in the cytoplasm.

6. *Band cell:* In band cells, the nucleus becomes coiled band or curved and the opposite sides of the nucleus are parallel.

7. *Segmented granulocyte:* In these cells the nuclues is lobulated and lobes are connected with filaments. The cytoplasmic granules are characteristic to differentiate neutrophils, eosinophils and basophils.

8. *Rubriblast:* The cytoplasm of rubriblast stains light blue or dark purplish blue in colour. The nucleus contains nucleoli and is round in shape.

9. *Prorubricyte:* Prorubricyte is smaller in size than rubriblast and nucleoli is absent. Cytoplasm takes blue basophilic stains. A reddish tint may be present in the cytoplasm of the prorubricyte which indicates the presence of hemoglobin. The nucleus is present in the center of the cell, surrounded by a narrow zone of blue staining cytoplasm.

10. *Rubricyte:* The rubricytes are smaller than prorubricytes. The cytoplasm is bluish red in colour and nuclear chromatin is arranged like spokes of a wheel.

11. *Metarubricyte:* The cytoplasm of metarubricytes is red with slight basophilic patches. The nucleus appears as a blue-black mass and is pyknotic.

12. *Reticulocyte:* In reticulocytes, nucleus is absent. It is larger than mature erythrocyte. In the cytoplasm a diffused network of fibrils is present.

13. *Erythrocytes:* It stains red and has crenation on the surface. It has no nucleus.

14. *Lymphoblast:* It is difficult to identify lymphoblast because lymphoblast and myeloblast have similar structure. But lympoblast is accompanied by other lymphocytic cells.

15. *Prolymphocyte:* It has blue cytoplasm and a large nucleus. The nuclear chromatin is coarser which has an indistinct nucleoli.

16. *Lymphocyte:* The cytoplasm of lymphocytes stains light blue and azurophilic granules are present in the cytoplasm. The nucleus is eccentrically placed and has coarse chromatin.

17. *Megakaryoblast:* It is also unidentifiable like other blast/stem cells. Cytoplasm stains light blue and outer lining of the cell is dark blue giving the appearance of a vaccuolated zone. The nucleus is large, red, round with fine chromatin and nucleoli.
18. *Promegakaryocyte:* The nucleus of promegakaryocyte is multilobed. The cytoplasm stains blue and contains blue granules. The cytoplasm has bud like projections on its surface.
19. *Megakaryocyte:* It is the largest cell present in bone marrow with about 100 micron diameter. Cytoplasm of megakaryocyte has coasrse granule, foams and clumps towards periphery. The nucleus is lobulated with no nucleoli.
20. *Thrombocyte:* Thrombocyte has non-nucleated fragments of megakaryocyte and cytoplasm has azurophilic granules.
21. *Plasma cells:* It has oval or elongated small nucleus which is eccentrically placed. The cytoplasm of plasma cells is dark purplish blue in colour and has foamy appearance. These cells are rare in bone marrow and their number increase due to plasmacytoma.
22. *Tissue eosinophils:* It is larger in size than blood eosinophils. It has irregular cytoplasmic projections with large nucleus and coarse chromatin.
23. *Tissue basophils:* It is deep staining cell having basophilic granules which are round, uniform in size, many in number and may hide the nucleus. The shape of cell is variable but it has lack of motility.
24. *Osteoblasts:* It is a fixed tissue cell and it resembles with plasma cells. It is oval in shape with dark blue cytoplasm. In smear it appears in clumps.
25. *Osteoclasts:* It is a multinuclear cell which has several small round nuclei. The cell has bluish, unevenly stained cytoplasm.

Interpretation of Bone Marrow Examination

In many disease conditions, gross and microscopic characteristics of bone marrow are altered, such as in anemia. The colour of bone marrow becomes unusual red. In leukemic conditions, the colour of marrow is grey. The gelatinous appearance of bone marrow is observed in starved animals or animals suffering from chronic wasting diseases like tuberculosis and Johne's disease.

In the microscopic examinations, the myeloid and erythroid ratio (ME ratio) is considered one of the main criteria of diagnostic importance. The ME ratio is calculated by dividing the total number of myeloid cells of the bone marrow by the total number of nucleated erythroid cells.

The ME ratio increases in the following conditions:

1. Infections
2. Leukemia
3. Leukemoid reaction
4. Hypoplasia of erythroid cells.

The ME ratio decreases in the following disease conditions:

$$\text{ME ratio} = \frac{\text{Myeloid cells of bone marrow}}{\text{Nucleated erythroid cells of the marrow}}$$

1. Depression of leucocytosis
2. Hyperplasia of erythroid series.

The alterations of ME ratio in different animals due to various diseases are described below.

1. *Leukemia:* In leukemia, the immature leucocytes, lymphocytes, monocytes and granulocytes increase in number. The erythroid series cells decrease in marrow and ME ratio increases.
2. *Canine malignant lymphoma:* In this disease, hyperplasia of myeloid cells is observed alongwith hypoplasia of erythroid cells and the ME ratio increases.
3. *Bovine lymphoma:* Lymphocyte increase over 30% due to bovine lymphoma with an increase in ME ratio.
4. *Granulocytic leukemia:* It is rare in bovines. In this the bone marrow activity suppresses and more than 70% cells are of blast type. On differential leucocytic count, large number of immature form of granulocytes are present in peripheral blood. In dogs, hyperplasia of bone marrow occurs due to granulocytic leukemia. The most characteristic cells are myeloblast, promyeloblast, myelocyte and metamyelocyte. In marrow the erythrocyte element decreases in percent.
5. *Myelomatosis:* Myelomatosis is common in cat and horses. In this condition the number of plasma cells increases.

6. *Monocytic leukemia:* It mostly occurs in cats and dogs. Immature monocytes increase in number in this condition.

7. *Agranulocytosis:* In this condition, there are mostly stem cells present in marrow due to maturation arrest. This condition may also occur due to depression of bone marrow due to certain medicines.

8. *Infectious mononucleosis:* In this disease condition, myeloid hyperplasia occurs and there is increase in number of immature cells in blood.

9. *Pernicius anemia:* In this condition, an increase in number of megaloblasts has been observed.

10. *Anemia:* In hemorrhagic, hemolytic and sickle cell anemia, the erythroblasts and normoblasts are increased in number.

11. *Aplastic anemia:* In this condition, all the cell types are reduced in number and differential leucocytic count is unaltered. If erythroid activity increases, it is a good sign of recovery.

12. *Active polycythemia:* In this disease, hyperplasia of ereythroid elements occur alongwith hyperplasia of granulocytes and megakaryocytes.

13. *Primary thrombocytopenic perpura:* In primary thrombocytopenic perpura, there is increase in number of megakaryocytes.

14. *Chronic pneumonia:* In chronic pneumonia, ME ratio increases alongwith increase in myeloid and lymphoid elements and decrease in erythroid series.

15. *Uremia:* In uremia, granulocytes and lymphocytes increase in number alongwith decrease in erythroid series cells.

16. *Traumatic pericarditis:* In traumatic pericarditis, increase in lymphocytes is seen alongwith decrease in myeloid and erythroid series cells.

17. *Pyelonephritis:* In pyelonephritis, there is increase in lymphocytes and myeloblasts while the erythroid cells are decreased in number.

18. *Liver abscess:* In this condition, erythrocytic series is depressed while lymphocytes increase alongwith slight increase in immature neutrophils.

19. *Pyometra:* In pyometra, megakaryocyte increases in number alongwith a disturbed maturation of neutrophilic cells.

20. *Canine distemper:* In canine distemper, the immature myeloid tissue increases in number in bone marrow.

21. *Filariasis:* Hyperplasia of erythroid cells along with decreased ME ratio has been reported in bone marrow of animals suffering from filariasis.

22. *Chronic kidney diseases:* In this condition, lymphocytes, monocytes and myeloid ratio increase with increase in band cells and immature neutrophils. There is decrease in erythroid elements.

23. *Osteomyelitis:* This is an inflammatory condition of bone. Infection gets access to marrow through local wound, fracture, etc. or by hematogenous route. It involves local bones and usually pyogenic infections cause purulent exudation. In this condition there is increase in number of neutrophilic cells.

24. *Fibrosis:* The fibrosis of bone marrow occurs as a sequel to hypoplasia or aplasia. It may occur with myxomatous degeneration due to starvation.

25. *Panmyelosis:* It is the cancerous growth of erythrocytic or granulocytic or megakaryocytic series. The tumour cells replace the bone marrow and also appears in blood. These cells can also be demonstrated in liver, spleen and lymph nodes.

26. *Myelofibrosis:* In this condition myeloid leukemia occurs which is followed by fibrosis of bone marrow.

4

Examination of Urine

- General considerations
- Collection
- Preservation
- Examination
- Physical examination
- Chemical examination
- Microscopic examination
- Organized sediment
- Unorganized sediment
- Cultural examination

General Considerations

Urine is the excretion of body fluid, filtered through kidneys and consists of waste substances, water and electrolytes. The urine maintains the body's water balance, pH of body fluids and electrolyte levels. It contains the waste products like urea, uric acid formed in body as a result of metabolism and dissolved in water. Urine is the end product of a complicated physiological process of body, the characteristics of which may be altered not only in kidney diseases but also in other systemic disorders.

The examinations of urine are indicated in renal disease, diabetes mellitus, urinary calculi in kidneys or at other places in tract, jaundice, ascites, edematous conditions of body, hematuria and hemoglobinuria. The examination of urine is not only helpful in concluding the diagnosis of disease but also useful in assessing the prognosis of condition.

Collection

The urine samples can be collected by following methods.

1. In large male animals, the polythene bags can be applied over the urethra and tied with the help of rope over the back. When animal urinates, the urine is collected in the polythene bag which should be removed from the animal at different intervals. It is the method of choice for quantitative examination of the urine sample.
2. In cows, buffaloes, sheep and goat one can stimulate the urethra through vulva, which allows the animal to urinate. Collect the urine sample in clean and dry container.
3. In large animals, urine can also be collected by applying pressure on urinary bladder through rectum.
4. In small animals, urine can be collected directly from the bladder through syringe and needle using aseptic conditions.
5. In some animals, urine is collected by catheterization. Catheter should be sterile. All aseptic conditions are followed. Clean the genitalia with soap and water and apply antiseptic solution. Dilate the vagina by using vaginal speculum with left hand and insert the catheter gently with right hand. Too much pressure should not be applied, if any obstruction is felt. When the catheter is inserted, slight pressure is applied on abdomen to press the urinary bladder and urine is collected through catheter. In bitch, the catheter is inserted at right angle to avoid the suburethral diverticulum. The external urethral opening is situated just ventral to clitoris. It is nearly 8 cm inside to the lower vulvar commissure. In cows, mare, sheep and goat the urinary orifice is just below the clitoris and 10 cm inside of the lower commissure of the vulva. In dogs, before the catheterization, clean the prepuce and glans penis with sterile gauze. Pass the catheter gently without applying much force. Collect the urine by just pressing the abdomen or applying a syringe and needle to the catheter.

Preservation

Normally, the urine sample is examined just after its collection. However, when delay is expected, it should be kept in refrigerator at 4^{0}C without adding any preservative. For longer storage, toluene can be added in urine to form a layer over urine; it suits for chemical examination. One drop of 40% formalin can also be used as preservative in urine but it may give false reaction for sugar examination. The addition thymol 0.1 gm/100 ml of urine is also recommended but it may give false reaction for albumin contents. One drop of phenol per 10 ml of urine can be used as preservative without much deterioration. The best way is to keep the urine sample at 4⁰C in refrigerator without addition of any preservative. All attempts should be made to examine the urine sample soon after its collection for a proper interpretation.

Examination

Physical Examination

Colour

The colour should be noted at the time of urine collection, by keeping it in a glass tube. Normally, the colour of urine is water colour to amber colour. However, in certain disease conditions the colour of urine alters:

- Hematuria: Red colour urine, cloudy (Fig. 4.1).
- Hemoglobinuria: Brown to red colour.
- Icterus: Yellow brown colour to greenish yellow.
- Pyogenic infections of kidneys: Yellowish green colour.
- High fever/dehydration due to diarrhoea/vomiting: Yellow orange to reddish colour.
- Azoturia in horses: Brown to black colour of urine.
- Phenothiazine phenolphthalein and/or azosulfamide treatments: Red colour urine.
- Methylene blue treatment: Blue to greenish urine.
- Acriflavin treatment: Green coloured urine
- Diabetes mellitus
- Diabetes insipidus pale colour urine
- Increased water uptake
- Chronic interstitial nephritis
- Pyometra

Odour

The normal odour of urine is uremic but in certain disease conditions it is altered. In case of ketosis, the odour of urine becomes sweetish or fruity while it becomes fetid in pyogenic infections of kidneys. The abnormal sample may give the odour of ammonia, acetone or fetid odour.

Turbidity

Normally the urine of equines is turbid and cloudy due to calcium carbonate and mucous while the urine of other animals is clear and transparent. Yellowish turbidity can be observed in pyogenic infections of kidneys. Kidney damage may be responsible for hematuria, albuminuria and proteinuria, which gives a turbid urine. Cloudiness in urine is due to presence of leucocytes, erythrocytes, epithelial cells, bacteria, mucous, fat and/or crystals. Of these, leucocytes give a white cloud while the red turbidity is seen due to erythrocytes and epithelial cells. Bacteria forms a uniform cloudiness in urine and fat forms cloud. On addition of chloroform or ether in the urine sample urine becomes transparent. On centrifugation, the fat comes at the top of urine while other turbid material settles down.

Foaming

On shaking, the normal urine produces white foams but in case of proteinuria, the amount of foam is in excess which remains for a longer duration. In icteric animals, the colour of foam may become green or yellow brown. The foams are red to brown in colour in case of hemoglobinuria.

Specific Gravity

The specific gravity of urine is measured by urinometer. The urine is filled in cylinder and urinometer is left in the urine which should not touch the wall of cylinder. The specific gravity should be read but it has little diagnostic value. The specific gravity increases in acute interstitial nephritis, cystitis, diabetes mellitus and dehydration and it decreases in chronic interstitial nephritis, pyometra and diabetes insipidus.

Chemical Examination

Reaction

The reaction of urine is determined by using pH strips or pH meter. Under normal conditions the urine of ruminants is alkaline while in canines it is acidic. The pH of alkaline urine is 7.4-8.4, while that of acidic urine is 6-7. Urine becomes acidic during starvation, fever, treatment of ammonium chloride, sodium chloride, calcium chloride and sodium acid phosphate. The alkaline urine occurs in cystitis and due to treatment of acetate, bicarbonate, citrate and nitrates of sodium or potassium.

Glucose

The urine sugar or glucose is measured by the following method using Benedict's reagent.

Take 0.5 ml of urine in a test tube and add 5.0 ml of Benedict's reagent and mix them thoroughly. Place this tube on a boiling water bath or flame for 5 min. Remove the tube from heating and keep on test tube stand for a few minutes and note the change of colour.

Blue	(-) No sugar
Blue to green sediment	(+) mild sugar
Yellow with heavy sediment	(++) moderate sugar
Orange with heavy sediment	(++++) highly positive for sugar.

Normally there should not be any glucose content in urine. Glycosuria occurs due to hyperglycemia and in diabetes mellitus, acute or chronic pancreatitis, hyperthyroidism, hyperadrenalism, hyperpituitarism, increased intracranial pressure, enterotoxemia. Certain drugs like streptomyclin, chlortetracycin, penicillin, tetracyclin and chloramphenicol may also lead to glycosuria.

Protein

The main protein in urine is albumin which comes under certain disease conditions. To test the presence of protein in urine, take 2 ml urine in a test tube and place 2 ml Robert's reagent over the urine. If albumin is present in the urine, a white ring will appear at the interjunction of two fluids which should be graded as follows.

Very heavy ring	+ + + +	Highly positive
Heavy ring	+ + +	Positive
A wide ring	+ +	Moderately positive
A narrow ring	+	Mild positive
No ring	(-)	Negative

In an another method take 2 ml urine in a test tube and add 0.5 ml of 20% sulfosalicylic, acid reagent and shake the tube; determine the turbidity as follows:

No turbidity	Negative
Slight turbidity	+
Moderate turbidity	+ +
Heavy turbidity	+ + +

Proteinuria may occur under some physiological conditions like excessive muscular exertion, stress, more protein in diet and convulsions which may disappear after removal of the factor. In disease conditions, proteinuria may occur in nephritis, acute interstitial nephritis, pyelonephritis and nephrosis. Phenol, arsenic, lead mercury, sulfonamides, phosphorus, turpentine and ether may cause proteinuria. Proteinuria may also occur in cystitis, prostatitis, pyelitis, urethritis, ureteritis, urolithiasis and due to mixing of vaginal and prepucial discharges in the urine.

Ketone Bodies

Ketone bodies are acetone, acetoacetic acid and beta hydroxy-butyric acid which are formed as a result of breakdown of fatty acids and accumulation of acetyl coenzymes.

1. *Acetone in urine* : Mix 1.0 gm of sodium nitropruside powder to 100 gm ammonium sulfate powder thoroughly and place 1 gm of mixed powder in a test tube. Add 5 ml urine and mix properly. To this overlay slowly 20% ammonium hydroxide solution. In case the acetone bodies are present, the colour becomes red to purple at the interjunction of the two fluids.
2. *Acetoacetic acid* : Take 10 ml urine in a test tube and add 5 drops of 30% acetic acid, 5 drops of Lugol's iodine and 3 ml of chloroform. Mix them properly and allow to stand. In case of a positive test, the chloroform will remain colourless while in negative test it may have a reddish violet colour.
3. *Betahydroxybutyric acid* : Take 20 ml urine sample in a small beaker and add 20 ml distilled water and a few drops of acetic acid. Boil the contents over flame till 10 ml. Add distilled water to make it 20 ml and place in test tubes, 10 ml each. In one tube add 1 ml hydrogen peroxide and warm it for 1 min and then cool it. Add 1 ml glacial acetic acid and 1 ml freshly prepared sodium nitroprusside solution and mix thoroughly. To this overlay strong ammonia water and allow to stand for 3-4 hours. In a positive test, purple colour ring is formed in test tube in which hydrogen peroxide was mixed, while the other tube remains the same without any ring.

Bile Salts

Take about 4-5 ml urine in a test tube and shake it. On shaking, persistent foams are produced if the bile salts are present in the urine. The presence of bile salts can also be determined by the Hay's sulfur test; in which the sulfur granules are sprinkled over the surface of urine in test tube. If urine contains bile salts, the sulfur granules sink through urine.

Bilirubin

Take about 4-5 ml urine sample in a test tube and boil it. Cool the tube and filter through filter paper. Add a few drops of acetic acid in the filtrate to make the urine acidic. Add 2 ml of 10% barium chloride in 4 ml filtrate, mix and filter through filter paper. Place a drop of trichloroacetic acid and ferric chloride solution on filter paper; the presence of bilirubin is indicated by the appearance of a green blue colour on the filter paper.

Indican

Take 5 ml urine in a test tube and add 5 ml of 0.2% ferric chloride solution and 2 ml chloroform. Mix well by inverting the tube and allow the contents to stand for some time. The chloroform settles; examine colour of chloroform. The presence of blue to violet colour is indication of presence of indican.

The indican level is increased in intestinal obstruction, constipation, rapid breakdown of protein, indigestion, gastritis, enteritis, intussusception and volvulus.

Chloride

Examination of urine for chloride is carried out in kidney diseases, shock, dehydration, prolonged diarrhoea and proteinuria. It also serves as a guide for a parenteral saline therapy. For the chloride test, take 10 drops of urine in a test tube and add one drop of 20% potassium dichromate solution. To this add drop by drop 2.9% silver nitrate and keep shaking the test tube constantly shaking till the colour changes from yellow to red brown. The number of drops of silver nitrate required to reach the end point is the chloride content of urine expressed as grains of sodium chloride per liter. Multiply by 0.171 to have mEq chloride/liter. A single sample of urine does not give the precise results of chloride content but a composite sample of 24 hours will provide more reliable results. The chloride content decreases in fasting, starvation, vomiting, severe diarrhoea, acute infections and glucose therapy. The increased chloride levels are observed in increased salt or water intake, ascites and administration of diuretics. Normally, the chloride content of urine of dog is 76 mEq/lit and in cattle 282 mEq/lit.

Blood

Take 2 ml urine in one test tube and in another tube 1 ml of saturated benzidine solution and 1 ml of 30% hydrogen peroxide and mix well. The contents of both the tubes are mixed thoroughly. If blood is present in urine, it is indicated by the development of a green to deep blue colour. The presence of blood in urine is known as hematuria which occurs in pyelonephritis, ureteritis, cystitis, urolithiasis, pyelitis, trauma in urethra, prostatitis, kidney neoplasms, acute nephritis, parasitic infection like *Dioctophyma renale, Dirofilaria immitis* and *Capillaria plica.* If whole urine is mixed with blood the possible source may be kidneys but if only last portion of urine is red and contains blood, it is from bladder.

Hemoglobin/Myoglobin

Take 5 ml urine in a test tube and add 2.8 gm ammonium sulfate, shake well and allow to stand for a few minutes. If the colour of urine becomes clear, it indicates the presence of hemoglobin in urine. If the colour remains the same, as before the test, it is myoglobin. Hemoglobinuria occurs in leptospirosis, piroplasmosis, photosensitization, post parturient hemoglobinuria and bacillary hemoglobinuria. The myoglobinuria occurs in azoturia.

Microscopic Examination

For microscopic examination, take 5-10 ml urine in a centrifuge tube and centrifuge it at 1000 rpm for 10 min. Discard the supernatant and place a drop of sediment in middle of a clean and dry glass slide. Cover it with a coverslip and examine under microscope for epithelial cells, leucocytes, erythrocytes, casts, bacteria and crystals. If the cells are not clear, the smear can be made from sediment and stained by Giemsa. The colour of sediment becomes red if red blood cells are present in urine while it becomes yellow if bile pigments are present in urine. The white colour sediment is seen in the presence of crystals in urine and fat is at the top of the contents on centrifugation.

If the urine sediment is more concentrated it should be diluted with supernatant and record this finding also. Under low power, hyaline castes are seen while high power objectives are used for cell types and bacteria. The urine sediment is of two types:

1. Organized sediment: It contains epithelial cells, leucocytes, erythrocytes, microorganisms, casts, parasites.
2. Unorganized sediment: It includes fat, crystals, pigments, etc.

Organized Sediment

Epithelial Cells

The epithelial cells are normally present in urine but in low number. The number of epithelial cells increases in cystitis or other inflammatory condition of urinary passage. Squamous epithelial cells in urine come from urethra, bladder and vagina. These are the largest cells in sediment and have small round nucleus. The epithelial cells of renal tubules are smaller, round or polyhedral in shape and these are larger than leucocytes.

Leucocytes

These are also normally present in urine but low in number. Presence of 10 leucocytes per high power field of 15 ml urine sediment are considered to be from any inflammatory condition; the genital system may also be a source for them. The number of leucocytes increases in nephritis, pyelonephritis, pyelitis, urethritis and cystitis. The leucocytes are also called ***pus cells***. These are larger than erythrocytes and have granular appearance. If urine is alkaline, the leucocytes are swollen and become very granular and appear in clumps.

Erythrocytes

Erythrocytes are spherical in shape, like a faint colourless ring "shadow cells"; these are not uniform in size and are smaller than leucocytes. If the urine is of low concentration with low specific gravity, the erythrocytes are ballooned. These have crenated periphery giving a distorted appearance. Presence of erythrocytes in urine is an indication of hemorrhage in the genitourinary system. If the blood comes during onset of urination, the source of hemorrhage is urethra. The bladder hemorrhage are characterized by blood mixed last portion of urine, while whole urine is mixed with blood in kidney hemorrhage. Hemorrhage also occur as a result of catheterization, bladder puncture and manipulation of bladder.

Microorganisms

Microorganisms are present during any infectious disease of the urinary tract. The bacteria, yeast, fungi or protozoa are the organisms which may be present in urine.

1. *Bacteria:* May be present in cystitis, pyelonephritis and can be identified after Gram's staining.
2. *Yeast:* These are colourless, round to ovoid bodies with double refractile walls and these are usually contaminants.
3. *Fungi:* Fungi have distinct segmented hyphae. Coloured fungi have no significance.
4. *Protozoa:* Protozoa are rare in urine; these are the contaminants of feces, Trichomonads are the contaminants of genital tract.

Casts

The presence of casts in urine is called ***cylindriuria***. The proteinous casts are formed in the distal tubules and collected in tubules of kidneys because of higher concentration of urine. Casts are of seven types.

1. *Hyaline casts:* It is composed of protein. It is homogenous, semitransparent, colourless, cylindrical having rounded ends. It is present in acidic urine. It indicates the mild form of renal irritation and is found in febrile conditions after anesthesia and exercise and in association with circulatory disturbances.
2. *Granular casts:* These are the hyaline casts containing granules which are formed as a result of disintegration of tubular epithelium. These are the most common casts seen in urine.
3. *Waxy casts:* These are similar to hyaline casts. These are homogeneous containing few granules and occasional cells. These are opaque, greyish or colourless, having dull and waxy appearance. These casts have blunt ends, broken and cigar shaped. These casts are seen in advanced nephritis and amyloid degeneration of kidneys.
4. *Epithelial casts:* These casts are formed from the desquamated epithelial cells of renal tubules. These contain oval, elongated or flat cells and such casts are seen in acute nephritis.
5. *Red cell casts:* These are homogeneous, cylindrical deep yellow to orange in colour and occur due to degeneration of red blood cells. These are the indication of hemorrhage in renal tubule.
6. *Fatty casts:* These casts occur as small droplets of fat as refractile bodies. These are colourless and indicative of degenerative tubular disease associated with lipid deposition and occur in diabetes mellitus.
7. *Leucocytic casts:* These casts are characterized by the presence of many pus cells adhered to hyaline casts. These casts are indicative of suppurative process and are seen in pyelonephritis and kidney abscess.

Mucous Threads

The mucous threads are seen in urine of horses but in other animals; these are the indications of urethral irritation. Most mucous threads are from genital tract secretions.

Parasites

In urine sediment, certain parasitic ova may also be seen; like.

1. *Capillaria plica* –bladder worm of dog and cat
2. *Stephanurus dentatus* – kidney worm of pig
3. *Dioctophyma renale* – kidney worm of dog.

Other worms/or ova if present in urine sediment may come as fecal contamination.

Spermatozoa

The spermatozoa can be seen in urine, when urine is mixed with semen. It is common in male dogs.

Unorganized Sediment

Fat Droplets

The fat droplets are present as round, refractile bodies of varying size. It stains orange to red by Sudan III. The source of fat in urine is extraneous such as lubricated material of catheter or contaminated vial. Lipuria commonly occurs in cats due to fatty metamorphosis of renal tubules, rupture of lymphatics, obesity, diabetes mellitus, hypothyroidism and high fat diet.

Crystals

Two types of crystals are seen in urine depending upon pH and solubility.

In alkaline urine, the crystals are triple and amorphous phosphates, calcium carbonates, ammonium urates. In acidic urine, the crystals present are amorphous urates, uric acid, calcium oxalates and hippuric acid. Leucine and tyrosine crystals are present in urine in case of calculi in kidney. Such crystals occur as a result of acute liver disease, carbon tetrachloride poisoning, chloroform or phosphorus. Cysteine crystals occur in urine due to disturbances in protein metabolism and may result in development of cysteine calculi.

Cultural Examination

For cultural examination, urine is collected in sterile container. It should be inoculated directly in culture media or after centrifugations. The details of cultural examination and antibiotic sensitivity test are described elsewhere in this book.

5

Examination of Feces

- General considerations
- Collection of feces
- Storage
- Examination of feces
    - Gross examination
    - Microscopic examination
    - Examination of feces for flukes
    - Examination of feces for blood
    - Culture of feces for nematode larvae
    - Sporulation of coccidia.

General Considerations

Fecal examination is indicated in diarrhoeic diseases, constipation, anorexia, jaundice, hepatitis, lungworm infection, anemia, weakness, low milk production and in dysentery. Examination of feces is mainly carried out for the detection of parasites, their ova/larva/oocyst, blood and other foreign material. Sometimes cultural examination of feces is performed for isolation of bacteria or virus in order to establish the etiology of diarrhoea/dysentry. The bacterial or viral antigens are also demonstrated in feces using immunological methods like immunofluorescence, enzyme linked immunosorbent assay and dot immunobinding assay. For proper examination of feces, its collection and storage is very important.

Collection of Feces

The fecal sample is collected directly from animal. In large animals, one should wear gloves and lubricate the hands with water and collect feces from rectum. If feces is not present in rectum, stimulate the mucosa of rectum with finger, the animal will defecate within few minutes. Collect 5-10 gm feces in a clear, dry glass container. If feces is to be collected for cultural examination, it should be collected in sterilized glass vials. In small animals like calves, sheep, goat and dogs, the feces is collected by using index finger. In poultry, the cloacal swabs are collected for examination. If the sample is collected from recently defecated feces, middle portion should be collected which should be free from mud, dirt and foreign material.

Storage

It is always preferred to examine the feces as early as possible after its collection. However, if the delay in examination is expected, then store the feces in refrigerator at 4^{0}C. If it is to be transported to laboratory from a distant place, it should be sealed and marked properly. For parasitic examination, 10% formalin can also be added as preservative in feces. The fecal samples collected for lungworm examination should be transferred in sealed containers without adding any preservative.

Examination of Feces

1. *Gross examination:* The fecal sample is kept in clean, dry petri dishes for gross examination. With the help of a spatula or clean glass rod, it should be spread properly and examined for its colour, consistency, odour, and presence of blood, parasite, segment of parasite, or any other foreign material.
2. *Microscopic examination:* Routinely the microscopic examination of feces is performed by following methods.

Direct Smear Method

In this method a clean and dry glass slide is used which should be free from scratches. Place a drop of distilled water in the middle of the slide and add small amount of feces on it. Mix with tooth pick or match stick and place a coverslip on it. Examine it under microscope for the presence of parasitic ova. In direct smear method, if no parasitic ova is detected then it should be examined by qualitative or quantitative methods before declaring it as negative.

Qualitative Concentration Method

In this method, the feces is mixed with either saturated sugar solution, saturated salt solution, saturated sodium nitrate solution, 41% magnesium sulfate solution or 33% zinc sulfate solution. The parasitic ova, being lighter, float on the top of fluid and thus can be concentrated for examination.

1. *Simple floatation:* In this method, about one gram of feces is taken and mixed with a few millilitres of distilled water and filtered through a fine sieve or muslin cloth. The filtrate is then mixed with 4-5 ml of saturated salt solution. It should be then placed in a tube or cylinder and filled up to the top with solution. A clean glass slide or coverslip is placed on the mouth of tube or cylinder. This is left for 30 to 60 min at room temperature without any disturbance. After that the coverslip or slide is removed and examined under microscope for the presence of parasitic ova. The unfiltered material left on sieve or muslin cloth is examined for tapeworm segments/parasite.

2. *Centrifugation floatation:* In this method, about one gram of feces is mixed with distilled water and filtered through a fine sieve or muslin cloth. The filtered material is mixed with saturated sugar solution in a ratio of 1:3 in a test tube. Mix the contents and centrifuge at 1500 rpm for 5 min, The tube is taken out and placed on stand without any disturbance. Transfer the small amount of superficial contents of tube on a clean and dry glass slide and examine under microscope for the presence of parasitic ova. The sediment of the floatation method is examined under microscope for eggs of liver flukes (Fig. 5.1).

Quantitative Concentration Method

1. *McMaster method:* In this method, 2 grams of feces is taken in a clean and dry beaker and 28 ml distilled water is added and mixed well. One ml of fecal suspension and 1 ml saturated sugar solution are mixed in another test tube. During mixing drain some fluid in a pipette and place in McMaster counting chamber to fill the marked area. Leave it for a few minutes. Place it on microscope and count the eggs in marked area. To calculate eggs per gram of feces, total count is multiplied with 200.

2. *Field method* : In this method, one gram of feces is mixed in 10 ml distilled water. Then 0.1 ml of this mixture is placed on a clean and dry glass slide, and covered with a coverslip. Count the parasitic ova under low power of microscope in all fields. Multiply with 100 to get the egg count per gram of feces.

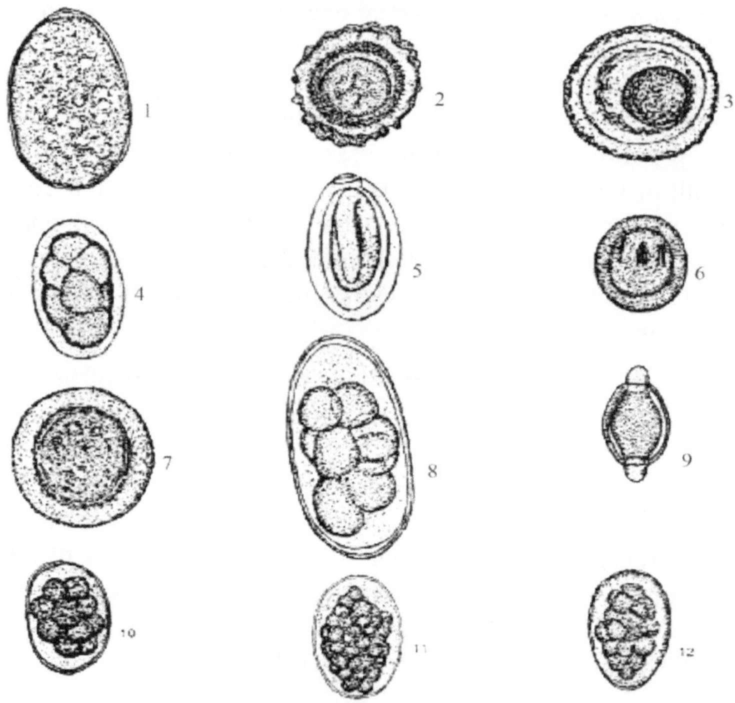

Fig. 5.1: Diagramatic illustrations of parasitic ova as observed in the feces on microscopic examination. **1.** *Fasciola hepatica,* **2.** *Ascaris lumbricodes,* **3.** *Ascaris equorum,* **4.** *Strongylus* sp., **5.** *Oxyuris equi,* **6.** *Taenia* sp., **7.** *Toxoscara canis,* **8.** *Nematodirus* sp., **9.** *Trichuris ovis,* **10.** *Haemonchus contortus,* **11.** *Ostertagia* sp and **12.** *Trichostronylus* sp.

Examination of Feces for Flukes

The eggs of liver flukes are heavy and do not float on water and settle in sediment. Two grams of feces is taken in a tube and mixed with distilled water. Put the mixture in a tube and leave it for 30-60 mins; discard the supernatant and repeat the process 2-3 times. Take small amount of sediment on slide and examine under microscope.

Examination of Feces for Blood

In a small test tube 2-3 ml of saturated solution of benzidine in glacial acetic acid is taken. To this equal amount of hydrogen peroxide is added. The feces (1-2 gm) is mixed with distilled water and the fecal suspension is poured in the benzidine solution drop by drop. The development of a blue colour is indication of the presence of blood in feces.

Culture of Feces for Nematode Larvae

Sometimes the identification of parasite becomes difficult by mere examination of eggs. For this one should cultivate the larvae from eggs. The feces is mixed with an equal amount of charcoal or granulated wood, moistened to make it damp. This mixture is stored on a filter paper in a covered container like glass jar and kept at room temperature (25^{0}C-30^{0}C) for one week. The moisture is maintained by addition of water. After one week, the larvae are separated by needle or brush. The larva which do not migrate should be separated by Baerman method (Fig. 5.2). In this method, a funnel is taken with a rubber tubing fitted in the narrow bottom. A clip is provided with tube to regulate the flow of fluid and the funnel is held in a stand. Now the feces is taken in gauze which is placed on a wire sieve in funnel. Place the normal saline solution in the funnel so that it is at the level just over the feces. Hold up the wire mesh and gauze. The larvae come in normal saline solution and accumulate at the bottom within hours due to gravitation force, and can be collected by releasing the stop cock. Examine the larvae under microscope. This method is best suited for the examination of lungworm larvae. The lukewarm temperature of the normal saline solution in the funnel stimulates the activity of larvae. The method is also suitable for separation of parasitic larvae from soil.

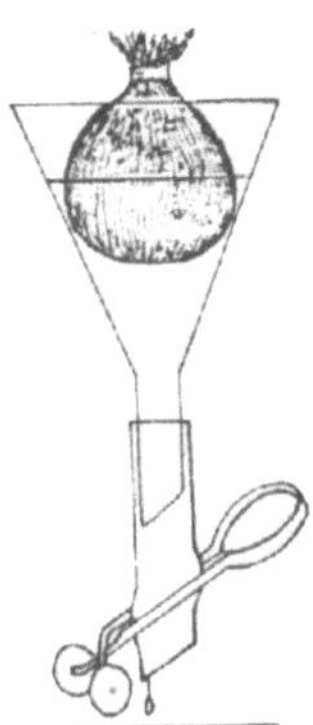

Fig. 5.2: Fig.5.2 Diagram of an equipment for the collection of larvae from feces

Sporulation of Coccidia

The identification of coccidia sometimes becomes difficult by the direct smear method. For proper identification, the fecal material is kept for sporulation of coccidia to the infective stage which is easily identifiable. The feces is mixed with 2.5% potassium dichromate solution in a ratio 1:5 or 1:10 and the suspension is transferred to petridish to make a thin layer (1-2 mm). The thin layer is necessary to coccidial sporulation because it provides requisite oxygen and potassium dichromate checks the oxygen utilization by bacteria. The sporulation occurs within a few days to week's time. The sporulated oocyst can be stored in refrigerator for long period also.

6

Examination of Milk

- General considerations
- Collection of milk sample
- Storage
- Examination of milk
  - Physical examination
  - Chemical examination
  - Cytological examination
  - Bacteriological examination

General Considerations

Milk is the secretion of mammary gland, meant for the young ones of the animals. It is nutritious and necessary for young growing animals for their development. It contains considerable quantities of protein, carbohydrate, fat, minerals and vitamins. The composition of milk of different animals is given in Table 6.1

Table 6.1: Composition of milk (percent)

Sr.no.	Species	Water	Protein	Fat	Carbohydrate	Minerals
1	Cattle	87.2	3.4	3.8	4.8	0.8
2	Buffalo	83.0	3.9	6.6	5.8	0.7
3	Mare	90.5	2.0	1.2	5.8	0.4
4	Sheep	81.9	5.8	6.5	4.8	0.9
5	Goat	84.1	4.0	6.0	5.0	0.8
6	Sow	84.6	6.3	4.8	3.4	0.9
7	Man	87.4	2.1	3.8	6.3	0.3

The examination of milk is indicated in udder ailments like mastitis. The milk examination is required to diagnose the mastitis which gives guidelines for treatment of a particular disease. One can make the prognosis of mastitis through examination of milk.

Collection of Milk Sample

The udder of the animal should be thoroughly cleaned with water and antiseptics like 1:1000 solution of potassium permanganate and dried with clean towel. The hands of clinician or person collecting milk should also be cleaned with soap and antiseptics. Disinfect the teats with swabs of 70% alcohol. Collect the milk sample from each teat in separate tubes. The first 3-4 streams of milk should be discarded and then 5-10 ml of milk sample is collected in tubes. Tubes should be sealed/stoppered properly immediately after collection of milk. It should be transported to laboratory for examination in ice.

Storage

The examination of milk should be performed immediately after its collection. But if delay is expected in examination, it should be kept in refrigerator at 4^0C.

Examination of Milk

Physical Examination

1. *Colour:* Normally, the colour of milk is white or creamy white but in acute mastitis it may become reddish due to presence of blood. In chronic mastitis or subacute mastitis it may become watery. The colour of milk becomes yellowish during colostral period, feeding of carrots, tetracycline therapy and therapy of acridine dyes. The pink to brown colour of milk is seen due to phenothiazine treatment.
2. *Specific gravity:* The specific gravity of normal milk is 1.015 to 1.037 which may get altered due to mastitis.
3. *Reaction:* The pH of normal milk is 6.4 to 6.6. But in mastitis it becomes alkaline upto 7.4 due to presence of sodium bicarbonate in the milk. The reaction can be determined by using pH strips.
4. *Odour:* Normally, the odour of milk is pleasant but it may turn obnoxious due to mastitis caused by *Actinomyces pyogenes*. In ketosis the odour of milk becomes sweet, stable and fruity.
5. *Consistency:* The colostrum or first milk of the animal just after parturition is viscous. The watery consistency occurs due to poor feeding and chronic mastitis. During mastitis (acute and subacute), the milk contains fine as well as large flakes. The consistency of milk is determined by using strip cups even under field conditions.
6. *Strip cup test:* This test is useful in field conditions for physical examination of milk. In this test, enamel plate divided in four strip cups

is used. The bottom of the plate is black coloured so that it gives a good contrast to easily observe the milk flakes. The comparison of milk from all four quarters can be carried out simultaneously. The milk flakes can be seen by tilting the cups at an angle. This test can be carried out by laymen at farm itself. If clots or flakes are observed in the milk, the animal is isolated from the herd for confirmatory diagnosis and treatment. This test is very useful in primary screening of animals for mastitis.

Chemical Examination

1. *Bromothymol blue test:* The reaction of milk is detected by this test. In this test, 1 ml of 0.2% bromothymol blue solution is taken and to this 5 ml of freshly collected milk sample is added. If sample is alkaline due to mastitis, it becomes blue to green. However, the test may give false positive reaction in later stage of lactation.

2. *Chloride test:* The presence of more than 0.14% chloride content in milk is considered abnormal. For this test, take 5 ml of 0.1341% silver nitrate solution in a test tube and add 2 drops of 10% potassium dichromate solution as indicator. To this add 1 ml of milk sample and mix it properly. If the chloride is less than 0.14% then it will remain brownish red while in positive case it will become yellow indicating more than 0.14% chloride content in milk. However, this test may give false positive reaction during early and late lactation.

3. *White slide test:* In this test, 4-5 drops of test milk sample are placed on a clean dry glass slide. To this add a drop of 4% sodium hydroxide and mix with a glass rod. If the milk is from animal having mastitis, it becomes thickened and flakes appear. While the negative milk sample remains the same. This test is based on the increased number of leucocytes in mastitic milk.

4. *California mastitis test:* This test is based on increased number of leucocytes and increased alkalinity in milk due to mastitis. Take 0.5 ml milk from each quarter in plastic peddle cups and add equal quantity of mast aid solution and mix well by circular movement of peddle on a horizontal plane. The results are read as follows.

a.	Liquid milk with no: negative for mastitis streaks or precipitation		
b.	Streaky fluid:	+	(weak positive cell count 500,000/ml)
c.	Slimy:	+ +	(Moderate positive)
d.	Gelatinous:	+ + +	(high positive)

This is an indirect measurement of cell count.

5. *Hotis test:* Take 0.5 ml of 0.5% bromocresol purple and sterilize it by autoclaving. Mix 9.5 ml milk sample after cooling and incubate it at 37^{0}C for 24 hours. The appearance of yellow colonies along the sides of tubes or on bottom indicates infection due to *Streptococcus agalactiae.*

Cytological Examination

Leucocyte count: Mix the milk sample thoroughly and take out 0.1 ml of mixed milk and place it on a clean, dry glass slide. Mark the area on central portion of slide (1 sq cm) and spread the milk sample with bacteriological loop in this area. Dry the smear and dissolve the fat by rinsing it in xylene for 2-5 min. Fix the smear with alcohol for 5 min and stain with methylene blue for 1 min. Remove the excess stain by immersing the slides in alcohol. Count the leucocytes under oil immersion of the microscope. The cells of 10 fields are counted and averaged and multiplied by 500,000 to get the total number of leucocytes per ml of milk.

Bacteriological Examination

1. *Direct microscopic examination:* This is rapid procedure to know the type of infection and total number of organism present in the milk. In this method, like leucocyte count, take 0.1 ml of properly mixed milk sample and place it on centre of a clean and dry glass slide. Mark the 1 sq cm central area of slide and spread the milk sample by bacteriological loop. Air dry the slide with gentle heat and fix it on flame. Stain the smear with Newmann's stain for 2 min, wash the stain and air dry the smear. Examine under oil immersion of the microscope. Count the single bacteria or isolated clumps in any 10 fields and average them. To get the bacterial count per ml, multiply the count with 500,000 and interpret as under in table 6.2.

Table. 6.2: Bacteriological quality of milk

Bacterial count	**Quality of milk**
<500,000	good
500,000 to 40,00,000	fair
40,00,000 to 20,000,000	poor
>20,000,000	very poor

As per the structures / morphology, the milk can be classified as under in table 6.3.

Table. 6.3: Morphology of bacteria and quality of milk

S.No	Structure /morphology	Interpretation
1.	Many cocci/rods in clumps/patches	Uncleaned utensils
2.	Excessive rod shaped bacteria spore forming	Dust mixed milk
3.	Large number of cocci in chains with large no. of leucocytes	mastitis.

2. *Cultural Examination:* The milk is collected in sterilized vials and stored in refrizerator. The milk sample is inoculated on bacteriological media (nutrient agar, blood agar or tryptose soya agar) for isolation of organism and antibiotic sensitivity test as described elsewhere in this book.

7

Examination of Skin Scrapings

- General considerations
- Examination of skin scrapings for mange
- Examination of skin scrapings for fungi
- Cultural examination

General Considerations

The skin scrapings are examined for the diagnosis of skin diseases, including parasitic, fungal and bacterial infections and infestations. The examination of skin scrapings differentiate and diagnose the type of mange present in animals. The confirmatory diagnosis of skin disease is made through microscopic examination of skin scrapings of animals. The skin lesions are mostly produced by mites or fungus; it is, therefore, necessary to describe the detailed method of examinations of skin scrapings for these ailments.

Examination of Skin Scrapings for Mange

Collection

The scrapings must be collected from the most affected part of the skin as there are more parasites on this part than in any other. The affected part should be moistened with mineral oil or 10% potassium hydroxide. The skin scrapings are collected with the help of scalpel dipped in mineral oil. Press the lesions on skin with thumb and index finger of left hand and scrap the skin with right hand using scalpel. Care must be taken to avoid any cut on skin. The scrapings should be collected so deep that some blood oozes out. The skin scrapings are collected in 10% potassium hydroxide or in glycerine and transported to laboratory after sealing and proper indentification.

Direct Smear Method

The potassium hydroxide treated skin scrapings are placed on clean and dry glass slide with one drop of 10% potassium hydroxide or sodium hydroxide. The scrapings are macerated with scalpel or spatula and covered with coverslip. Examine the slide under low power of the microscope (Fig 7.1 to Fig.7.4).

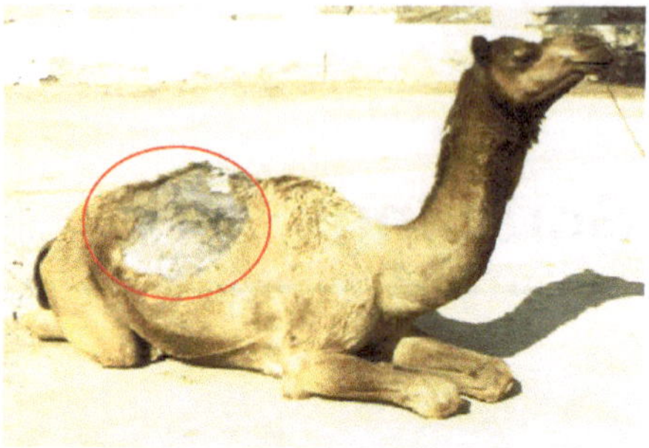

Fig. 7.1: Photograph showing mange due to *S. scabei* in a camel

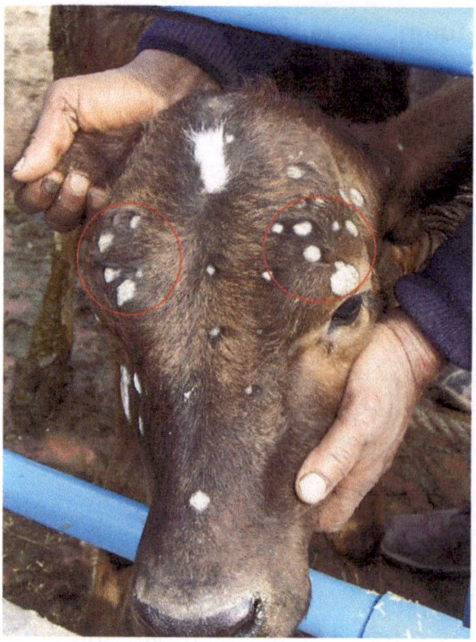

Fig. 7.2: Photograph showing demodectic mange in cattle

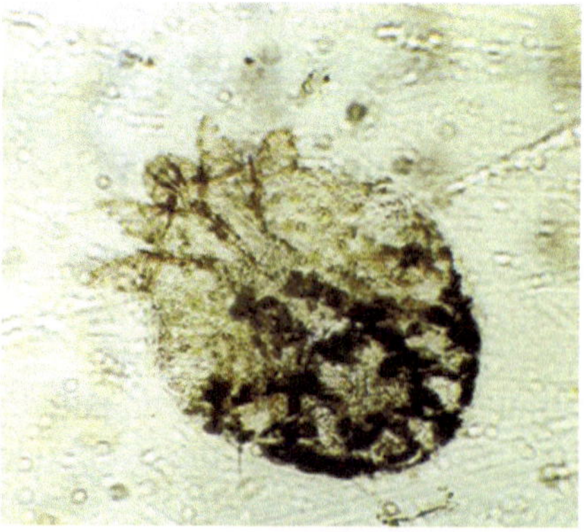

Fig. 7.3: Photomicrograph of skin scraping showing Sarcoptes scabei

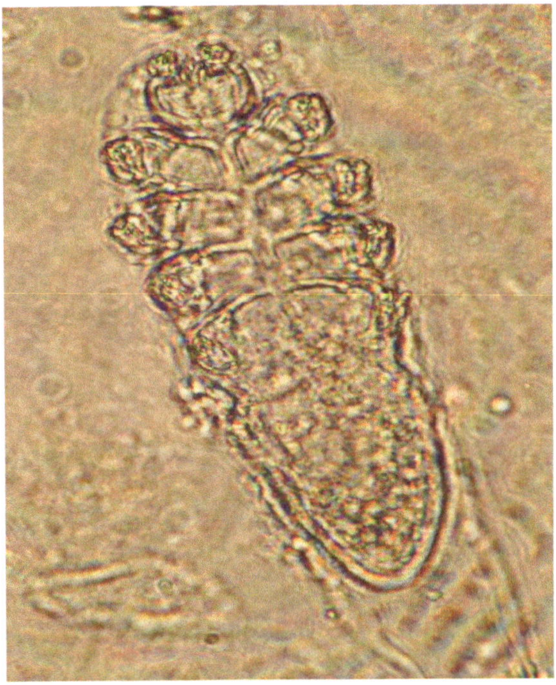

Fig. 7.4: Photomicrograph of skin scraping showing demodectic mange

Sedimentation Method

The skin scrapings are kept in 10% potassium hydroxide or sodium hydroxide for 2-4 hours to digest the debris; the digestion process may be expedited by providing the gentle heat to the sample. The scrapings should be transferred to centrifuge tube and centrifuge at 3000 rpm for 10 min. The supernatent is discarded and one drop of sediment is placed on middle of a clean and dry glass slide, cover it with coverslip and examine under low power of the microscope.

Sugar Floatation Method

The skin scrapings are kept 2-4 hours in 10% potassium hydroxide for digestion of debris; then tansfered to a centrifuge tube and centrifuged at 3000 rpm for 10 min. Discard the supernatent and add distilled water in the centrifuge tube to fill it half and mix the contents. Centrifuge tube is filled with saturated sugar solution. Centrifuge it for 10-15 min at 3000 rpm. By the gravitational force, parasites of mange mites will come over the contents of the centrifuge tube. Take one drop of fluid from top of the centrifuge tube and place on middle of clean and dry glass slide. Cover it with a coverslip and examine under microscope.

Examination of Skin Scrapings for Fungi

Fungal examination of skin scrapings is indicated when fungal infection of skin is suspected. The site of collection of scrapings should be the most active lesion at skin. Since some fungal infections spread towards the periphery, it is advisable to collect the scrapings from centre as well as from periphery of the lesion. Before collection of the scrapings, skin is swabed with 95% alcohol or spirit to remove any saprophytic organism. The scalpel should be moistened with mineral oil and the skin scrapped deeply to include hairs. The skin scrapings are collected in sterilized petridishes containing 10% potassium hydroxide or sodium hydroxide.

Gross Examination

The gross examination is performed on the intact skin to detect the presence of ringworm. In this test, chloroform is applied on the affected part of skin with the help of a swab. After a few mintues, the chloroform gets evaporated and the hair of the ringworm affected area becomes white in colour. If there is no ringworm, the hairs remain the same. This test is directly performed on the skin of animal, suitably at the time of collection of skin scrapings.

Examination by Wood's Lamp

The Wood's lamp has UV light, which is directed on the intact skin or on the scrapings collected in petridishes. If the fungus microsporum is present, it gives yellow-green fluorescence while no fluorescence is observed in negative or trichophyton fungal infection of skin.

Microscopic Examination

1. *Direct examination*: The skin scrapings collected in petri dishes are placed on slide with one drop of 10% potassium hydroxide. Cover it with coverslip and apply vaseline around the rim of cover slip. The slide is warmed gently over spirit lamp or gas burner for a few seonds. Examine the slide under microscope for fungus, which looks like chain of hyphae and sproes (Fig 7.5).

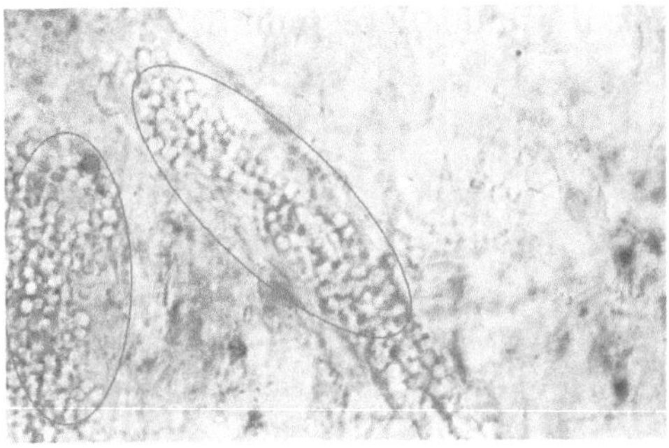

Fig. 7.5: Photomicrograph of skin scraping showing presence of fungus (Ttrichophyton metagraphite)

2. *PAS staining method:* The skin scrapings are placed on glass slides coated with egg albumin and the slides are gently heated. Before proceeding to staining, one should check that the scrapings are properly fixed on slide; then follow the staining procedure in following way.

    a. Place the slides in 95% alcohol for 1 min.

    b. Transfer the slides to 5% periodic acid for 5 min.

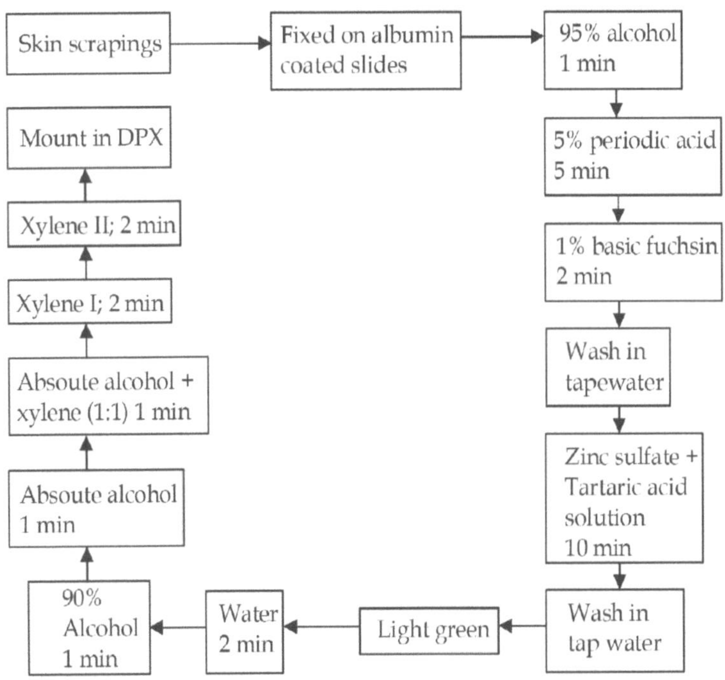

Fig. 7.6: Line drawing showing PAS staining

c. Place the slides in 0.1 % basic fuchsin solution for 2 min.
d. Wash the slides in tap water.
e. Place the slides in zinc sulfate-tartaric acid solution for 10 min.
f. Rinse the slides in tap water.
g. Counter stain with 1 % light green for 2 min.
h. Rinse quickly in running tap water.
i. Dehydrate in 90% alcohol; absolute alcohol for 1 min each.
j. Place the slides in absolute alcohol + xylene (1:1) mixture for 1 min.
k. Clear the slides in xylene I and II for 2 min in each.
l. Mount in DPX and examine under microscope.
m. Interpretation—the fungi will take a bright red or purplish red colour.

The entire method of PAS staining has been shown in Fig. 7.6.

Cultural Examination

The skin of the affected area is cleared with 70% alcohol or spirit. The skin scrapings are collected in sterilized petridishes. These skin scrapings are inoculated on Sabouraud's dextrose agar media and are incubated for at least one week at 37^{0}C. The plates of culture are examined daily for fungal growth. On appearance of fungal growth it should be examined under microscope. Cultural examination of the skin scrapings is not rountinely carried out. However, it is required for the confirmation of the disease and identification of the fungus. For cultural examination of bacteria, refer to Chapter -11.

8

Examination of Synovial Fluid

- General considerations
- Collection of synovial fluid
- Examination of synoival fluid
  - Physical examination
  - Chemical examination
  - Cytological examination
  - Microbiological examination
  - Examination for immune complexes
  - Miscellaneous examination
- Inflammatory conditions of joints
  - Non-infectious arthritis
  - Infectious arthritis
  - Immune complex mediated arthritis

General Considerations

Synovial fluid is a tissue fluid found in the joints (intra-articular space) and contains protein, mucin, secreted by synovial membrane and dialysate of plasma. The non-electrolytes of joint fluid passes readily in either direction between blood and synovial fluid while the electrolytes are present in accordance with Gibbs-Donnon theory of membrane equilibrium. Normally the synovial fluid is clear, viscous, pale or straw coloured and does not clot due to the absence of fibrinogen. The specific gravity of synovial fluid is 1.010-1.015 and some leucocytes are present in normal fluid.

Synovial fluid is formed from the components of blood supplied by synovial membrane and vascular network and is modified by endothelial lining, connective tissue and synovial lining cells. The normal constituents of synovial fluid are to nourish the avascular articular cartilage. Normal exchange of constituents occurs between synovial fluid and blood-lymphatic network of the synovial membrane. Synovial fluid also provides cushion and lubrication for movements of joints to minimize the frictional movements within the joints.

In joint disease, the characteristics of synovial fluid changes with altered metabolism in intra-articular space leading to a disturbed exchange of substances between vascular and lymphatic system and synovial fluid. The synovial fluid formation, destruction and utilization of various components within the joints are also altered. The analysis of synovial fluid is performed for the diagnosis of joint diseases which may yield information about degree and type of changes in joints.

Collection of Synovial Fluid

The synovial fluid is collected by joint puncture and aspiration by syringe; 5-10 ml synovial fluid is collected from large animals (cattle, buffaloes, horse, camels, etc.) while 0.5-1.0 ml synovial fluid is taken from joints of small animals (dog, cat, sheep, goat). The synovial fluid should be collected aseptically using appropriate sterile needle and syringe. The site of joint puncture must be shaved and usual antiseptics should be applied on the surface. It is usually collected under local anesthesia and short needles of 18 gauge alongwith stylet are used for synovial fluid collection. The synovial fluid is collected in an anticoagulant like 3.8% sodium citrate (0.1 ml/ml of synovial fluid) and mixed properly to prevent coagulation. Care must be taken to avoid the contamination of red blood cells or blood at the time of joint puncture.

The synovial fluid is collected from the affected joints. The procedure of collection of synovial fluid and site of joint puncture for various joints of the body are as follows.

1. *Hip joint* : The puncture is made in the nick between the anterior and posterior trochanter major. A needle of 12 cm length with stylet is inserted at the right angle to the skin and then it is directed horizontally to puncture the joint capsule.
2. *Stifle joint* : In large animals, the stifle joint (femoro-patellar articulation) is punctured by inserting a needle at right angle between middle and medial patellar ligament about 4 cm above the tibia. For puncture of lateral sac of femoro-tibial articulation, the needle is inserted in an obliquely cranial position between the tibial tuberosity and the lateral condyle of tibia on either side of the tendon of the long digital extensor. The medial sac of femoro tibial joint is punctured by inserting the needle

2-3 cm above the middle condyle of tibia in the groove between the median patellar ligament and the medial femoro tibial ligament.

In small animals, the fixed joint is punctured by inserting a needle medial or lateral to the pateller ligament half way between patella and tibial crest.

3. *Hock joint* : The joint is punctured from the anterior side. The needle is inserted on the medial side of area bounded by tendon of insertion of tibialis anterior muscle and long medial ligament.
4. *Shoulder joint* : A 10 cm long needle is inserted just anterior to the tendon of the infraspinatus muscle about 2 cm proximal to the lateral tuberosity of the humerus to a depth till joint capsule is priced which is felt by slight tremor in needle.
5. *Elbow joint* : In cattle and buffaloes, the needle is inserted obliquely in the cranio-distal direction in the angle formed by the lateral epicondyle of the humerus and olecranon.

   In horse, the needle is penetrated in the middle of the space between lateral epicondyle of the humerus and the lateral tuberosity of the radius.

   In dogs, the needle is directed obliquely to disto-medial position in the anterior part of the lateral surface of the limb, a few millimeter below the lateral condyle of the humerus in the flexed joints.
6. *Knee joint* : Knee joint is also known as carpal joint. It has three joints together; radiocarpal, intercarpal and metacarpal. The radiocarpal joint is flexed and the needle is inserted horizontally 3 cm deep between the tendon of common digital extensor and the extensor carpi radialis. For intercarpal joint, the needle is inserted into the intercarpal sac just medial to the tendon of extensor carpi radialis by keeping the joint flexed.
7. *Fetlock joint* : The needle is inserted just above the fetlock joint on the medial and lateral side of the extensor-tendon in ventral direction till the joint is punctured.
8. *Pastern joint* : The needle is inserted in the space between the common digital extensor and the lateral or medial digital extensor into the joint capsule.
9. *Coffin joint* : The needle is pierced 1-2 cm above the coronet medial or lateral from the midline through the common extensor tendon till the penetration of joint capsule.

After the joint puncture and collection of synovial fluid, the needle is withdrawn and the joint is sealed with wound adhesive or a sticking plaster to prevent the joint from infections.

Examination of Synovial Fluid

The synovial fluid should be examined for its physical, chemical and cytological characteristics.

1. *Physical Examination*: The physical examination of synovial fluid includes its quantity, colour, odour, specific gravity, clot formation, viscosity and turbidity.
2. *Chemical Examination*: The characteristics of mucin, glucose, protein and alkaline phosphatase activity are detected in chemical examination of synovial fluid.
3. *Cytological Examination*: The cytological examination is conducted for total cell count, including both leucocytes and erythrocytes, and for differential leucocyte count in which the percent distribution of polymorphonuclear and mononuclear cells is determined.
4. *Microbiological Examination:* The smears of synovial fluid are stained with Gram's staining and examined for the presence of bacteria. The synovial fluid is inoculated on suitable culture media for isolation and identification of the organism.
5. *Examination for Immune Complexes*: The synovial fluid is examined for the presence of ragocytes, immune complexes and antinuclear antibody in order to diagnose the joint diseases related to altered immune functions of the body.

Physical Examination

Quantity

Normally, the synovial fluid is in small quantity in any joint and sometimes it may become difficult to collect the desired quantity for examination. But in joint diseases, the amount is increased as the inflammatory fluid also accumulates in the joint. In some infections, however, the joint is swollen and enlarged enough, which can be clinically palpable, and sufficient amount of synovial fluid can be withdrawn for analysis.

Colour
The normal synovial fluid is colourless or sometimes it is slightly yellow tinged. But in inflammatory conditions of joint, it may become yellow, red, or greenish depending upon the type and severity of infection.

Turbidity
Normally, the synovial fluid is clear and transparent while in joint diseases it becomes cloudy and turbid owing to the presence of cells, inflammatory exudate and micro-ogransims. The turbidity due to cells in synovial fluid depends on the type and severity of infection. In severe inflamamtory conditions the joint fluid may become very cloudy with increased cellular count; if such fluid is centrifuged it becomes clear with considerable amount of sediment.

Odour
Usually the synovial fluid is odourless. It may become foul smelling in pyogenic infections of joint or the conditions in which saprophytes invade the joint due to repeated rupture of joint capsule for collection of synovial fluid and/or administration of medicines.

Viscosity
Synovial fluid collected from normal joints is viscous and stringy; which may be judged by rubbing a drop of fluid between thumb and forefinger. If one does not evaluate the viscosity by this method then a glass rod is dipped in fluid and the length of thread is measured upon withdrawal of glass rod. Usually a 3-4 cm thread is formed in normal synovial fluid while in joint ailments, the thread would break before reaching this height. For more precise measurements of viscosity, the use of viscometer is indicated.

Specific Gravity
The specific gravity of normal synovial fluid varies between 1.010 to 1.015. In joint diseases, the specific gravity of synovial fluid increases but has little diagnostic value.

Coagulation
The synovial fluid does not clot upto two days under normal conditions at 4^0C. However, in pathological conditions of joints, it may clot within 15 min to 3 hours depending on the severity of inflammation. To prevent the coagulation, certain anticoagulants are added in the synovial fluid. An early coagulation is an indication of serious joint disease.

Chemical Examination

Mucin

Synovial mucin is an acido-glycoprotein which can be precipitated by acetic acid. For the mucin precipitation, take 0.8 ml distilled water and one drop of 7 N acetic acid in a small test tube and mix thorughly. To this add 0.2 ml synovial fluid in such a way that the fluid does not come in contact with glass of test tube. Mix the fluid thoroughly by swirling and allow to stand for one hour at room temperature. It should be interpreted as under.

I. A tight ropy clump in a clear solution - normal (N)

II. A soft mass in a slight turbid solution - fair (F)

III. A small friable mass in a turbid solution-poor (P)

IV. A few flakes present in a turbid solution-very poor (VP).

The quality of mucin clot of synovial fluid is considered representative of quality of hyaluronic acid present in synovial fluid. In articular diseases, the process of hyaluronic acid polymerization is reduced resulting in a poor clot or varying degree of flocculation appearing in a cloudly reaction. In non-infectious articular diseases the mucin clot is usually normal.

Protein

Normally the synovial fluid in bovines contain albumin and alpha 1, beta and gamma 2 globulins with an albumin-globulin ratio as 1:2. Protein content of synovial fluid is determined by using Biuret method.

Table 8.1: Normal protein content in synovial fluid of animals

Sr.No.	Animal species	Protein content (G/100 ml)
1.	Bovine	0.8
2.	Horse	1.48
3.	Pig	3.9

The normal protein content (Table 8.1) varies from joint to joint. In cattle, the synovial fluid protein content usually present less than 2 G/100 ml while in joint diseases, it increases most of the time upto 5 G/100 ml and sometimes upto 8.5 G/100 ml. The protein content of synovial fluid increases in inflammation of joint or tendon sheath, which is of special diagnostic significance.

In acute non-infectious joint inflammation, the albumin content decreases while in chronic non-infectious joint inflammation the decrease in albumin is associated with increases in beta globulins. Non-mucin protein level may become double in concentration in traumatic and degenerative conditions of joint.

Glucose

The glucose level of synovial fluid is estimated as in case of blood by Folin and Wu method. In cattle, the blood and synovial fluid glucose level has a ratio of 1.3:1.0 in off fed animals; while it is 1.0:5.0 in animals fed prior to sampling. In early intra-articular diseases, the synovial fluid glucose level increases significantly, and is followed by decrease in the glucose level due to the glycoytic activity of certain bacteria and neutrophils. In non-inflammatory joint conditions, the glucose level remains normal in synovial fluid. However, it may be lowered due to high cellularity and glycolysis in inflammatory conditions. Sometimes the level of glucose may become zero due to the presence of inflammatory cells and microorganisms.

Alkaline Phosphatase and Other Enzymes

The level of alkaline phosphatase in synovial fluid is much lower in comparison to its serum levels. In synovial fluid, the alkaline phosphatase is 0.53-0.93 sigma unit/ml. In cattle and horses, the injection of 6-methyl predinisolone acetate markedly reduces the alkaline phosphatase activity in synovial fluid while the serum alkaline phosphatase remains normal. The high activity of alkaline phosphatase in synovial fluid is associated with depolymerization for hyaluronic acid responsible for poor mucin clot formation on acetic acid test.

In horses, synovial fluid is also examined for the activity of lactic dehydrogenase (LDH) enzyme. In normal joints, the level of LDH is 50 –109 units/lit which may increase in articular diseases. The increase in enzyme level of synovial fluid is an indication of tissue damage in joint structures.

Cytological Examination

A. Total Cell Count

The total cell count per cubic mm is done in undiluted synovial fluid using hemocytometer and WBC pipette. If the dilution is required, then it should be diluted in normal saline solution containing one percent cresyl blue or crystal violet as the WBC diluent have acetic acid which may form clot in synovial fluid. The addition of cresyl blue or crystal violet makes the nucleated cells more visible. The cell count may vary from one joint to another and it depends on the type of reaction in the joints (Table 8.2). The cellular count must be interpreted considering the normal count of that joint.

Table 8.2: Cell count in synovial fluid

Sr.No.	Animal	Cell count in normal synovial fluid (per cumm)	Cell count in joint diseases (per cumm)
1.	Bovine	65-250	36250
2.	Equine	390-1638	10800
3.	Canine	430+ 60	19000
4.	Porcine	30 - 450	2000-56750

The leucocytes are normally present in synovial fluid which increases in joint diseases. The early cells present in synovial fluid are neutrophils while in chronic cases variable number of mononuclear cells are present. The differential leucocyte count is done in same way as in the blood but if the total cell count is low then it is advisable to centrifuge the sample and then do differential count is using the smears of sediment stained with Giemsa or Leishman stain. About 200 cells should be counted in a sample. Usually, in synovial fluids, the lymphocytes and monocytes account for 80% and the neutrophils are present only about 10% in bovines. In horses, the neutrophils are less than 7% while the majority of cells are lymphocytes. In pigs, however, the neutrophils are 25-37% and lymphocytes are 40-60%.

The inflammation of joints leads to alteration of cellular content of synovial fluid. In mild cases, the neutrophilic content increases while in severe cases the increase of mononuclear cells is also present. In some severe cases, erythrocytes may also be present in synovial fluid.

In cattle, the total cell count has been reported to be 355 + 220 per cumm in arthritis cases in comparison to 65 cumm of normal joints. The differential leucocyte count reveals 85% neutrophils in synovial fluid of affected joints. The absolute count in synovial fluid of joints having severe inflammation has been reported as neutrophils 167 + 150, lymphocytes 59 + 36, monocyte 86 + 34, macrophage 41 + 29, and eosinophils 1 + 0.

Microbiological Examination

For microbiological examination, the smears of synovial fluid are prepared on clean glass slides and stained with Gram's staining for the presence of bacteria. The smears can also be prepared with sediment of centrifuged synovial fluid. The cultural examination, if required, can be carried out in suitable culture media for bacteria and mycoplasma. However, the culture of chlamydial agent and virus suspected synovial fluids are done in eggs and cell cultures, respectively.

Examination for Immune Complexes

The synovial fluid is examined for the presence of ragocytes by preparing smears and staining with Giemsa. The ***ragocytes*** are the neutrophils containing variable sized pinkish red granules within the cytoplasm; these are the phagocitized immune complexes. For demonstration of free immune complexes, the method is described elsewhere in this book.

Miscellaneous Examination

The synovial fluid should be examined for the presence of crystals in case of gout in animals. The synovial fluid contains the crystals of calcium phosphate associated with calcific lesions, cholesterol crystals and crystals due to repeated intra-articular injections of corticosteroids. The crystals of gout can be demonstrated in wet mount preparation using light microscopy. However, the phase contrast microscopy is better for demonstration of crystals. Such crystals can also be observed by using electronmicroscopy, scanning electron microscopy and X-ray examination which is considered very useful method in identification of crystals.

Inflammatory Conditions of Joints

The inflammatory conditions of joints are of three types: (i) non-infectious, (ii) infectious and, (iii) immune complex mediated. Earlier, the immune complex mediate arthritis was included in the non- infectious joint inflammations but in this book, it has been described in a separate class for a better understanding of immune mediated arthritis.

Non-Infectious Arthritis

The non-infectious arthritis includes degenerative and traumatic types of joint inflammations. In this, the synovial fluid is clear with good or fair mucin clot, normal glucose and protein contents with a cellular content of 100-1000/ cumm.

Infectious Arthritis

The infectious arthritis is caused by bacteria, mycoplasma, chlamydia or viral agents either in single or in combination. The synovial fluid is less viscous, coloured, foul smelling, turbid, thick, opaque, and often clots on standing with poor mucin test. The glucose content is lowered with increased protein contents. Micro-organisms can be demonstrated or isolated from the synovial fluid.

Immune Complex Mediated Arthritis

Usually the immune complex mediated arthritis is non-infectious in nature which may affect more than one joint. The synovial fluid may become purulent having increased number of neutrophils. In such synovial fluids, the enzyme collagenase is increased due to its increased production by neutrophils. The collagenase is responsible for invasiveness of immune complexes. Besides, prostaglandin level is also increased in immune mediated arthritis, which promotes bone resorption and articular cartilage destruction. The complement activity of normal synovial fluid is 10% of the serum activity. In case of immune mediated arthritis, the synovial fluid complement becomes low indicating its utilization in immune complex formation. The complement level measurement in synovial fluid may be of importance in immune mediated arthritis. The immune mediated arthritis is of two types.

Erosive

In this type of arthritis, the articular cartilage is destroyed and the fragments of cartilage can be seen in synovial fluid. Besides, the subchondral bone material may also come in synovial fluid, e.g. rheumatoid arthritis in dogs. The rheumatoid arthritis in dogs is characterized by a poor mucin clot, increased cellular content, increased neutrophil count and presence of ragocytes. The ragocytes are characteristic neutrophils containing variable sized pinkish red granules within the cytoplasm consisting of phagocitized immune complexes. The synovial fluid of such arthritis is sterile and does not yield any micro-organism on cultural examination.

Non-erosive

In the non-erosive arthritis, the articular cartilage damage is less and the condition resembles with systemic lupus erythmatous of men. The synovial fluid contains large number of erythrocytes, leucocytes with at least 50% neutrophils. The viscosity of such synovial fluid is decreased; mucin clot is fair to poor with neutrophils having phagocitized debris of scavanged DNA.

Characteristics of synovial fluid in various joint disease conditions is shown in table 8.3.

Table 8.3: Characteristics of synovial fluid in various joint disease conditions

Sr.No.	Test	Degenerative Arthritis	Traumatic Arthritis	Infectious Arthritis	Immune Mediated Arthritis	Neoplastic condition of joints
1.	Colour	Pale yellow	Red	Yellow	Pale Yellow	Pale Yellow
2.	Turbidity	Clear to slight turbid	Blood tinged	Turbid	Clear/ slig -ht turbed	Clear/ slig-ht turbid
3.	Viscosity	Normal	Reduced	Reduced	Not much affected	Normal
4.	Mucin clot	Normal	Fair	Poor	Poor	Normal
5.	Erythrocytes	Few	Many	Moderate	Few	Moderate
6.	Leucocytes	Few	Moderate	Many	Many	Moderate
7.	Neutrophils	Few	Moderate	Many	Many	Moderate
a.	Toxic neutrophils	Nil	Nil	Prominent	Nil	Nil
b.	Ragocytes	Nil	Nil	Nil	Many	Nil
8.	Lymphocytes	Moderate	Few	Few	Few	Few
9.	Macrophages	Moderate	Few	Few	Few	Few
10.	Synovial cells	Moderate	Rare	Rare	Moderate	Few
11.	Neoplastic cells	Nil	Nil	Nil	Nil	Many
12.	Microorganisms	Absent	Absent	Present	Absent	Absent
13.	Protein	<2	<2	6-8.5	2-4	2-4
14.	Coagulation	No	No	15-30 min	Within 2 hrs	Within 2 hrs
15.	Odour	Nil	Nil	Present	Nil	Nil

9

Examination of Cerebrospinal Fluid

- General considerations
- Indications
- Collection of cerebrospinal fluid
  - Sub-occipital puncture
  - Lumbar puncture
- Examination
  - Physical examination
  - Chemical examination
  - Cytological examination
  - Microbiological examination

General Considerations

Cerebrospinal fluid is found in the ventricles, cistern of brain, canal of spinal cord and in space between piamater and arachnoid. The fluid is formed by the active secretions and through a highly selective filtration of blood. The main source of cerebrospinal fluid is choroid plexus in the ventricles of brain; where two processes occur. The cerebrospinal fluid slowly flows from ventricles to subarachnoid space from where the venus sinuses of duramater reabsorb it. The main functions of cerebrospinal fluid are:

1. It acts as medium for transfer of nutrients and metabolites from brain and spinal cord to blood stream.
2. It provides protection to the brain and spinal cord and acts as fluid buffer against injury.
3. In conjunction with cerebral blood flow, it maintains the intracranial pressure and regulates the contents of cranium.
4. It works as space compensate mechanism; the volume of cerebrospinal fluid may change due to any change of blood volume within the cranium.

5. It provides protection and nourishment to the parenchyma.
6. It serves as medium of transport for neuroendocrine substances and neurotransmitters.

In normal animals, the cerebrospinal fluid is clear, colourless and does not have tendency to coagulate outside the body. The cellular contents are also negligible being 0-25 cells per cumm and most of them are lymphocytes. During the diseases of brain and spinal cord; the composition, appearance, quantity and quality of cerebrospinal fluid is altered. The normal production and its reabsorption is disrupted. Therefore, in suspected pathological conditions of brain and spinal cord, the examination of cerebrospinal fluid is advised.

Indications

1. The examination of cerebrospinal fluid is indicated for the diagnosis of diseases of central nervous system.
2. In the evaluation of clinical signs associated with central nervous system, the cerebrospinal fluid is examined.
3. For the evaluation of prognosis and effect of therapy, the examination of cerebrospinal fluid is advised.
4. Cerebrospinal fluid is used for radiographic procedures employed to demonstrate the shape of cerebrospinal fluid containing system and to reveal the changes due to disease.

Collection of Cerebrospinal Fluid

In horses, sheep, goats, pigs and dogs, the cerebrospinal fluid is collected from suboccipital region while in cattle and buffaloes, the lumbo-sacral site is preferred.

Sub-Occipital Puncture

The animal should be anesthetized and head is bent towards brisket making a 90 degree angle from neck. The site of puncture is the mid-line, a hand breadth behind the poll. Before puncture, the site must be shaved and cleaned using disinfectant. The sterile needle of about 10-15 cm length and 1.5 mm diameter along with stylet is inserted in the direction of the occipital bone. As the needle reaches the bone, withdraw a little and reinsert at a more acute angle so that the tip of the needle passes below the occipital bone into foramen magnum; the animal may feel a pain reaction and may jump when needle penetrates the duramater. Now the stylet is removed and the cerebrospinal fluid is aspirated using a syringe. In normal cerebrospinal fluid pressure, a drip may come out on application of syringe while in case of increased cerebrospinal fluid pressure, the fluid comes out with speed.

Lumbar Puncture

The cerebrospinal fluid may either be collected under local or general anesthesia by lumbar puncture. A 12 cm long needle with stylet is inserted vertically in the midline of soft depression between the dorsal process of lumbar vertebrae and the anterior end of median sacral crest, the point at the level of line joining anterior border of tuber coxae. As the needle penetrates duramater, animal may show some signs of pain and may jump. The stylet is removed and the cerebrospinal fluid is collected by syringe.

For estimation of glucose, the cerebrospinal fluid should be collected in sodium fluoride containing vials while for other examinations it should be collected without any preservative. However, if delay is expected in examination, any anticoagulant can be added as described elsewhere in this book.

Examination

Physical Examination

Pressure

The pressure of cerebrospinal fluid is determined by manometer and is expressed in mm H_2O. The pressure is measured at the time of collection of cerebrospinal fluid. After the needle penetrates the duramater and stylet is removed, the manometer is fitted over the needle to measure the pressure. Thereafter, the cerebrospinal fluid is collected by applying syringe. The normal cerebrospinal fluid pressure is given in Table 9.1. The pressure is increased in many disease conditions.

1. The cerebrospinal fluid pressure increases in space occupying lesions of central nervous system such as neoplasms, abscess, hemorrhage and hydrocephalus. The venous sinuses are compressed by these lesions preventing the absorption of fluid through arachnoid villi.
2. Vitamin A deficiency may also interfere with cerebrospinal fluid absorption from arachnoid villi. This condition is observed in young cattle kept on dry and vitamin A deficient diet. The elevation of cerebrospinal fluid pressure is related with plasma vitamin A deficiency which can be corrected with vitamin A feeding.
3. The increase in cerebrospinal fluid is observed in cerebral edema as a result of brain injury.

Table 9.1: Normal characteristics of cerebrospinal fluid in domestic animals

Sr. No.	Characters	Cattle	Sheep	Goat	Horse	Pig	Dog	Cat
1.	Pressure (mmHzO)	200	270	-	400	145	170	100
2.	Specific gravity	1.005-1.008		--	1.004-1.008	-	1.003-1.010	-
3.	Viscosity	1.01-1.02	-	-	1.0-1.05	-	-	-
4.	Protein (mg/ dl)	16-33	29-42	12.0	29-72	24-29	11-55	20
5.	Albumin (mg/dl)	-	-	-	23-68	17-24	-	-
6.	Globulin							
	a. Nonne-Apelt	Negative	Negative	Negative	+	Negative	Traces	Negative
	b. Pandy's	Negative	Negative	-	+	Negative	Traces	-
	c. Ross-Jones	Negative	Negative	-	+	Negative	Negative	-
7.	Reaction (pH)	7.22-7.26	7.35	-	7.13-7.36	-	7.42	-
8.	Calcium (mg/ dl)	5.1-6.3	5.77	4.6	5.55-6.98	-	6.56	5.2
9.	Chloride (mg/dl)	390-435	450-521	460	414-475	-	485	540
10.	Glucose (mg/ dl)	35-70	52-85	70	57.2	48-87	74	85
11.	Magnesium (mg/dl)	2.17	2.86	2.28	1.98	-	3.09	1.60
12.	Phosphorus (mg/dl)	1.6-1.9	-	-	1.44	-	-	-
13.	Potassium (mg/dl)	11.2-13.8	-	11.6	12.66	-	11.6	11.6
14.	Cells/ (Cumm)	0-10	0-15	1-11	4-23	1-20	0-25	0-1
	a. Small lymphocyte	-	-	-	-	-	65%	-
	b. Large lymphocytes	-	-	-	-	-	21%	-
	c. Degenerative cells	-	-	-	-	-	14%	-
15.	Sodium chloride (mg/dl)	650-725	750-868	766	690-792	-	808	900
16.	Urea (mg/ dl)	9.2	-	-	3.28	-	10.7	20.2
17.	Urea nitrogen (mg/dl)	4.4	-	-	1.68	-	5.1	9.7

Cerebral fluid pressure in various disease conditions of domestic animals is given in Table 9.2.

Table 9.2: Cerebrospinal fluid pressure in various disease conditions of domestic animals

Sr.No.	Disease	CSF Presure
1.	Canine distemper	120
2.	Canine cryptococcal meningitis	364
3.	Canine toxoplasma encephalitis	256
4.	Suppurative meningoencephalitis in calves	168
5.	Polioencephalomalacia in cows	220
6.	Brain tumours	170-410
7.	Polioencephalomalacia in goats	210

Colour

Normally the cerebrospinal fluid is clear like distilled water. However, it may turn to a bright red colour if at the time of puncture, fresh blood is mixed. Such red colour can be removed by centrifugation. The colour of cerebrospinal fluid becomes dull red to brown in intracranial hemorrhage due to chronic hemorrhagic pachymeningitis or previous trauma. Yellowish-white colour of cerebrospinal fluid with a tendency towards redishness is observed in infectious septicemic thromboembolic meningoencephalitis. Yellow colour of cerebrospinal fluid may occur due to the presence of bilirubin, which is also known as xanthochromic as, a result of destruction of erythrocytes in subarachnoid space and may occur in subarachnoid hemorrhage, extradural and subpial hematoma, spinal block, brain tumours, abscess, keutonemia and in acute toxoplasmosis. In servere and chronic jaundice the cerebrospinal fluid may contain bile. Greenish or greyish colour may occur due to presence of pus cells which may appear during acute inflammation.

Turbidity

Normally the cerebrospinal fluid should be transparent, without any turbidity. It may become turbid due to the presence of cellular components which give it a cloudy appearance in purulent infections. In purulent encephalomyelitis, the cerebrospinal fluid becomes cloudly with fibrinous strings with a tendency to coagulate. Red turbidity may be seen due to hemorrhage and mixing of erythrocytes.

Reaction

In general, the reaction of cerebrospinal fluid is alkaline. An alteration is an indication of any illness or disease condition of brain and spinal cord.

Specific Gravity

Specific gravity of cerebrospinal fluid in normal animals ranges from 1.003 to 1.008 which may be increased during inflammatory conditions of brain and spinal cord.

Coagulation

The cerebrospinal fluid from normal animals does not have the tendency to coagulate. The early coagulation of cerebrospinal fluid may occur due to increase in protein fibrinogen content. Heavy coagulation and sedimentation occurs in acute suppurative meningitis. In tuberculous meningitis, 'cob-web' or pine tree like coagulation occur from surface of fluid down to the middle of the tube. In such cerebrospinal fluid, anticoagulant should be added which will facilitate its further examination.

Chemical Examination

Protein

The cerebrospinal fluid proteins are precipitated by trichloroacetic acid and the resultant turbidity is measured by spectrophotometer. In a test tube, 0.6 ml of cerebrospinal fluid is taken, in which 2.4 ml of 3% trichloroacetic acid is added and mixed thoroughly. The mixture is kept on stand for 10-15 minutes and mixed again and examined against distilled water blank at 450 nm. For standardization, use bovine serum albumin and plot a standard curve for calculation of total protein level in cerebrospinal fluid.

Normally cerebrospinal fluid consists of only albumin but in pathological conditions, the level of globulin increases which affects the total protein contents. The cerebrospinal fluid protein level in disease conditions of domestic animals is shown in Table 9.3.

Table 9.3 : The cerebrospinal fluid protein level in disease conditions of domestic animals

Sr.No.	Species	Disease	Protein level
1.	Dog	Canine distemper	45-88 mg / dl
2.	Dog	Canine cryptococcal meningoencephalitis	501 mg / dl
3.	Dog	Canine toxoplasmosis	94 mg / dl
4.	Horse	Equine rhinopneumonitis	278 mg / dl
5.	Goat	Polioencephalomalacia	52 mg / dl
6.	Bovines	Listeriosis	79 mg / dl
7.	Bovines	Meningoencephalitis	110-143 mg / dl
8.	Bovines	Brain tumours	19-214 mg / dl
9.	Bovines	Polioencephalomalacia	135 mg / dl

Increased globulin in cerebrospinal fluid has also been reported in abscesses of brain and spinal cord, pneumonia, convulsive state, uremia, hemorrhage and extensive non-inflammatory degeneration of brain parenchyma with brain tissue necrosis.

The globulin level in cerebrospinal fluid can be determined by the following methods.

1. *Pandy's test* : In this, Pandy's reagent is used which contains 10% carbolic acid crystals in distilled water. One ml of Pandy's reagent is taken in a test tube, in which few drops of cerebrospinal fluid is added and mixed properly; the turbidity is then observed. In normal cerebrospinal fluid there should not be any turbidity while in inflammatory conditions of brain and spinal cord, it becomes turbid and may be scored as +, ++, +++, ++++ and +++++. The Pandy's reaction is +++ in case of meningoencephalities of bacterial or viral origin.
2. *Ross-Jones test* : In this test, the saturated ammonium sulfate solution is used for the precipitation of proteins. One milliliter of saturated ammonium sulfate solution is taken in a test tube, in which one ml cerebrospinal fluid is overlaid. The test tube is allowed to stand for 10-15 min. If the cerebrospinal fluid contains globulins, a greyish ring would be formed at the interjunction of two fluids. Such ring will not occur in normal cerebrospinal fluid.
3. *Nonne-Appelt test :* In this test, one ml saturated solution of ammonium sulfate is taken in a test tube and to this one ml cerebrospinal fluid is added. Mix the contents thoroughly and keep on stand for 5 min. The normal cerebrospinal fluid remains same, while it becomes turbid with a cloudly precipitate if the protein is in excess in cerebrospinal fluid. The None-Appelt reaction is usually ++ in viral encephalomyelitis while in bacterial encephalitis it is +++ reaction.
4. *Foam test :* Take about one ml cerebrospinal fluid in a test tube and shake well, the foam will appear which would disappear within a few minutes in case of normal cerebrospinal fluid. The extent of foams would be more and for longer duration occurs in cerebrospinal fluid having high protein content.
5. *Sulfosalicylic acid test* : In this test, one ml cerebrospinal fluid is taken in a test tube. Add 3 ml of 3% sulfosalicylic acid and mix them properly. Keep on stand for 5-10 min. In case of high protein content the turbidity will appear which should be graded as +, ++, +++ and ++++.

Glucose

In normal cerebrospinal fluid the glucose concerntration is 60-70% of the blood glucose concentration. Normally it is 40-80 mg/100 ml in cerebrospinal fluid. The glucose concentration of cerebrospinal fluid depends on the blood glucose concentration, permeability of blood cerebrospinal fluid barrier, and the presence of glycolytic micro-organisms. The decreased level of glucose in cerebrospinal fluid is known as ***hypoglycorrhachia*** while the increased level is called as ***hyperglycorrhachia***. The hypoglycorrhachia is mostly found to be associated with hypoglycemia. However, the glucose level of cerebrospinal fluid may be lowered due to the glycolytic activity of micro-organism present in acute pyogenic infections, suppurative meningitis and meningeal neoplasms. In canine cryptococcal meningoencephalitis, the glucose level falls to 21 mg/dl in cerebrospinal fluid while the blood glucose level comes down to 67 mg/dl. The hyperglycorrhachia is found to be associated with hyperglycemia due to diabetes mellitus, encephalitis, spinal cord compression, brain tumour and brain abscess. The level of glucose in cerebrospinal fluid is measured as in case of blood. It is advisable that blood glucose level should also be tested along with cerebrospinal fluid glucose level for a better and proper interpretation.

Chloride

The cerebrospinal fluid chloride level, normally, is higher than the blood chloride levels. The chloride level of cerebrospinal fluid has been recorded to have decreased in meningitis associated with high protein level in cerebrospinal fluid, protected vomiting, and in advance cases of pneumonia. The level of chlorides in cerebrospinal fluid is inversely related to protein content of cerebrospinal fluid. The chloride levels in cerebrospinal fluid are measured in same way as in case of blood.

Calcium

Usually the cerebrospinal fluid calcium level is lower than serum calcium levels due to its binding with serum proteins. However, the concentration of calcium in cerebrospinal fluid is independent of serum calcium levels.

Magnesium

Normally, the magnesium level of cerebrospinal fluid is higher than the blood magnesium levels. The cerebrospinal fluid magnesium is independent of serum magnesium levels. In grass tetany or magnesium deficient diets in sheep, the cerebrospinal fluid magnesium level decreases.

Urea Nitrogen

The urea nitrogen levels are slightly lower than blood urea levels. In case of uremia, the urea nitrogen of cerebrospinal fluid also increases. The rate of increase of urea nitrogen level in cerebrospinal fluid is somewhat similar to that of blood urea levels.

Cholesterol

In cerebrospinal fluid, there is no cholesterol. However, in case of hemorrhage in central nervous system, brain tumours, meningitis and brain abscess, the level of cholesterol increases in cerebrospinal fluid.

Enzymes

The elevation of GOT and GPT levels in cerebrospinal fluid has been observed in canine distemper induced clinical signs in dogs. Creatinine kinase (CK) level increases in cerebrospinal fluid in central nervous system diseases and is indicative of a guarded or poor prognosis. Lactic dehydrogenase (LDH) may increase in lymphosarcoma while aspartate aminotransferase (AST) level increases in cerebrospinal fluid due to myelin degeneration. In meningeal carcinoma, the increase in LDH, aldolase, AST and CK has been reported.

Other Examinations

In case of brain tumour, carcino-embryonic antigen, alpha fetoproteins and glial fibrocillary acetic proteins are useful markers for diagnosis and prognosis.

Cytological Examination

The total and differential leucocyte counts are mostly performed in cerebrospinal fluid examination. The cell counts of cerebrospinal fluid must be made within an hour of its collection as the cells start disintegrating on standing. The diluting fluid for total cell count should contain 1.0 gm crystal violet, 50 ml glacial acetic acid and 450 ml distilled water. This fluid must be filtered before use. The total cell counts are carried out in hemocytometer using the leucocyte pipette. For this, draw diluting fluid upto mark 1 of the pipette and cerebrospinal fluid up to mark 11 of the pipette. Remove the rubber from the pipette and shake well by rotating the pipette. Discard few initial drops and fill the chamber as in case of blood cell counts. Leave the chamber for 2-5 min and count the cells in entire ruled area (9 primary squares) and multiply by 1.22 to obtain the total cells per cubic mm of the cerebrospinal fluid. The differential counts are made by making the smear from cerebrospinal fluid. If the total cell count is less than 500/cumm; then prepare smear from sediment of centrifuged cerebrospinal fluid for differential cell counts. The smear is fixed and stained with Giemsa as in case of blood smears.

Normally, there are 0-25 cells in the cerebrospinal fluid of domestic animals, which may increase to 400 cells/cumm in non-purulent encephalomyelitis. In non-purulent encephalomyelitis, lymphocytes are mainly (70%) present in the cerebrospinal fluid. Increase of leucocytes in cerebrospinal fluid is known as ***pleocytosis*** which may occcur in acute pyogenic meningitis, neoplasms with chronic focal degenerative changes, abscess of brain and spinal cord and in encephalitis.

Increased number of neutrophils is observed in pyogenic bacterial infections, abscess, bacterial encephalitis, bacterial meningitis and in hemorrhage; while the increased lymphocyte count in seen in viral infections, chronic diseases of brain and spinal cord, toxic conditions, fungal infections and in uremia. In case of neoplastic condition of brain and spinal cord, the neoplastic cells may also be present in the cerebrospinal fluid.

A continuous increase in number of neutrophils may be a sign of progressive lesions which may be considered as unfavourable prognosis. If the cell pattern changes and rise in lymphocyte count is observed then it can be considered as a favourable sign of prognosis.

Microbiological Examination

The cerebrospinal fluid smear is stained by Gram's staining for the demonstration of Gram positive and Gram negative bacteria, while for demonstration of mycobacteria, the smear is stained with acid fast stain of Zeil-Neelson. For fungus, the smear should be stained with India ink. The bacteria can also be seen inside the leucocytes in case of suppurative meningitis; such cells should also be stained with Gram's staining. For further identification of causative organism, the cerebrospinal fluid is cultured in suitable media.

Characteristics of cerebrospinal fluid in central nervous system disorders of cattle is shown in Table 9.4.

Table 9.4: Characteristics of cerebrospinal fluid in central nervous system disorders of cattle

Sr.No.	CSF examination	Tuberculous meningitis	Purulent meningitis	Non-purulent meningiits
1.	Pressure	Increased	Normal to slight increase	Normal
2.	Turbidity	Turbid flakes	Fibrinous strings	Clear
3.	Colour	No change	Whitish yellow	No change
4.	Coagulation	Within few minutes	-	-
5.	Protein (mg / dl)	300-500	200	300
6.	Pandy's test	+++ to ++++	++++	- to +++
7.	Nonne-Appelt test	Cloudy to precipitate +++ to ++++	+++	+ to +++
8.	Glucose (mg%)	27-59	50-78	34-57
9.	Chloride (mg%)	650	-	-
10.	Cells/cumm	500-5000	-	30-400
11.	Neutrophils	-	6000	30%
12.	Lymphocytes	-	-	70%
13.	Microbial organisms sp.	*Mycobacterium*	Present	Absent

10

Examination of Semen

- General considerations
- Volume
- Colour
- Reaction
- Concentration of spermatozoa
- Motility
- Live and dead count
- Microbiological examination

General Considerations

The semen of bulls used for natural services should be examined regularly for the presence of live spermatozoa, their motility and for the presence of any infection such as bacteria, virus etc. Such regular examination of semen results in good fertility rate and health maintenance of herd.

Semen of animals, particularly in artificial insemination and infertility cases, is examined for its quality and quantity. The quality of semen determines its ability to fertilize the ovum. In brief, the following observations should be made for the examination of semen:

1. Volume

The volume of semen during normal ejaculation is given as under:

Bull	4.0 ml
Horse	7.0 ml
Goat	1.0 ml
Boar	250 ml
Dog	1.0 ml
Cat	0.04 ml

The decreased amount of semen indicates the aspermatogenesis or oligospermia.

2. Colour

Normally the colour of semen is pearly white to grey or creamy white and translucent. It may become brownish due to blood pigment. The colour of semen is yellowish due to presence of riboflavin secreted by accessary glands. The yellowish green colour o semen might occur due to presence of *Pseudomonas aeruginosa* in the semen. The addition of blood in semen gives it dark red or pink colour which comes due to hemorrhage in penis or urethra.

3. Reaction

Normally, the pH of semen is neutral or slight alkaline. The pH of bull's semen is 7.0 or 6.7 while it is 7.4 of the semen of stallion, boar and cat.

4. Concentration of Spermatozoa

The concentration of sperms in semen is important as a particular amount is needed for fertilization; without which infertility may occur. Normally in bull's semen, 3 lakh to 20 lakh sperms per cumm are present and at times below 6 lakh sperms in semen are considered poor. In oligospermia the number of sperms decreases in semen while in testicular hypoplasia, it becomes very low like 25000/cumm. The counting of sperms can be done like erythrocyte count of blood using hemocytometer. For the purpose, the RBC diluting pipette is used and the semen is sucked upto 0.5 mark. Then suck 3% chlorazene upto 101 mark and remove the rubber tubing, mix the contents by rotating the pipette in between palms. The chlorazene acts as dilutent for semen and also kills the sperms. Discard the first few drops and charge the Neubauer's chamber on both sides; keeping all precautions in mind as given in total erythrocyte count. Leave it for 1-2 min and count the sperms in 5 secondary squares of central large square of the Neubauer's chamber. For total sperm count multiply the number by 10000 to get the sperm count per cumm.

5. Motility

The motility of sperms can be observed by diluting the semen in 2.9% sodium citrate solution or in Ringer's solution. Place one drop of diluted semen on slide and examine under microscope for movements of sperms. Record the finding in the following manner.

a. Immotile	'0'
b. Weak rotary movements	'1'
c. Less than 50% sperms move progressively but no waves	'2'
d. Progressive rapid movement with slow waves	'3'
e. Vigorous progressive movements	'4'
f. Very vigorous forward motion	'5'

6. Live and Dead Count

For counting of live and dead sperms, the following stain can be used.

Sodium citrate	3.0 gm
DW (sterile)	100 ml
Eosin B	1.0 gm
Nigrosin	5.0 gm

One drop of semen is placed on clean and dry glass slide and a drop of above stain is added. Mix them properly with bacteriological loop or glass rod. Dry the smear on flame of spirit lamp or burner. Count sperms on the smear under microscope. The dead sperms will take pink or red colour while live sperms will remain as such with a blue or black background. At the time of counting of live and dead sperms, one should also note the morphological abnormality in the sperms.

7. Microbiological Examination

The semen can be examined for the presence of bacteria by direct smear staining with Gram's staining. Indirectly it is cultured on suitable media for isolation of the organisms as given elsewhere in the book.

11

Clinical Microbiology

- General considerations
- Direct examination
- Culture methods
- Some important tests used in identification of bacteria
- Characteristics of some organisms
    - Gram positive cocci
    - Gram positive rods
    - Gram negative rods
    - Mycobacteria
    - Leptospira/spirochete
    - Rickettsia
    - Chlamydia
    - Mycoplasma
    - Fungi
    - Virus
- Antibacterial sensitivity testing

General Considerations

The microbiological examination of clinical samples is required to establish the etiology and line of treatment to be followed through antibacterial sensitivity testing. In certain cases, it is advisable to start the treatment with antibiotics only after sensitivity test. In the recent past, with the extensive and indiscriminate use of antibiotics, resistance is developed in the microorganisms leading to ineffectiveness of treatment. Therefore, it becomes very important to a veterinarian the he should go for antibacterial sensitivity test before start of treatment with antibacterial drugs. In some situations, however, this may not be possible. In such situations one should start the treatment after collecting the samples for laboratory examination while simultaneously the antibacterial sensitivity testing is done and result utilized to follow a further line of treatments.

The microbiological examination of clinical samples, sometimes, does not yield the desired results because certain organisms are very difficult to isolate or in some cases, the collected material is not proper. Besides, some procedures are difficult and it is not possible to carry them out in a diagnostic laboratory; such cases may be referred to well established laboratories. The clinical samples are examined by two ways:

1. Direct examination
2. By culturing on media and isolation of organism.

Direct Examination

The clinical samples which can be directly examined are tissues or organ swabs (nasal/fecal/vaginal/prepucial/conjunctival), urine, blood and exudate. The impression smear of tissue or organ can be prepared on clean and dry glass slide. Thin smears are prepared from blood or exudate or swabs; air dried and fixed on flame for a few seconds. The smears are stained by methylene blue or Gram's staining or acid fast staining.

Gram's Staining

1. Place the slides on gention violet stain for 2 min.
2. Wash with water.
3. Place the slides in Gram's iodine for 1 min.
4. Wash with water.
5. Decolourize with 95% alcohol (ethanol) or with a mixture of alcohol and acetone.
6. Wash with water.
7. Counter stain with safranin for 30 sec.
8. Wash with water, blot dry and examine under oil immersion microscope.

Interpretation

Gram positive- Blue, black or violet colour organism

Gram negative - Pink or red colour organism

Acid Fast Staining

1. Stain the smears with Zeihl-Neelson carbol fuchsin and heat the slides on burner or spirit lamp for 5-10 min to boil the stain over the slide.
2. Wash with running tap water.
3. Decolourize with acid alcohol till the smear becomes colourless.
4. Counter stain with methylene blue for 15 sec and wash with water and blot dry the smear. Examine it under oil immersion for acid fast bacilli.

Interpretation

Acid fast bacilli- Pink or red coloured organisms

Other background-Blue in colour.

Methylene Blue Staining

1. The smears are stained with methylene blue for 1 min. Wash in running tap water and blot dry.
2. Examine under oil immersion microscope for the presence of organism.

It stains well the capsule of *Bacillus anthracis* which takes amorphous purplish colour. The causative organism of hemorrhagic septicemia, pasteurella organism show bipolarity. It is a fast test and useful in diagnosis of hemorrhagic septicemia and can be performed before opening the carcass to determine the presence of *Bacillus anthracis* in suspected anthrax cases.

Culture Methods

The clinical samples are inoculated in culture media mainly for two purposes:

1. To cultivate the organisms.
2. To obtain the discrete colonies for isolation of organisms in pure culture.

The inoculation on bacteriological media is done by a number of ways depending on the type of clinical sample and type of media used. The culture media are classified into four major groups.

a. *Simple media:* Which are used for routine bacteriological examinations of the clinical specimens. These are also suitable for antibacterial sensitivity tests, e.g. nutrient agar.

b. *Enriched media:* The culture media is enriched with certain materials for growth of certain fastidious organism, e.g. blood agar, serum agar.

c. *Selective media:* These media permit the growth of certain type of organisms and prevent the others to grow, e.g. McConkey agar.

d. *Biochemical media:* These media are used for carrying out the biochemical tests of the organisms for their identification.

The routine bacteriological examinations are carried out by using blood agar or tryptose soya agar plates/McConkey agar plates. The clinical material is directly inoculated on the plates but in some cases it requires broth culture before being inoculated on solid media, e.g. fecal swabs are incubated in McConkey broth or tetrathionate broth or selenite broth and then one loop of material is transferred to McConkey agar plates or blood agar plates. The different types of clinical specimens are inoculated on culture media for cultural and antibacterial sensitivity tests as follows.

Blood

The blood is collected in sterile pasteur pipettes directly from heart puncture from dead chickens at the time of post mortem and is inoculated on solid meda like McConkey agar or blood agar or tryptose soya agar. The diagnosis of colisepticemia, fowl typhoid and fowl cholera can be made by this method. In large animals, the blood is collected from jugular vein (cephalic vein in dogs) using sterile syringe and needle with all aseptic conditions. One drop of blood is inoculated on McConkey agar/blood agar/tryptose soya agar or nutrient agar plates for growth of bacteria. The drop is placed at one point in plate and then is spreaded by using bacteriological loop by streaking method (Fig 11.1).

Tissues or Organ

The tissues are collected in sterile petri dishes from animal or bird at the time of necropsy examination . The tissue surface is sterilized by touching with hot spatula or knife; then the surface is cut with sterile sharp knife or blade. The freshly cut surface is touched with solid media on plate which is further spread by bacteriological loop. Alternatively, by using bacteriological loop, some material from freshly cut surface is inoculated on plate or broth. In some cases the tissues are as such inoculated in broth culture and organisms are allowed to grow. After broth culture, these are inoculated on plate for isolation and further characterization (Fig.11.1).

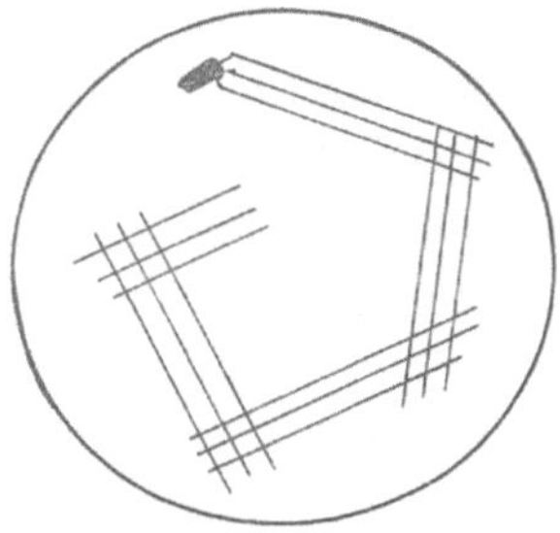

Fig. 11.1: Diagramatic illustration of petri dish showing streaking method of inoculation

Swabs

The swabs (fecal, pus, nasal, vaginal, prepucial, conjunctival) are directly inoculated on solid media, if freshly collected. If the swabs are transported after collection, these should be kept in liquid like nutrient broth/normal saline/ phosphate buffered saline / McConkey broth / selenite broth / tetrathionate broth, so that they do not dry up during transportation and storage. The swabs are incubated in the broth and then inoculated on agar plates for isolation and characterization.

Urine

Urine is collected in sterile vials for cultural examination. The mid portion of urine is always preferred. However, the urine samples are collected directly from bladder through syringe and needle or catheterization. The urine is directly inoculated on agar plates by using bacteriological loop for isolation and identification of bacteria.

Feces

The fecal samples are first inoculated in broth (tetrathionate/selenite/ McConkey broth) and after 24 hours of incubation, they should be inoculated on solid media in plates for isolation and identification of the bacteria.

Cerebrospinal Fluid/Synovial Fluid/Semen

These are directly inoculated on solid media by using bacteriological loop.

Milk or Water

These can be directly inoculated on solid media by bacteriological loop or for colony count, the dilutions are made and these are inoculated in the plates at the time of pouring of media.

Incubation

After inoculation, the agar plates or broth tubes are incubated at 370C for 24 hours (or at specified temperature for a specified period). After 24 hours incubation, if no colony is observed it should be further incubated for 72 hours before being declared as negative. The cuture plates are carefully examined for the presence of colonies of bacteria. The charcteristics of colony may guide the diagnostician about the further course of action for identification of the organisms. The size, colour and shape of colonies are recorded. The contaminants are mostly from bacilli and diphtheroids group; their colonies are relatively large, dry, hemolytic on blood agar, with rough and irregular edges. The colonies of diphtheroids are smaller, white to tan in colour and non-hemoloytic on blood agar.

Most of the pyogenic organisms have a colony size from 1 mm to 5 mm which are smooth, moist, entire, slightly raised and some are hemolytic.

Staining Characteristics

The suspected colonies are selected for Gram's staining by making smear on clean and dry glass slide. For this, take a drop of normal saline solution or phosphate buffer saline on middle of the slide. Using bacteriological loop, touch one colony on plate and rub it with NSS or PBS on slide and make smear by spreading the drop on slide. Care should be taken that one smear is prepared by only one colony. Dry the smear in air and fix on flame of burner of spirit lamp. The smears is then stained with Grams's staining.

Interpretation

1. *Staining* (a) Blue/Violet/black- Gram positive. (b) Pink/red-Gram negative.
2. *Morphology* (a) Round or spherical- Cocci. (b) Rod shaped – Bacilli. (c) Short rod shaped with rounded ends- Coccobacilli, (d) Spores at both ends- Bipolar.
3. *Arrangements* (a) Bunches, e.g. Staphylococci, (b) Chains, e.g. Streptococci, (c) In two or duplicate, e.g. Diplococci, (d) In four pairs, e.g. Tetracocci.

Pure Culture and Identification

From the growth of culture on agar plates, a single colony is further inoculated on nutrient agar or tryptose agar slants in duplicate for preservation and further identification of the organisms. The selected colony should be representative of majority of the colonies as identified by Gram's staining and colongy characteristics. After incubation at 37°C for 24 hour, the slants are stored at 4°C in refrigerator. One slant is used for identification of the organism including different biochemical tests.

Some Important Tests used in Identification of Bacteria

1. *Catalase test* : On a clean and dry glass slide, place a drop of 30% hydrogen peroxide. Take bacterial culture with loop from a slant or colony of plates and mix it with hydrogen peroxide on glass slide. The production of gas characterized by appearance of bubbles is indication of a positive reaction.

2. *Coagulase test:* Take 0.5 ml of rabbit plasma diluted (1:5) with sterile normal saline solution. Add 2-3 drops of overnight incubated broth culture and mix well. Incubate at 37°C a positive reaction is indicated by coagulation of plasma within 2-3 hrs.

3. *Oxidase test:* Prepare a 0.5% solution of N, N, N', -N Tetramethyl-p-phenylenediamine dihydrochloride and put a drop of this on suspected colony on the plate . The colour of colony will become dark purple in case the oxidase test is positive.

4. *Nitrate reduction test:* In a test tube, take 5 ml trypticase broth culture and add 1 ml of 0.8% sulfanilic acid in 5N acetic acid. Add drop by drop 0.5% alpha naphthylamine in 5N acetic acid. Development of red/pink/maroon colour is an indication for the positive nitrate utilization reaction. However, in negative test reaction add zinc dust in the tube of test culture as well as in broth for control. The colour of positive reaction is characterized as red or pink while the control will remain the same.

5. *Indole test:* Take a 48 hour growth of organism in brain heart infusion (BHI) broth. Add 1 ml ether in 5 ml culture and mix well. Keep the tube on stand for a few minutes. Add 0.5 ml of Kovac's reagent slowly on the top of the test tube contents. If indole is present, a red colour ring is formed just below the ether layer in the culture.

6. *MR Test:* Take 5 ml growth of organism in MR-VP broth and incubate for 4-5 days. To this add a few drops of MR reagent. In positive test, red colour will develop in the culture. Yellow colour is indication of a negative reaction.

7. *VP test:* Take 2 ml growth of organism in MR-VP broth incubated for 2 days and to this add 0.6 ml of 5% alpha naphthol in ethanol and 0.2 ml

of 40% potassium hydroxide containing 0.3% creatine and shake well. Place the test tube on stand for 5-10 min. In positive reaction, orange red colour will develop.

8. *Urease test:* Inoculate the organism on urea agar slants under sterile conditions. Incubate for 12 hours at 37°C. In case of positive test, the media turns into pink colour.

9. *Citrate utilization test:* Inoculate the organisms on Simmon's citrate agar slants and incubate for 24 hours at 37°C. The development of a blue colour is indication of citrate utilization.

10. *Hydrogen sulfide gas production test:* The organism is inoculated on TSI agar slants with a straight wire of the bacteriological loop. Inoculate the slant as well as butt and incubate the culture for 18-24 hours at 37°C. Observe the TSI reaction and interpret the reaction as follows:

Butt and slant yellowish	only lactose fermented
Slant red	Lactose not fermented
Slant red, butt yellow	Dextrose fermented
Slant black	H_2S (hydrogen sulfide) production
Bubbles in butt	Gas from dextrose

11. *Hemolysis:* Inoculate the organism in pure culture on blood agar plate in straight line and incubate for 24 hours at 37°C. If there is greenish narrow zone around the colony, it is alpha hemolytic. Clear zone indicates beta hemolysis and no zone indicates gammahemolysis.

12. *Sugar fermentation tests:* The organisms are inoculated in the sugar fermentation media (sugar + peptone water) (Appendix). The fermentation of sugar is indicated by development of pink colour in the sugar tube. The development of gas is detected by placing Durham's tube in the sugar tube. The sugars which are generally used for fermentation tests are glucos, lactose, fructose, mannose, mannitol, dulcitol, sucrose, rhamnose, etc.

Characteristics of Some Organisms

Some important characteristics of the organisms are given in each genera which may serve as key for their identification.

Gram Positive Cocci

1. *Staphylococci:* Gram positive cocci arranged in bunches, catalase positive, acid from glucose. Pathogenic staphylococci are coagulase positive.

2. *Streptococci:* Gram positive cocci, arranged in chains, catalase negative, beta hemolytic.

3. *Micrococcus:* Gram positive cocci, single or small clusters, catalase positive, maltose (-), mannitol (-), coagulase (-), nonhemolytic.

Gram Positive Rods

1. *Bacillus anthracis:* Gram positive rods, cylindrical rods, spores are centrally located, short chains, square ends of rods, capsulated, reduce methylene blue, non-hemolytic, produces dull, opaque, greyish colour colonies.

2. *Listeria:* Beta hemolytic, catalase (+), nitrate not reduced, motile at 250C, acid from glucose. Single or short chains, non-capsulated, on blood agar circular, transparent colonies, pathogenic for guinea pigs leading to death in 3-4 days.

3. *Erysipelothrix:* Alpha hemolytic, small round, translucent, discrete colonies with entire edge, 1 mm dia, organisms are short rods, thickened filament, non-motile, guinea pigs are resistant, glucose fermented, catalase negative, nitrate not reduced.

4. *Actinomyces:* Gram positive coccoid, branching filaments in media; in tissues sulfure granules, club like process.

5. *Corynebacteria:* Gram positive, coccoid or pleomorphic, non-motile, clumps or single, on blood agar minute pin point colony, beta hemolytic, cream to orange coloured colonies.

6. *Lactobacillus:* Long, slender, Gram positive rods, motile, catalase negative.

7. *Nocardia:* Gram positive rod, acid fast, branching filaments, rod or coccoid, catalase positive.

8. *Clostridium:* This group consists of anaerobic bacilli with rounded ends, spore formers, Gram positive rods.

   a. *Clostridium chauvoei:* Gram positive rods with rounded ends, single or short chains, long filament, spores are elongated or oval and subterminally or terminally located and are wider then width of organism which gives it a tennis racket like appearance.

b. *Cl. septicum:* Cylindrical Gram positive rod, single filaments.

c. *Cl. novyi:* Largest size, parallel edge, rounded ends, long jointed filaments, Gram positive.

d. *Cl. perfringenes:* Gram positive rods with square ends, non-motile.

e. *Cl. botulinum:* Gram positive large rods with rounded ends, short chains, oval spores and terminally located.

f. *Cl. tetani:* Gram positive large slender rod, short chains, rounded ends; spore 2-3 times larger than diameter of rod, located terminally giving the organism drum stick like appearance.

g. *Cl. hemolyticum:* Gram positive rods, oval or elongated, spore terminally situated.

Gram Negative Rods

1. *Yersinia:* Small, Gram negative rods or coccobacilli, catalase (+), oxidase (-), motile at 25^{0}C , urease (+), reduces nitrate.
2. *Pasteurella:* Small Gram negative rods or coccobacilli, oxidase (+), opaque whitish colonies on blood agar, bipolar staining from blood or tissues.
3. *Brucella:* Gram negative coccobacilli, non-motile, non-capsulated, oxidase positive (*Br. ovis* oxidase (-)),. urease positive (*Br. ovis* urease (-)), produces small delicate semi-transparent colonies on tryptose soya agar.
4. *Pseudomonas:* Gram negative rods, catalase positive, oxidase positive, motile (*Pseudomonas mallei* non-motile), produces translucent large, irregular and spread colonies, blue-green water soluble pigment in media.
5. *Actinobacillus:* Gram negative rods, oxidase positive, catalase positive, non-motile, produces flat colonies, transparent, slightly bluish in colour.
6. *Moraxella:* Gram negative rods, non-motile, catalase positive, oxidase (+), does not grow on McConkey agar, short, diplococcoid rods, produces small, round, greyish white colonies, translucent, beta hemolytic.

7. *Escherichia coli:* Produces circular, convex, smooth translucent colonies having wet appearance, lactose fermenter, non-motile, Gram negative coccobacilli, Indole (+), MR (+), VP (-), citrate not utilized, produces metallic sheen in EMB agar.
8. *Salmonella:* Gram negative rods, non-lactose fermenter, produces white colonies on McConkey agar and pink on brilliant green agar (BGA), produces homogenous, smooth, glistening, greyish colonies.
9. *Proteus:* Gram negative rod, motile, thin tansparent colonies, swarming on agar plates, MR (+), VP (-), citrate not utilized, H2S (+), urease positive.
10. *Klebsiella:* Gram negative, coccobacilli, mucoid colonies, indole (+), MR (+), VP (+), citrate utilization (+),H2S (-), ureases (+).
11. *Shigella:* Gram negative rod, non-motile, pleomorphic, long filaments, occurs in chain, rough, dry, circular, mucoid colonies, opaque, raised colony on agar surface.
12. *Aeromonas:* Gram negative rod, lysin (-), acid butt and slant, H2S negative on TSI.
13. *Citrobactor:* Gram negative rod, indole (+), MR (+), VP (-), citrate utilization (+), H_2S (-),and urease (+).
14. *Hemophilus:* Gram negative rod or coccobacilli, non-motile, semitranslucent, flattened, circular, greyish colony with sharp edges.
15. *Vibrio or Campylobacter:* Gram negative, non-capsulted, 's' shaped, bluish pin point size colonies, slightly raised on thiol medium or blood agar.

Mycobacteria

Acid fast bacilli, capsulated, slow growth, takes at least a week's incubation period for growth.

Leptospira or Spirochete

Long spiral rods, having many curves, ends look like hook, demonstrated in dark field microscope, difficult to grow.

Rickettsia

Rod shaped, coccoid or pleomorphic, Gram negative, intracellular organism, does not grow on artifical media. Grows well in yolk sac of 5-7 days old chicken embryo; after 4-5 days' incubation inclusions in yolk sac smears stained with Geimsa or Macchiavello stain. Intra-cytoplasmic inclusions can be demonstrated in liver impression smears of guinea pig inoculated I/P with rickettsia.

Chlamydia

Intra-cellular organisms, produce intracellular inclusions, do not grow in artificial media, grow in seven day old chicken embryo through yolk sac route, inclusion in yolk sac membrane.

Mycoplasma

Pleomorphic, small coccobacilli, ring form, filamentus, produces fried egg colony, grows on PPLO broth or agar containing horse serum, produces nipple shaped colonies, small colonies seen by stereoscope, for cultivation incubated at 2-3^{0}C for 24-48 hours in PPLO broth, then transferred 0.1 ml to solid media. Incubated in humid chambers at 37.5^{0}C. Growth occurs in 2-4 days, flood the plate with 1-2 ml PPLO broth, incubate further for 2-3 days , if no growth for 14 days then declare as negative.

Fungi

Skin scrapings or suspected clinical samples are inoculated on Sabouraud's dextrose agar containing anti-bacterial drugs and cycloheximide in order to prevent the growth of bacteria and saprophytic fungi. Media may be placed in plates or tubes. Incubate the culture media at room temperature for several days and examine this daily for fungal growth.

1. *Trichophyton:* It takes 7-10 days to grow on Sabouraud's dextrose agar. Colonies are white which become tanned after sometime and have a granular pigment. Smear made from the colonies may show the presence of numerous microconidia with some macroconidia; these can be stained with lactophenol cotton blue which enhances the visibility of fungus.
2. *Microsporum:* It grows well in 3-4 days and produces flat colony, white or yellow. Microscopically, few microconidia and numerous macroconidia seen; macroconidia are large, spindle shaped, multiseptate, thick walled bodies having a knob at the tip.
3. *Candida:* It produces soft, cream coloured colonies, with yeasty odour.
4. *Blastomyces:* White colonies which turn brown after some time. Branching septate hyphae containing lateral oval conidia.

5. *Cryptococcus:* Thick walled, oval to spherical budding cells surrounded by gelatinous capsule, growth in 10-15 days, colonies are white, glistening, mucoid, which turn brown with age.
6. *Histoplasma:* On Sabouraud's dextrose agar, it produces white, cottony colonies which become brownish after some time. Branching septate hyphae having microconidia; in older cultures macroconidia are seen.
7. *Coccidioids:* It produces fluffy white colonies on Sabouraud's dextrose agar. The hyphae contain rectangular arthrospores, which float in the air. It should be grown only in sophisticated laboratories because there is danger of air transmission.

Virus

The isolation and cultivation of virus can be undertaken in diagnostic laboratories but it requires trained and specialized personnel. It is difficult to carry out the virus culture in a small diagnositc laboratory. Here, some of the preliminary methods used in culture of virus are described. The culture of virus can be done in embryonated chicken eggs or in cell culture systems.

Chicken Eggs

The clinical samples (feces/tissues/secretion/excretion) are collected in sterile containers. These are processed in order to prepare bacteria free filtrate for inoculation in chicken eggs or cell culture. For this, prepare 1:5 or 1:10 suspension of clinical samples in HBSS, which is centrifuged at 10000Xg for 30 min at 4^0C. The supernatant is collected and filtered through EK grade seitz filter. If the material is less in quantity (5-10 ml), it can be filtered through nitrocellulse membrane filter having 0.22 µm pore size. The filtrate is stored at -20^0C till use. It can be inoculated (0.1ml) in embryonated chicken eggs through following routes:

1. Chorioallantoic membrane (CAM)
2. Yolk Sac
3. Allantoic cavity

The eggs are inoculated under aseptic conditions preferably in laminar flow or sterile hoods. The inoculated eggs are incubated for 2-5 days at 37^0C in incubator. During incubation, the eggs are seen daily through candling and dead embryos (within 24 hrs) are discarded. The growth of virus on CAM is observed by appearance of thickening, congestion, hemorrhage, pock lesions, and necrosis (Fig.11.2). The allantoic or yolk sac fluid is examined for the presence of virus by using indirect tests like HA or HI. The growth of embryos and lesions on various organs of embryo are also observed.

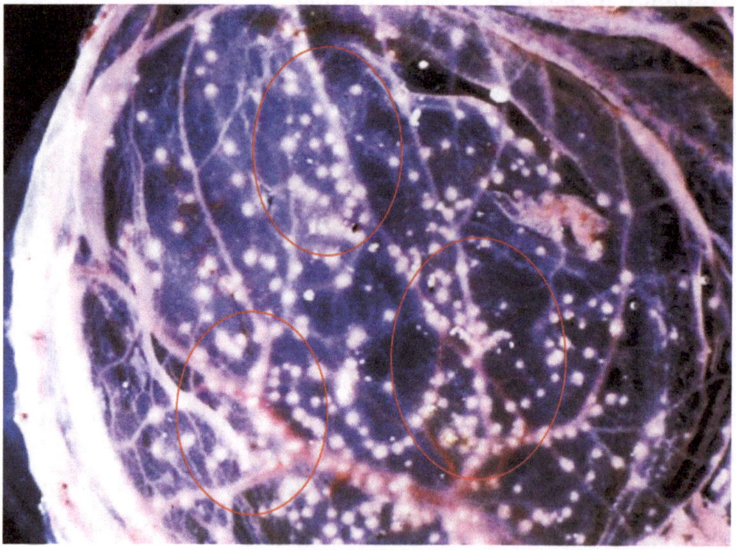

Fig. 11.2: Photograph of CAM showing pock lesions

Cell culture

The cell cultures are primary or continuous cell lines. The primary-cell culture can be prepared from chicken fibroblasts, calf kidneys, calf testes, lamb kidneys and lamb testes. For this the tissues or organs are collected under sterile conditions in HBSS. These are cut into small pieces with sterile scissors and forceps. The cell suspension is kept on magnetic stirrer with a bar after addition of trypsin which dissociate the cells. After stirring, the cell suspension filtered through gauze or muslin cloth and the cells are washed with HBSS three times and one time with culture medium (Eagles MEM or medium 199) having 10% fetal calf serum . A 10% cell suspension is prepared and is poured in cell culture bottles. The bottles are incubated at 37^0C to form a sheet on flat surface of glass bottle; it is ready within 2-3 days. Check the cell culture for contamination. After completion of sheet, clinical sample can be inoculated on the cell culture. The presence of virus in cell culture can be detected by appearance of cytopathic effects, including necrosis, desquamation, aggregation, syncytia formation, plaques and presence of inclusions in the cell. The growth of virus is also observed by immunofluorescent-staining, immunoperoxidase staining and cell culture fluid can be examined for the presence of virus by ELISA, DIA or CIEP. Electromicroscopically, one can demonstrate the virus in cells or in cell culture fluid.

Continuous Cell Lines

These are immortal cancerous cells, which grow fast if proper nutrition is provided. Now a days, these cells are available commercially or in some developed institutes which supply them on request free of cost or with some nominal charge. The cells are maintained and cultured in same way as in primary cell culture. The relevant details of media and/or other growth requirements are supplied with the cells which should be followed for their culture.

Antibacterial Sensitivity Testing

The antibacterial sensitivity testing is performed to make a proper choice of therapy. With the extensive and indiscriminate use of antibiotics, the organisms become resistant to most of the antibacterial drugs. It, therefore, becomes necessary to carry out sensitivity test so that proper medication is initiated. To test the sensitivity of bacterial cultures, antibiotic discs are used. The pure culture is prepared in broth (nutrient broth or brain heart infusion broth) and with the help of sterile cotton swabs it is layered on agar plates (nutrient agar/ tryptose soya agar). Plate is then kept for a few minutes for drying and antibiotic discs are placed with the help of forceps. Usually 5-6 discs can be placed in one plate. The plate is then incubated at 37^{0}C for 24 hours. After incubation the size of zone of inhibition is measured using a scale and compared with the scale/ standard provided in the literature of antibiotic discs. A clear and wider zone that the bacteria is sensitive to that particular antibiotic. Presence of a single colony in zone area indicates that few organisms are resistant and if this is the same organism, it may be a resistant mutant.

Based on the results of antibacterial sensitivity tests, the therapy should be advised.

12

Cytopathology

- General considerations
- Scope
- Exfoliative cytopathology
- Interventional cytopathology (Biopsy)
    - FNAC
    - Imprint cytopathology
    - Crush smear cytopathology

General Consideration

Cytopathology deals with interpretation of cells from animal body that either exfoliate/desquamate spontaneously from epithelial surfaces or are obtained from organs/tissues through biopsy. Histopathology is based on interpretation of distortions in tissue architecture, and the cytopathologic diagnosis rests upon alterations in morphology of a single or group of cells.

Scope

Cytopathologic diagnosis has numerous applications in diagnosis of animal diseases.

1. Diagnosis and prognosis of Neoplasm: Cytopathologic interpretations are helpful is diagnosis and prognosis of cancer in animals specially in urinary tract neoplasms, lymphoma, ovarian cancer, mammary gland tumour, horn cancer and tumours of reproductive tract.
2. Identification of benign neoplasms: With the help of imprint smears or exfoliative cells, one may diagnose and identify the extent of alterations in tumour cells e.g. fibroadenoma versus carcinoma of eyes.
3. Diagnosis of infectious diseases : It is helpful in diagnosis of various infectious diseases of animals, including bacterial and viral diseases

e.g. infection in calves. One can demonstrate rotavirus antigen in desquamated cells in diarrhoeic feces.

4. Cytogenetics: Cytopathologic diagnostic procedures can be employed for chromosomal studies, including karyotyping and abberations in chromosomes.

Cytopathologic diagnosis can be performed through two methods viz. exfoliative and interventional cytopathologoy.

1. Exfoliative Cytopathology

It includes the examination and interpretation of cells spontaneously shed off from epithelial surfaces in body cavities of body fluids. Cells obtained through scraping, brushing and/or washing of mucosal surfaces are also included in exfoliative cytopathologic diagnosis. Exfoliative cytopathology is based on the fact that the rate of exfoliation is enhanced in disease states there by yielding a larger number of cells for study. Samples from different organs that can be obtained for exfoliative cytopathological diagnosis are listed in table 12.1.

Table12.1: Types of samples from different organs/body site for exfoliative cytopathologic diagnosis in animals.

	Site		**Sample**
1.	Urinary tract	—	Urinary sediment
		—	Bladder washing
		—	Prostatic massage-secretions
			in dogs
2.	Gastrointestinal tract	—	Endoscopic lavage
		—	Fecal sediment (Fig.12.1)
		—	Rectal washings
		—	Rectal pintch.
		—	Buccal smears
3.	Respiratory tract	—	Sputum
		—	Bronchial washings
4.	Female genital tract	—	Vaginal smears
		—	Cervical smears
		—	Vaginal discharges
		—	Endometrial washings
5.	Body fluids	—	Cersebrospinal fluid
		—	Synovial fluid
		—	Amniotic fluid
		—	Seminal fluid

2. Interventional Cytopathology (Biopsy)

Interventional cytopathology includes the samples obtained from aspiration or surgical biopsy. In veterinary sciences, however, there is limited scope of aspiration interventional cytopathology except in a few diseases such as in theileriosis lymph node aspirate is useful in diagnosis. But surgical biopsy is comparatively common in the diagnosis of tumours in animals. It includes fine needle aspiration cytology (FNAC), imprint cytology and crush smear cytology.

(A) Fine Needle Aspiration Cytology (FNAC)

Fine needle aspiration cytologic procedures are useful in palpable lesions in animals e.g. enlargement and hardness of superficial lymph nodes. The FNAC technique is quick, safe and painless and carried out without any anesthesia, However, it should be performed by a trained personnel otherwise multiple attempts or repeated procedure may cause inconvenience and pain to animal. This method of diagnosis is cost effective and provides first hand information to the veterinary clinician.

Fine needle ranges from 25 (0.6mm) to 20 (0.9mm) guage for aspiration of cells. The standard size of needle is 21 guage disposable needle of about 40 mm length. For lymph node biopsy, 24 guage needle of 25 mm length may be used. Needles of up to 200 mm length are used for aspiration from internal organs. Syringes of 10-20 ml capacity are suitable but the grip of syringe and needle should be such that it does not leak during aspiration. The needle is inserted into the targeted area through skin puncture. On reaching the lesion, the plunger of syringe is retracted and at least 10 ml of suction is applied while moving the needle back and forth within the lesion. The angle of the needle may be changed to access different areas of the lesion. Aspiration is terminated when aspirated material or blood becomes visible at the the base/hub of the needle. For diagnostic purpose cells obtained within the needle are more than adequate and the material drawn into the barrel of the syringe is sometimes not recoverable and thus becomes useless for cytopathological diagnosis.

Aspirated material is recovered by detaching the needle from syringe and filling the syringe with air. The syringe and needle are then reconnected and the aspirate is placed on one end of a glass slide. Aspirate deposits on the slide are inspected with naked eyes. Semisolid particulate aspirates are crush-smeared by pressing between two glass slides. Other material may be pulled just like blood smears on to slide. These smears are either wet fixed or air dried. Most cytopathologists use both type of smears. Wet fixation in done in 95% ethanol for 10-15 min and then transported to laboratoy while air-dried smears are rapped and directly sent to laboratory (Fig. 12.2).

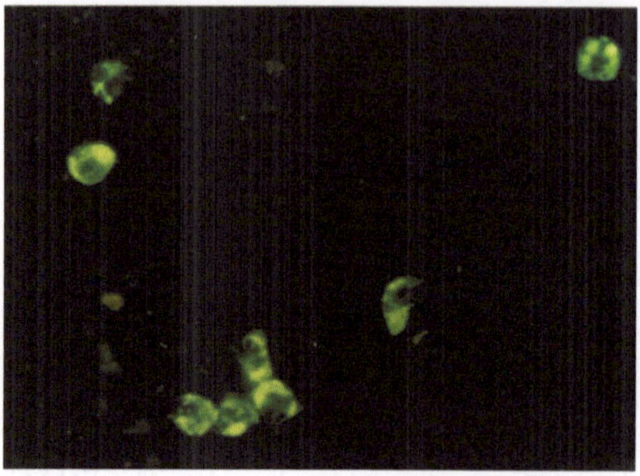

Fig. 12.1: Photomicrograph showing immunofluorescence for demonstration of antigen in exfoliated cells

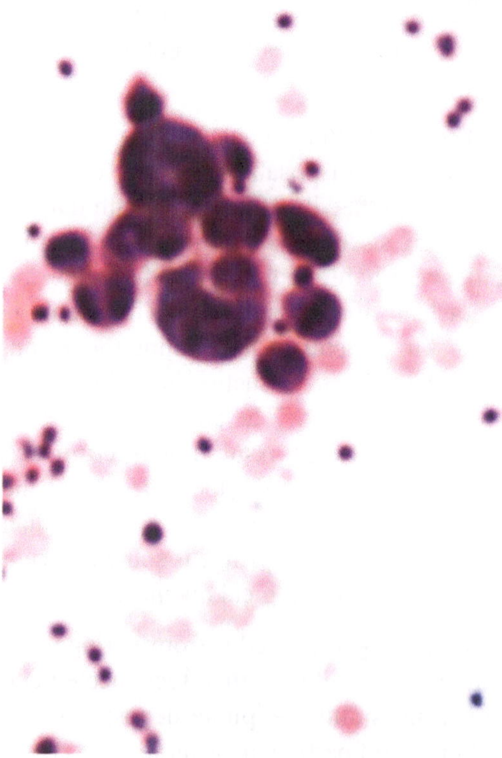

Fig.12.2: FNAC of abdominal fluid showing neoplastic cells

B. Imprint Cytology

In this, touch preparations from cut surfaces of superficial cut/excised lesions are prepared. Imprints are also prepared from draining sinuses and/or ulcerated areas. The main advantage of imprint smear examination is that the cell distribution reflects the tissue architecture thus aiding in interpretation. It is useful in quick diagnosis of several animal and poultry diseases.

C. Crush Smear Cytology

Crush smear preparations of particulate tissue material are help ful in diagnosis of tumours. It provides the recognition of tissue architecture in addition to better cytological details.

13

Necropsy

- General Consideration
- Post-mortem examination of large animals
- Post-mortem examination of poultry
- Steps in post-mortem examination
- Writing of post-mortem report
- Collection, preservation and dispatch of specimens for laboratory diagnosis

General Consideration

Necropsy is examination of animal after death also known as post mortem examination. It helps in diagnosis of diseases and their control. It is said that ***"Necropsy is a message of wisdom from dead to living"***. Necropsy include systemic examination of dead animal, recording of pathological lesions, their interpretation to make diagnosis of disease. Sometimes it is difficult to arrive any conclusion merely based on gross examination of dead animal. Then one should seek the help of laboratory examinations such as Histopathology, Microbiology, Immunology and Toxicology for confirmation.

Necropsy examination is an integral part of disease investigation. Therefore, veterinarian must have the knowledge of the techniques of post-mortem examination, recording of lesions, collection of proper material for laboratory and most importantly their correlation to arrive at conclusive diagnosis. The technique of post-mortem examination is as under:

Post-mortem Examination of Large Animal

- Place animal on left side (Ruminants) (Fig. 13.1).
- Place horse on right side and dog on vertebral column (Figs. 13.2 & 13.3).
- Make midventral incision with knife from chin to anus.
- Surround the prepuce, scrotum/mammary gland.

- Remove skin dorsoventrally. Remove skin at face, neck, thorax and abdomen.
- Cut the muscles and fascia in between scapula and body; remove fore legs.
- Raise hind legs, cut the coxo femoral ligament.
- Examine caps tissue, muscles, superficial lymph nodes- pre scapular, pre femoral supra mammary, etc.
- Open abdominal cavity by cutting muscles and peritoneum
- Open thoracic cavity by cutting xiphoid cartilage at sternum; lift ribs and press them to break at joints with vertebral column.
- Examine the visceral organs in both cavities:

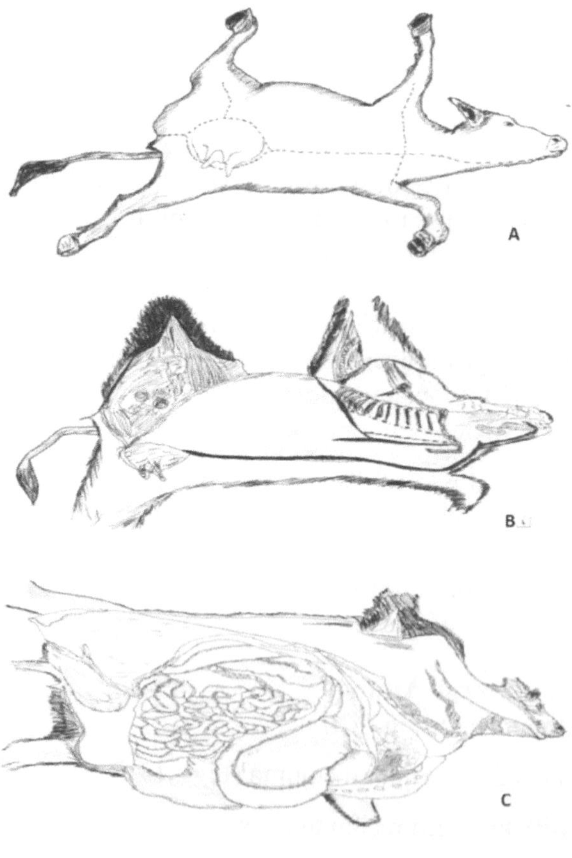

Fig.13.1: Diagram showing post-mortem examination of ruminant **(A)** position of cow and the marking for incision **(B)** after removal of skin and **(C)** after exposure of abdominal cavity

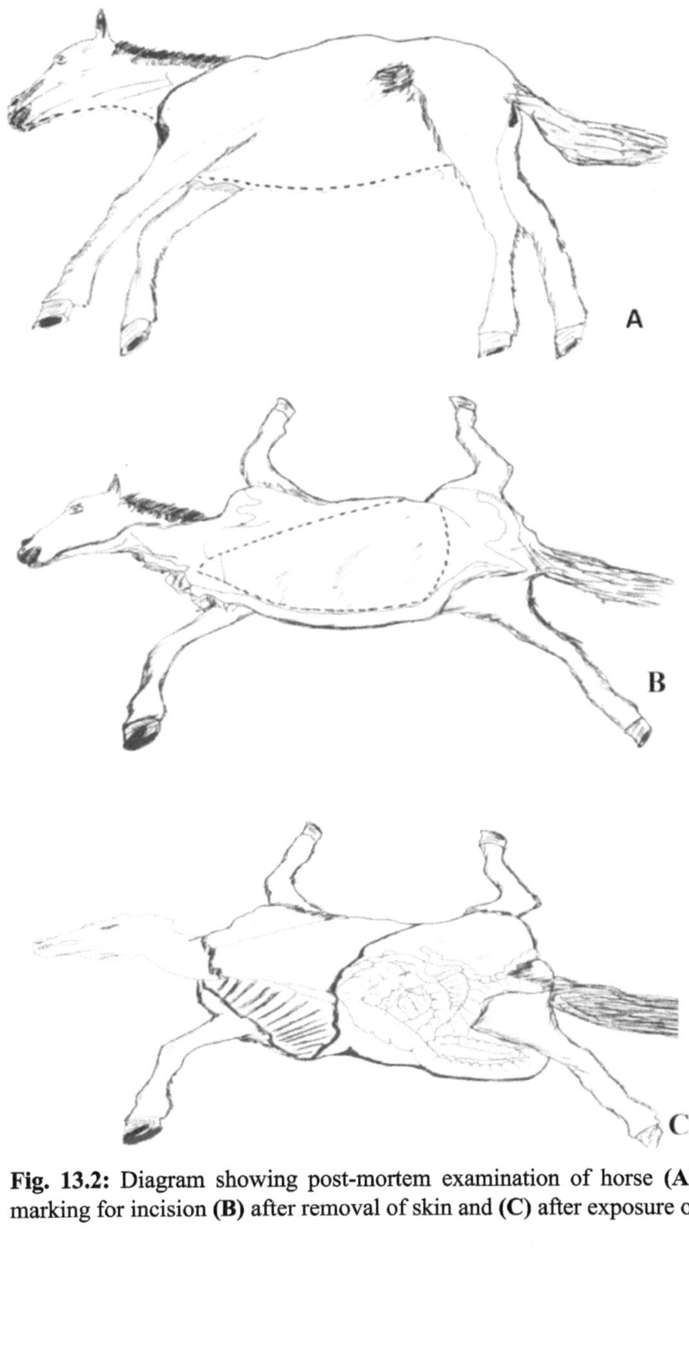

Fig. 13.2: Diagram showing post-mortem examination of horse **(A)** position of horse and marking for incision **(B)** after removal of skin and **(C)** after exposure of abdominal cavity

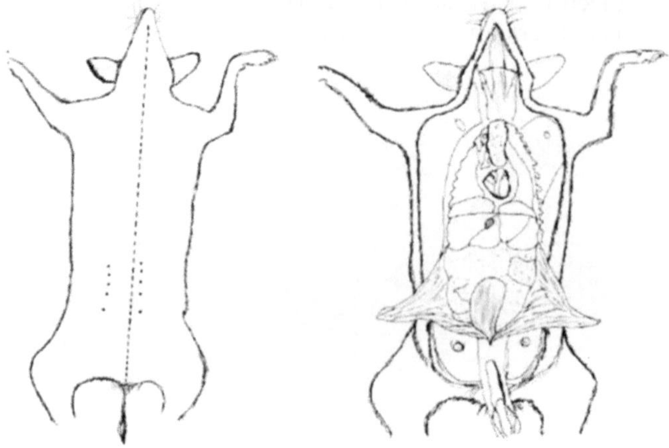

Fig.13.3: Post mortem examination of dog (A) Incision and exposure of abdominal cavity

Thorax	:	**Heart, Lungs, Trachea, Oesophagus, Mediastinal lymph nodes, Diaphragm**
Abdominal cavity	:	
Ruminants	:	Rumen, Reticulum, Omasum, Abomasum
Other animals	:	Stomach
In all animals	:	Liver, Pancreas, Intestines, Mesenteric lymph nodes, Spleen, Kidneys, Ureter
Pelvic cavity	:	Urinary bladder, uterus

Post-mortem Examination (Poultry, fig. 13.4 to 13.22)

- Dip the dead bird in antiseptic solution or in water; to avoid feather contamination.
- Keep the bird on post-mortem table at vertebral column and look for any lesion or parasite on skin.
- Examine the eyes, face and vent.
- Remove skin through a cut with knife and with the help of fingers. Expose thymus, trachea, esophagus in neck.
- Break the coxofemoral joint by lifting the legs. Examine the chest and thigh muscles.
- Cut on lateral side of chest muscles. Lift the chest muscle dorsally and break bones at joints with thorax. Cut bones at both sides and remove muscles, bones to expose thorax, abdomen.
- Examine different organs.

- Cut proventriculus and pull the organs of digestive tract out. Separate liver, spleen, intestines, caecum, proventriculus, gizzard, etc.
- Expose bursa just beneath the cloaca.
- Cut beak at joint, examine mouth cavity and expose esophagus and trachea.
- Remove skin of head and make a square cut on skull to expose brain.
- Take a forceps and place in between thigh muscles, remove fascia and expose the sciatic nerve.
- Separate each organ, examine them for the presence of lesion.

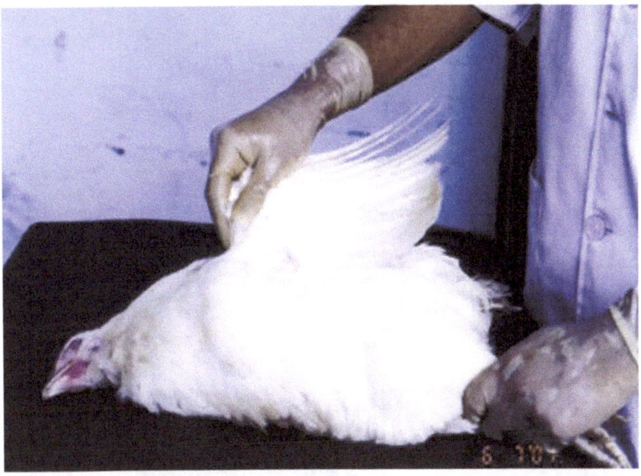

Fig.13.4: Post mortem examination of poultry- Position of bird on pm table

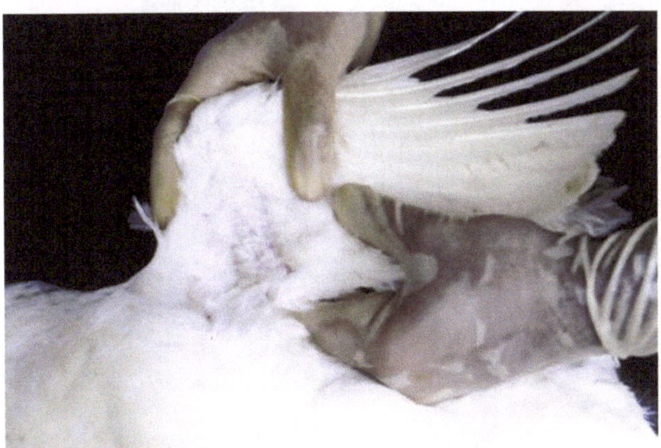

Fig.13.5: Post mortem examination of poultry- External examination

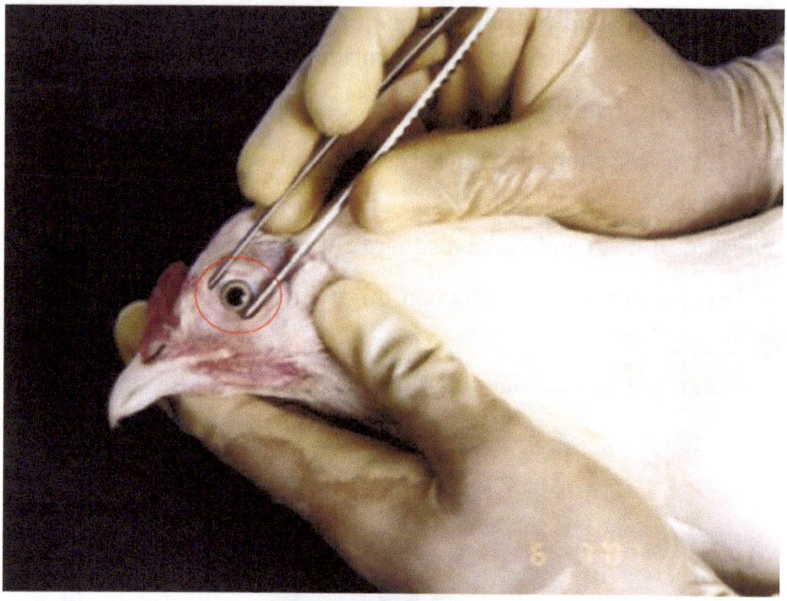

Fig.13.6: Post mortem examination of poultry- Examination of eye

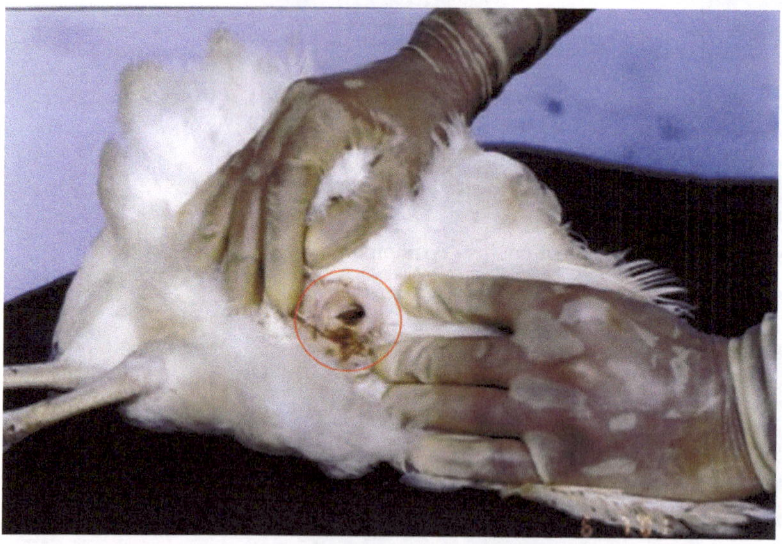

Fig.13.7: Post mortem examination of poultry- Examination of vent

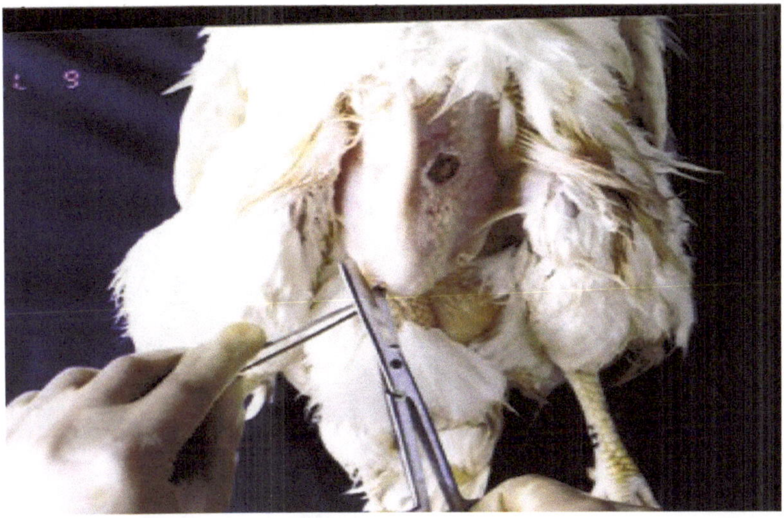

Fig.13.8: Post mortem examination of poultry- Removal of skin

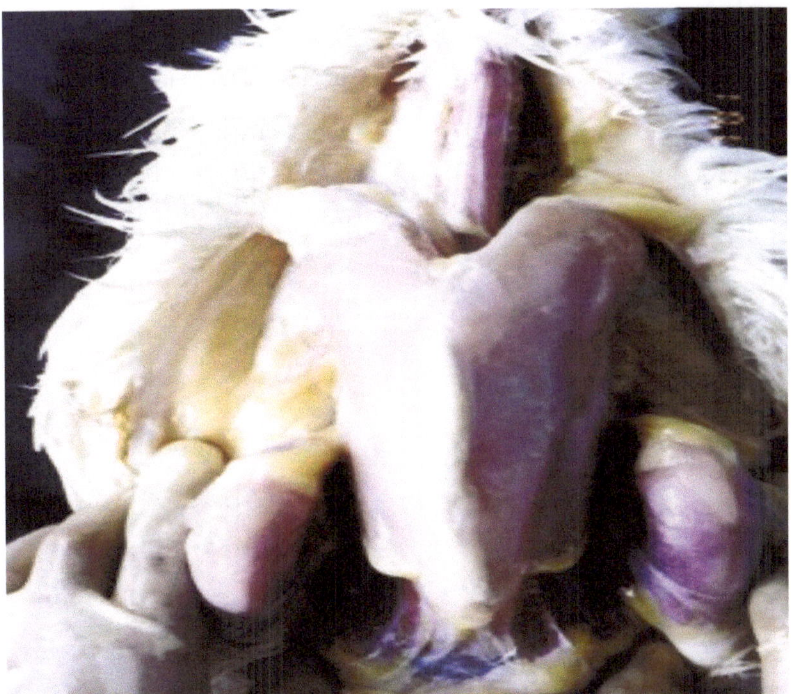

Fig. 13.9: Post mortem examination of poultry- Coxo-femoral joint break

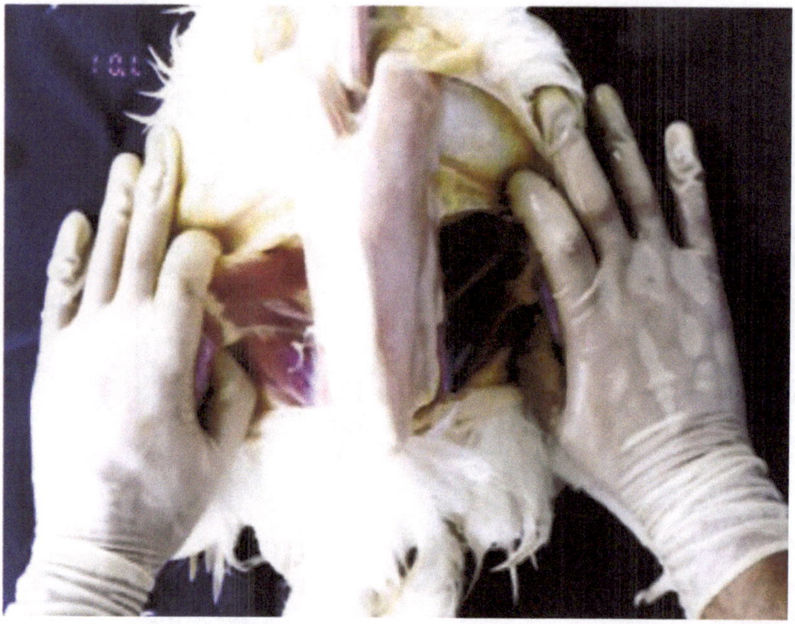

Fig.13.10: Post mortem examination of poultry- Exposure of muscles for examination

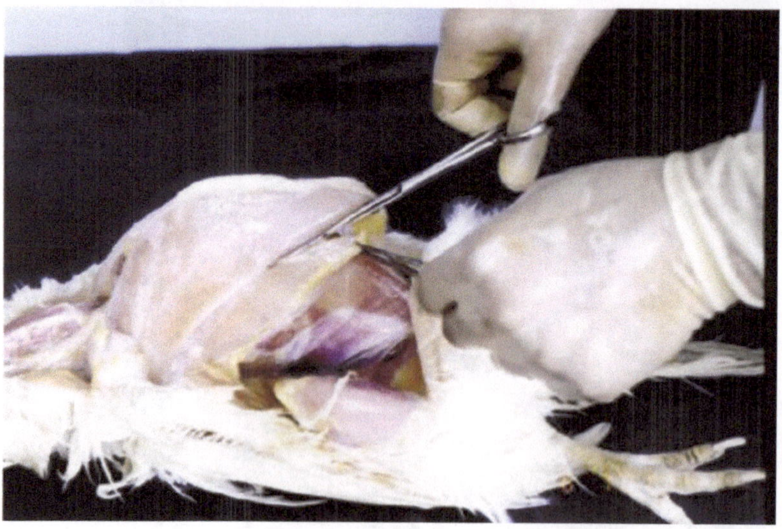

Fig.13.11: Post mortem examination of poultry- Removal of breast muscles

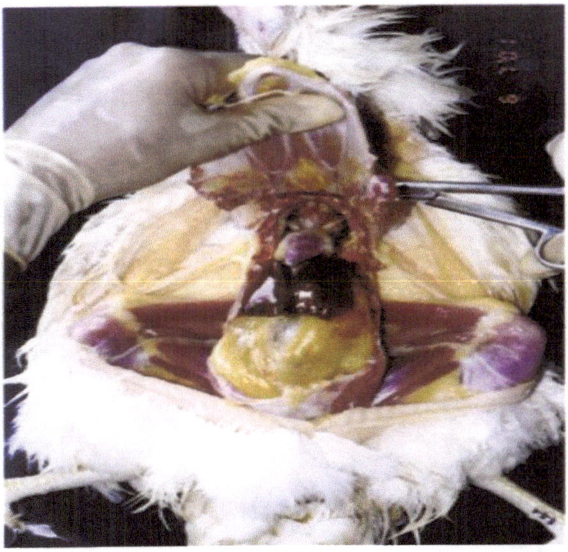

Fig.13.12: Post mortem examination of poultry- Cutting of neck bones

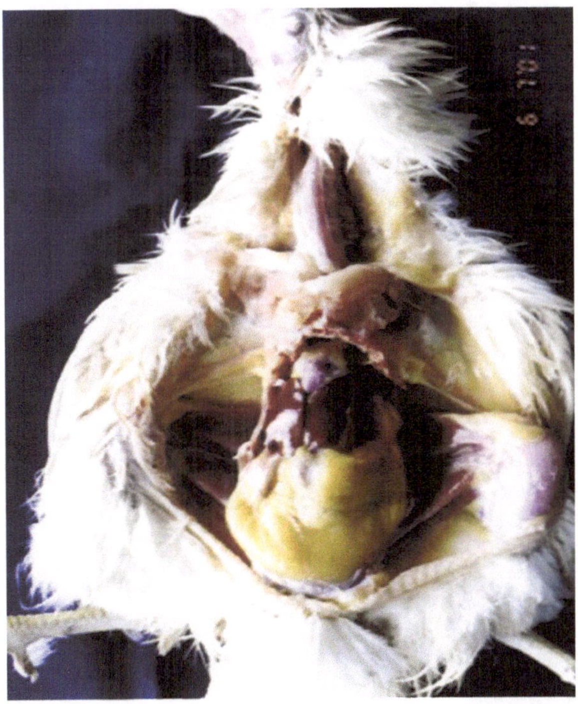

Fig.13.13: Post mortem examination of poultry- Exposure of internal organs

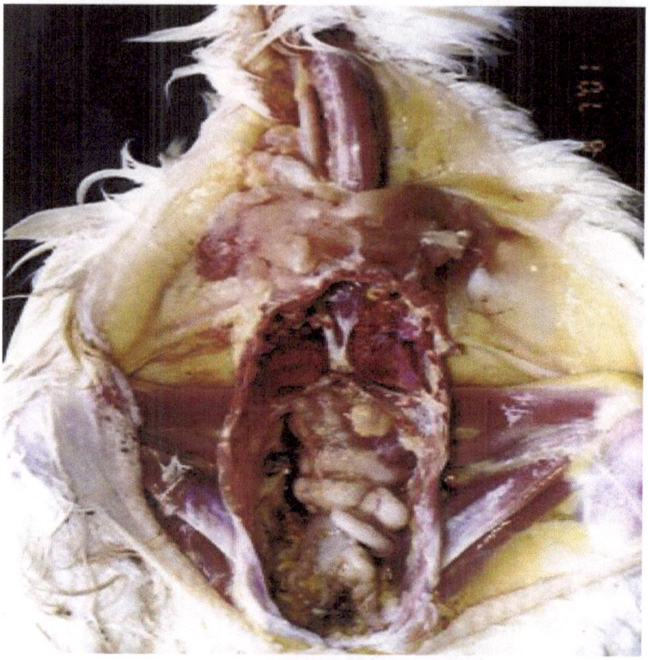

Fig.13.14: Post mortem examination of poultry- Exposure of kidneys, ovary, oviduct after removal of digestive tract

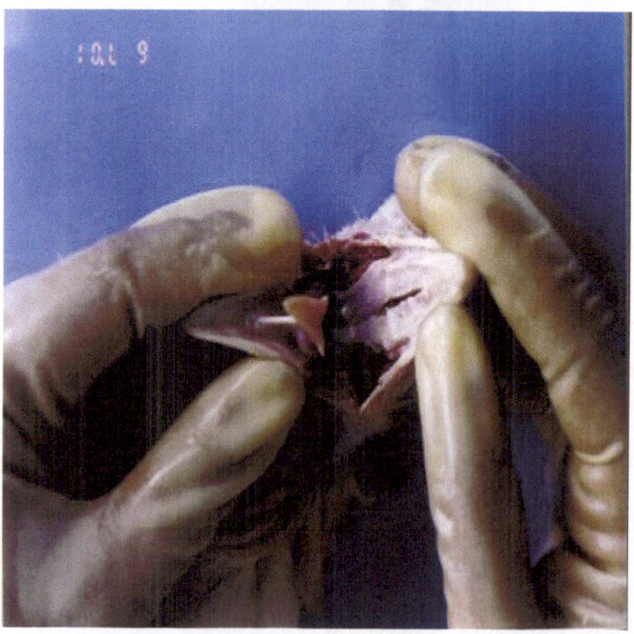

Fig.13.15: Post mortem examination of poultry-Examination of mouth cavity

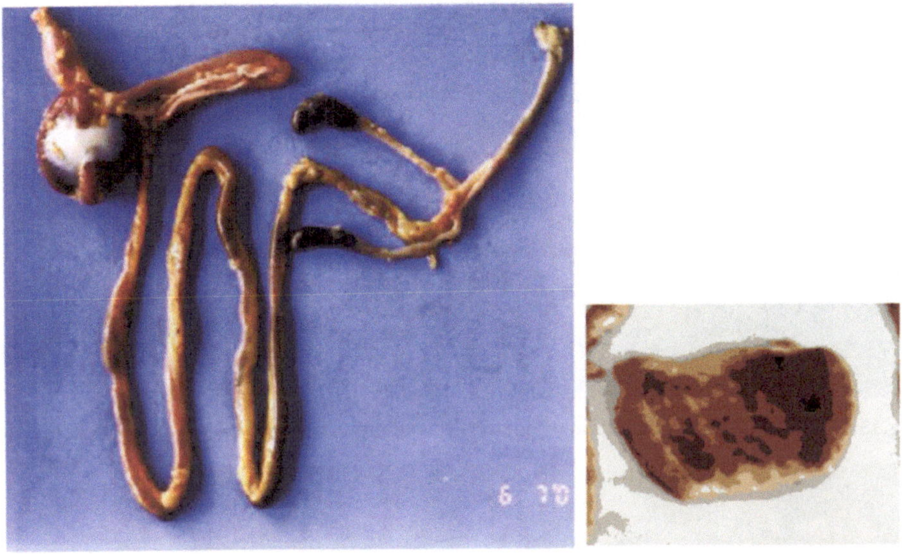

Fig.13.16: Post mortem examination of poultry- Examination of intestine, caecum, proventriculous

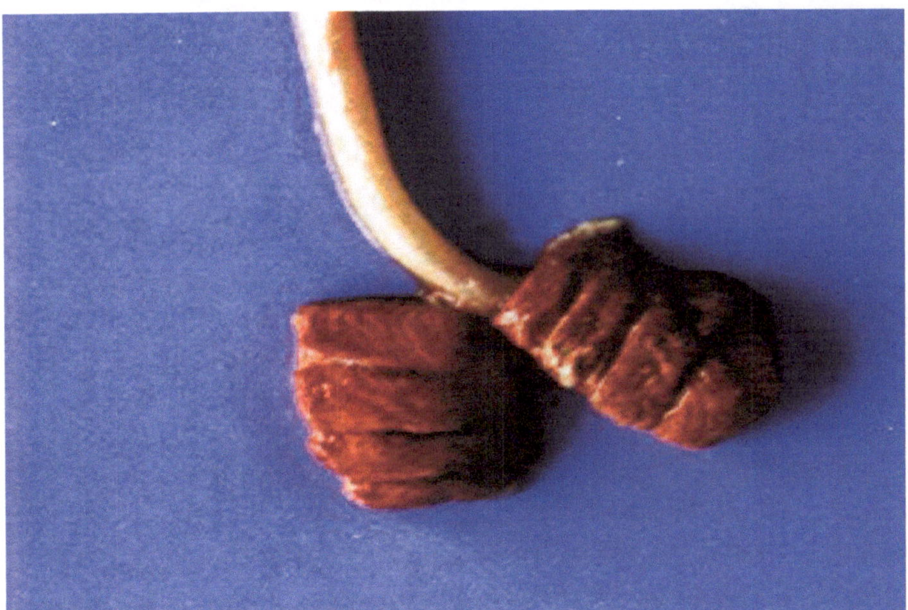

Fig.13.17: Post mortem examination of poultry- Examination of lungs, trachea and bronchi

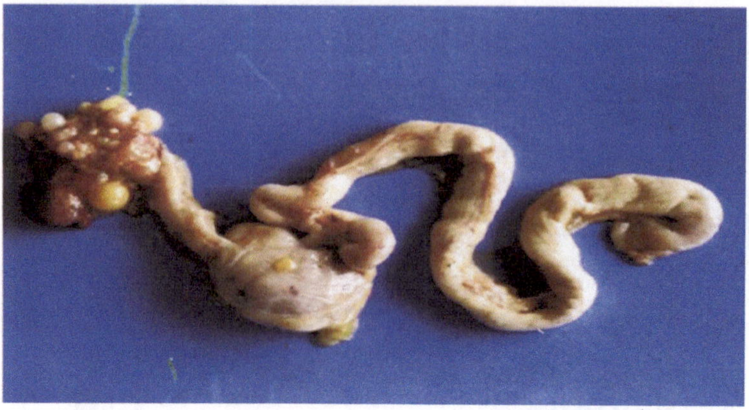

Fig.13.18: Post mortem examination of poultry- Examination of female reproductive tract

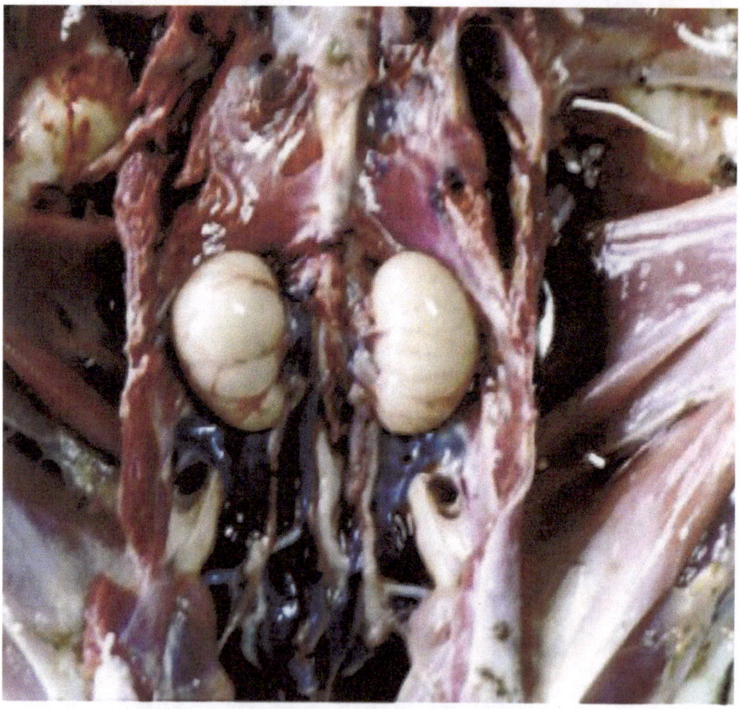

Fig.13.19: Post mortem examination of poultry- Examination of testes

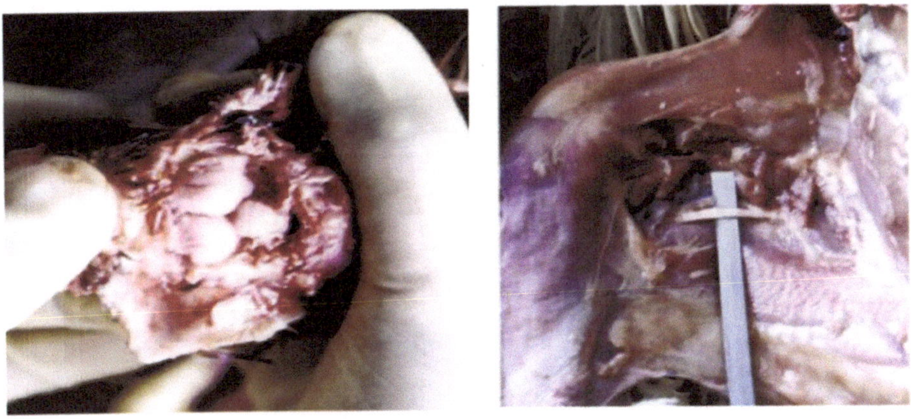

Fig.13.20: Post mortem examination of poultry- Examination of nervous system

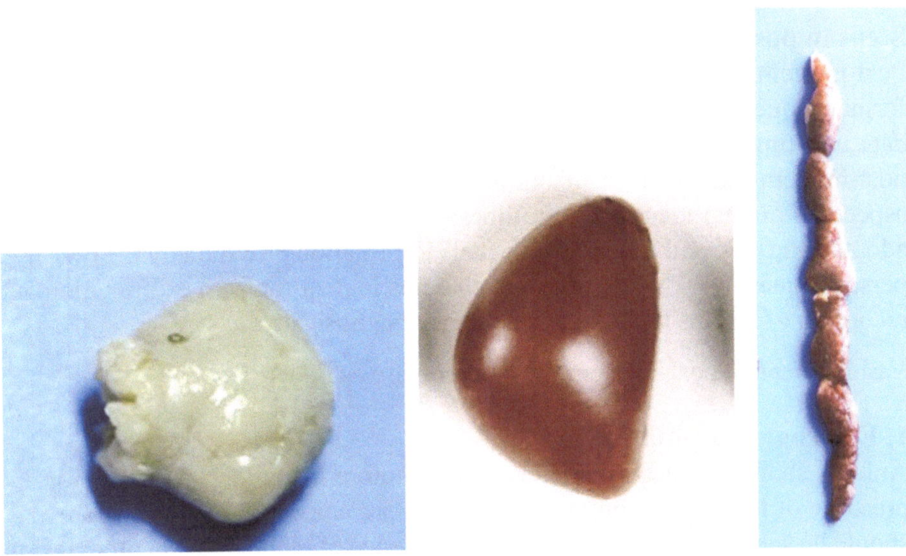

Fig.13.21: Post mortem examination of poultry- Examination of immune system

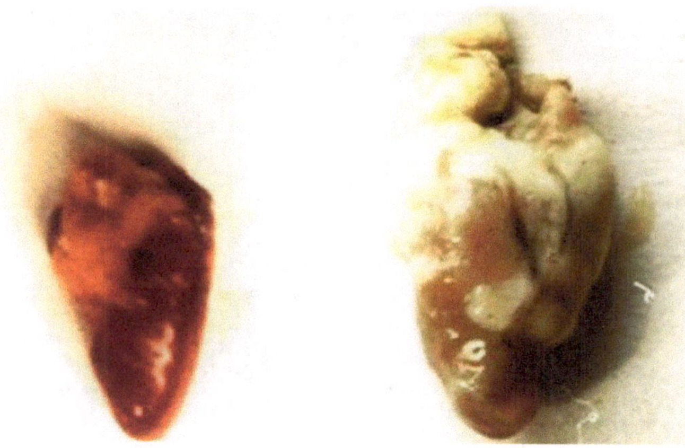

Fig.13.22: Post mortem examination of poultry- Examination of Heart

Steps in post-mortem examination

Post-mortem examination should be conducted only after receiving of a formal request from the owner of animal having details of anamnesis and date and time of death. Without formal written request, one should not do post-mortem examination of animal. The post-mortem record includes the aspects of animal identification, illness, therapeutic and preventive measures adopted and date and time of death. This information provided by the owner or person requesting post-mortem, which helps in post-mortem examination and recording of lesions to make a conclusive diagnosis.

Various steps in post-mortem examination are as under:

1. External Examination

Animal should be examined externally before opening the body for the presence of lesions on body surface. Eyes, ear, anus, vulva, mouth, nares etc. should be specifically examined for the presence of blood and any other lesion. If the blood is coming out from natural orifices, it should be examined for the presence of anthrax bacilli and such carcasses must not be opened for post-mortem examination. Following points should be taken into consideration while conducting external examination.

- Trauma, wound, fracture, cuts, etc.
- Fungal infection *e.g.* ringworm
- Parasitic infestation *e.g.* mange, lice, ticks
- Side of animal is lying down on earth.

- Discharges from openings.
- Burn, ulcers, erosions etc.

2. Subcutaneous Tissue and Musculature

Examine the subcutaneous tissue and musculature after removal of skin for the presence of lesions such as:

- Congestion, hemorrhage, oedema, nodule, anemia, icterus.
- Fat deposits
- Necrosis on muscles, hardening, calcification.

3. Abdominal and Thoracic Cavity

Just after opening the carcass, one should observe the presence of any lesion in abdominal and thoracic cavity and following points must be kept in mind.

- Accumulation of fluid (serus, serosanguinous, blood, pus etc.)
- Fibrinous or fibrous adhesions.
- Parasites
- Abscess, tumor etc.

4. Respiratory System

Organs/Tissues to be Examined

External nares, nasal passage, larynx, trachea, bronchi, lungs, air sacs (poultry) mediastinal lymph nodes.

Lesions to be Observed

- Discharge from external nares.
- Growth (granuloma/polyp) in nasal passage if there is blood mixed nasal discharge.
- *Trachea and Bronchi*- Congestion, hemorrhage, presence of caseous exudate, frothy exudate etc.
- *Lungs*- Congestion, consolidation, nodules, presence of exudate on cut surfaces, oedema, atelectasis, emphysema, hemorrhage, necrosis.
- *Mediastinal lymph nodes*- Oedema, hardening, calcification, congestion, hemorrhage.

5. Cardiovascular System

Organs/tissues to be examined
Heart, aorta, arteries, veins and lymphatics

Lesions to be observed

- Fluid, blood, pus etc. in pericardial sac
- Adhesions, fibrin, fibrosis
- Congestion, hemorrhage, necrotic foci
- Hardening of blood vessel, obstruction, thrombi
- Presence of parasites
- Post-mortem clot/thrombi.

6. Digestive System

Organs/tissue to be examined
Mouth cavity, esophagus, crop, proventriculus, gizzard (poultry), rumen reticulum, omasum, abomasum (ruminants), stomach, intestine (duodenum, jejunum, ileum, caecum, colon, rectum), cloaca, vent (poultry), anus, liver, pancreas, gall bladder, mesenteric lymph nodes etc.

Lesions to be observed

- Erosions, ulcers, vesicles
- Congestion, hemorrhage, oedema
- Necrosis
- Icterus
- Abscess/pus
- Perforation, needles or hard objects in reticulum.
- Intussusception, torsion, volvulus
- Parasites
- Atrophy, hardening, nodules
- Contents, catarrhal, blood mixed, digested/ undigested feed material, thickening of wall of intestines.
- Cut surface of liver for parasites, lesions in bile duct.

7. Cardiovascular System

Organs/tissue to be examined

- Kidneys, ureter, urinary bladder, urethra

Lesions to be observed

- Congestion, hemorrhage, infarction, oedema.
- Necrosis, hardening, nodules
- Deposition of salts, calculi
- Obstruction

8. Genital System

Organs/tissue (female)

- Ovaries, oviduct, uterus, cervix, vagina

Male

- Testicles, Epididymis, penis, prepuce

Lesions to be observed

- Cysts in ovary
- Congestion, hemorrhage, oedema
- Foetus in uterus, pus, fluid
- Necrosis, overgrowth, nodules
- Atrophy, adhesions, granularity

9. Immune system

Organs/tissue to be examined

- Spleen, lymph nodes, bursa and thymus (poultry), bone marrow
- Peyer's patches, GALT, RALT

Lesions to be observed

- Size, shape, atrophy, hardening.
- Oedema, congestion, hemorrhage

10. Nervous System

Organs/tissue to be examined

- Brain, spinal cord, nerves, meninges

Lesions to be observed

- Congestion, haemorrhage, hematoma
- Oedema, swelling
- Abscess
- Hypoplasia

11. Miscellaneous Observation

- Adhesions in pleural/peritoneal cavity
- Any other left over information pertinent to post-mortem examination/ diagnosis

12. Post-mortem Diagnosis

- Diagnosis should be made on the basis of above findings which involve any system or organ. The most involved organ based diagnosis should be written with suggestion of etiological factors or etiology based diagnosis.

Writing of Post-mortem Report

Post-mortem report consists of two parts post-mortem record and post-mortem examination as given in the format on next page. The first part *i.e.* post-mortem record is having information related to animal and is supplied by the owner or person requesting post-mortem examination. Actually, it is a part of request form of the case for post-mortem examination. This is necessary for the identification of animal. It should be filled in before conducting post-mortem examination. The proper record will be helpful in establishing accurate diagnosis based on post-mortem examination.

Post-Mortem Record

1. **Species:** Here one should write the species of animal such as bovine, porcine, equine, poultry, etc.
2. **Date:** Date of the post-mortem examination.
3. **Case no.:** The serial number of your post-mortem book. It shows cumulatively how many animals are examined by you in necropsy.

4. **Breed:** Mention the breed of animal, if known or supplied in the request form, such as Murrah buffalo, Jersey cattle, etc.
5. **Age/Born:** Age of animal or its date of birth. In case the exact age is not known then mention young, adult or chick, grower, adult in case of poultry.
6. **Sex:** Sex of animal (male or female).
7. **Identification number/mark:** It must be filled with utmost care; the number (tattoo number or brand number) should be the same as on animal. If the identification number is not available/illegible then write the characteristic mark of animal.
8. **Owner:** Here, the name of owner with complete address must be filled clearly. The address should be complete enough so that the report can reach the owner through post also.
9. **Referred by:** In this column, the name of Veterinary Officer/any other officer who referred the case for post-mortem examination should be written. Sometimes owner himself/herself is interested in post-mortem examination of animal; in such case the name of owner should be written.
10. **History of the case:** This includes the clinical illness of animal, duration of illness, epidemiological data, tentative diagnosis, therapeutic and preventive measures adopted. This is very important and information of this column has an important role in making the diagnosis.
11. **Reported date and time of death:** It should have the exact date and time of death of animal. Sometimes, it is difficult to note the exact time then one can write morning, noon, evening, midnight etc. to approximate the timings of death of animal. In some large farms, it is very difficult to record information with regard to each individual animal/bird so here one can write "previous night" as time of death.
12. **Date and time of post-mortem examination:** Pathologist conducting post-mortem examination should write here the exact time and date of the post-mortem examination.

The above information is very important to arrive any conclusive diagnosis. The correct information enhances the specificity of post-mortem diagnosis. Some points might be looking like insignificant but one should not overlook them and write as correct as information he/she can gather from the owner's request letter/form.

Post-Mortem Report

Post-Mortem Record

1. Species:
2. Date:
3. Case No.:
4. Breed:
5. Age/Born:
6. Sex:
7. Identification No.:
8. Owner with address:
9. Referred by:
10. History of the case:
11. Reported date & Time of Death:
12. Date and Time of post-mortem examination:

Post-Mortem Examination

1. External appearance
2. Subcutaneous tissue and musculature
3. General observations after opening the carcass
4. Respiratory system
5. Cardiovascular system
6. Digestive system
7. Urinary system
8. Genital system
9. Immune system
10. Nervous system
11. Miscellaneous observations
12. Post-mortem diagnosis Signature of officer conducting post-mortem

    Date:
    Place:

Post-Mortem Examination

It includes the observations made by the pathologist conducting post-mortem examination. This part of report should be filled in as soon as possible after the post-mortem examination. It is advisable that one should record some points on a small paper or diary during post-mortem examination and fill them in report after the conduct of post-mortem examination.

1. **External appearance:** Record the lesions observed in intact animal before its opening. One should place on record the side of animal lying down, lesions on skin, external parasites, trauma etc.
2. **Subcutaneous tissue and musculature:** The observations made after removal of skin, on subcutaneous tissue and muscle should be included in this column.
3. **General observations after opening the carcass:** It contains the general information or lesions present in abdominal and thoracic cavity such as accumulation of fluid, pus, blood, clot of blood, post-mortem changes such as pseudomelanosis, etc.
4. **Respiratory system:** Record the lesions observed in respiratory system right from external nares, nasal passage, trachea, bronchi and lungs along with mediastinal lymph nodes.
5. **Cardiovascular system:** Record the lesions present in heart, aorta, arteries, veins and lymphatics.
6. **Digestive system:** Record the lesions observed in digestive tract from month cavity, esophagus, crop, proventriculus, gizzard (poultry), rumen, reticulum, omasum abomasum (ruminants), stomach, intestines, rectum, anus, cloaca, vent (poultry), liver, pancreas, gall bladder etc.
7. **Urinary system:** Place on record the lesions present on kidneys, ureter and urethra.
8. **Genital system:** Record the lesions present in ovaries, uterus, oviduct, cervix and vagina in females and testes, penis etc. in males. Be careful in recording lesions in this column as it should match with the sex of animal written in post-mortem record section.
9. **Immune system:** Record the lesions present in spleen, bursa, thymus, lymph nodes, respiratory associated lymphoid tissue (RALT), gut associated lymphoid tissue (GALT) etc. Careful recording of lesions in these organs will be helpful in diagnosis.

10. **Nervous system:** Place on record the lesions present in brain, spinal cord and nerves. Most of the pathologists overlook this system and often not taken pain to examine the brain. It should not be done and every effort should be made to examine and place on record the lesions present in this system.
11. **Miscellaneous observations:** Here one can record any missing observation which has not been covered above.
12. **Post-mortem diagnosis:** This is very important. Based on the history and lesions present in different systems, pathologists by using his experience and conscience conclude the diagnosis. He/she may also write suggestions along with diagnosis or some points to suggest the diagnosis and/or contain the disease in other animals.
13. **Signature of officer conducting post-mortem:** Each and every report must be signed by the officer doing post-mortem examination. Without signature of competent officer, it has no validity.
14. **Place and date:** The person signing the post-mortem report must also write date and place of post-mortem examination.

Collection, Preservation and Dispatch of Specimens for Laboratory diagnosis

Tissue samples are collected from dead or live animals for laboratory examination to confirm the tentative diagnosis.

Purpose

- Diagnosis of disease or for identification of new disease.
- Confirmation of tentative diagnosis.
- Prognosis
- To observe the effect of treatment and give directions for future therapy.

Precautions

- Collect the tissues as early as possible after death of animal.
- Representative tissue/sample should be collected.
- Sharp knife should be used for cutting
- Collect the tissues directly in fixative.

- Size of tissue should not be more than 1 cm for histopathology in 10% formalin.
- Hollow organs should be taken on paper to avoid shrinkage.
- Hard organs like liver, kidneys etc. should be collected along with capsule.

Collection of Specimens for Bacteriological Examination

- Collect the tissues under sterile condition.
- Sterilize knife/ scalpel/ spatula on flame or in boiling water.
- Surface sterilized by hot spatula
- Cut with knife and collect sample from inner tissue.
- Body fluids/blood should be collected in sterilized syringe or in Pasteur pipette.
- Specimens should be collected directly in media (liquid media-nutrient broth, peptone water, tetrathionate broth or even in normal saline solution/phosphate buffer saline).
- Seal, pack and transport the collected material to laboratory in ice/under refrigeration conditions.

Bacterial Diseases

Abscesses

- Swab in sterile conditions/pus in vials
- Collect material from margin of abscess

Actinobacillosis/ Actinomycosis

- Tissues from affected parts in 10% formalin.
- Pus in sterile test tube/from edge of lesion
- Slides from Pus for sulfur granules.

Anthrax

- Blood smear from tip of the ear
- Blood for cultural examination
- Muzzle piece for biological test.
- Mark the specimen as "***Anthrax suspect***"

Black Quarter/Black leg

- Smear from swelling
- Affected muscle piece in ice.

Brucellosis

- Serum after 3 weeks of abortion
- Foetal stomach tied off
- Swabs from uterine discharge
- 5 to 10 ml milk in ice

Glanders

- Smear from discharge
- Lung, liver and spleen in 10% formalin
- Serum

Johne's disease

- Bowel washings in sterile bottle
- Smear from rectal mucosa
- Mesenteric lymph node in 10% formol saline

Leptospirosis

- Serum 21 days after abortion
- Milk/urine in vials (1 drop of formalin in 20 ml)
- Liver, kidney tissue in 10% formalin

Listeriosis

- Half brain in ice
- Half brain in 10% formalin

Mastitis

- 10 ml milk in sterile vial in ice

Pasteurellosis

- Heart blood

- Lung, spleen and mediastinal lymph nodes in ice.
- Affected tissues in 10% formalin.

Salmonellosis

- Liver, spleen, kidney and intestine tied off in ice.

Strangles

- Smear, swab of pus in ice.

Erysipelas

- Blood
- Spleen, kidney, liver in ice.

Campylobacteriosis

- Foetal stomach tied off
- Vaginal mucosa in ice.
- Preputial washings
- In pig, intestine and liver in 10% formalin.

Colibacillosis

- Heart blood in sterile vial.
- Tissues from intestine and lymph nodes in 10% formol saline.

Tuberculosis

- Lungs, mediastinal and bronchial lymph nodes in ice and in 10% formalin.

Collection of Specimens for Virological Examination

- Collect tissue under sterilized condition
- Body fluids/ blood in sterilized syringe or in Pasteur pipette
- Tissues in buffered glycerin
    - PBS pH 7.2- 50%
    - Glycerin- 50%
- Avoid samples in glycerin from sensitive viruses *e.g.* Rinderpest, canine distemper
- Seal and mark the specimen bottle and transport to laboratory.

Viral Diseases

Foot and mouth disease

- Tongue epithelium, vesicular fluid, saliva, pancreas in 50% buffered glycerin
- Serum

Hog cholera/ swine fever

- Serum under refrigeration
- Spleen, liver, kidney in 50% glycerin/ice
- Tissues from intestine, mesenteric lymph node and half of the brain stem in 10% formol saline.

Infectious Canine Hepatitis

- Several pieces of liver, gall bladder and kidney in 10% formol saline.

Pox

- Scabs in ice and in 10% formol saline.

Rabies

- Intact head should be soaked in 1% carbolic acid.
- Fracture the skull with hammer.
- Remove skin and bones
- Half brain in 10% formalin
- Half brain in 50% neutral glycerin.
- Tissues from cerebellum and hippocampus in Zenkers fluid for 20 hrs, wash in tape water for 24 hr and keep in 80% ethyl alcohol for Negri bodies.

Ranikhet disease

- Liver, spleen in 50% neutral glycerin
- Proventriculus in 10% formalin
- Brain in ice.

Rotaviral enteritis

- Faecal sample
- Intestinal tissue in 10% formol saline.

Gumboro disease

- Bursa of Fabricious, kidney, muscles in 10% formol saline.
- Bursa, kidney in 50% buffered glycerin.

Systemic diseases

Diarrhoea/Enteritis

- Faecal sample in sterile vial
- Serum
- Tissues of intestine, mesenteric lymph nodes in 10% formol saline.

Abortion/Metritis

- Faetal stomach content tide off or in sterile vials.
- Serum of dam after 21 days of abortion.
- Vaginal discharges in sterile conditions.
- Tissues of placenta, foetal liver, stomach, kidney in 10% formol saline.

Pneumonia

- Nasal discharge/nasal swabs.
- Lung tissue/pieces in sterile vials.
- Lung tissue and mediastinal lymph node in 10% formol saline.

Dermatitis

- Skin scrapings in 10% KOH.
- Skin tissue in 10% formol saline.

Encephalitis

- Cerebrospinal fluid in heparinised vials.
- Brain tissue in 10% formol saline.
- Brain tissue in 50% glycerol.

Nephritis

- Urine sample in sterile vial.
- Kidney tissue in 10% formol saline.

Collection of Specimens for Toxicological Examination

- Stomach/ intestinal contents
- Liver, kidneys, heart blood
- Urine
- In clean glass jars
- In ice/refrigeration without any preservative
- Seal, label, transport to laboratory.
- In veterolegal cases all specimens must be collected in presence of police.
- Type of poison suspected along with detailed history, signs, lesions/ treatment etc. should be written on letter with specimens.

Toxicosis/Poisoning

Heavy metal Poisoning

- Hg, Pb, Bi, Ag
- Liver, kidney, stomach content in ice in separate containers.

Alkaloids

- Liver, stomach contents and brain tissue in ice.

Nitrate

- Fodder
- Stomach contents, blood in ice

Strychnine Poisoning

- Stomach contents, intestinal contents, urine, liver, kidney in ice.

Hydrocyanic acid

- Plants
- Stomach contents, blood, liver
- Preserved in 1% solution of mercuric chloride.

Pesticides

- Fatty tissue, liver, stomach contents, blood in ice.
- Subcutaneous, omental, mesenteric fat.

Collection of Specimens for Immunological Examination

- Heart blood in syringe/ Pasteur pipette
- CSF/Synovial fluid /peritonial fluid
- Tissues in formol sublimate or in buffered formalin
- Blood/serum/others should be sent to laboratory under refrigeration conditions.
- Add one drop of 1:10000 merthiolate in 5 ml serum as preservative.

Dispatch of material

Following points must be kept in mind while dispatching the material to laboratory for diagnosis.

1. Describe the clinical signs, lesions, tentative diagnosis and treatment given to animal in your letter. Also mention the type of test you want with your tentative diagnosis.
2. Write correct address on letter as well as on the parcel preferably with pin code, if the material is sent through post.
3. Mark the parcel 'Biological Material', 'Handle with care', 'Glass material', 'Fragile' etc. in order to avoid damage in parcel. Also mark the side to be kept on upper side with arrows.
4. Seal the container so that it should not leak in transit.
5. Try to send the material as soon as after its collection from animal.
6. Keep one copy of cover letter inside the parcel and send another copy by hand or post in a separate cover.
7. Keep adequate material like thermocol etc. in the parcel which will save the material from outside pressures/jerks.
8. Use dry ice, if available otherwise use ice in sealed containers.

14

Histopathological Techniques

- General considerations
- Scope
- Microscopic examination techniques
- Smear
- Vital staining
- Routine histopathological techniques of sectioning
    - Collection of tissues
    - Fixation
    - Washing
    - Dehydration
    - Clearing
    - Impregnation
    - Casting of blocks
    - Trimming
    - Section cutting
- Staining
- Routine procedures
- Special procedures
    - Demonstration of Acid Fast Bacilli
    - Demonstration of Gram positive/Gram negative bacteria
    - Demonstration of Spirochetes
    - Demonstration of Fungi

- Demonstration of Rickettsia
- Demonstration of Inclusion Bodies

- Electron microscopic procedures

General Considerations

Histopathology is the branch of pathology which concerns with the demonstration of minute structural alterations in tissues as a result of disease. Most of histopathological techniques simulate to those applied for study of normal histological structures. For the demonstration of minute histological changes, the tissue must be process, in such a manner that it will provide maximum information. The histopathological diagnosis is an overlooked area especially in veterinary sciences. Many times it has been observed that the procedures are not properly followed or the qualified person trained for histopathology is not available, which in turn affects the interpretation and/or diagnosis. Histopathological procedures are, thus, described here not only for the benefit of students but also for those engaged in histopathological diagnosis in various diagnostic laboratories.

Scope

Though the histopathological techniques are labour intensive, cumbersome and time consuming, particularly when the automation equipment are not available; their use in diagnosis of diseases is unequivocal. Some of the areas where histopathological diagnosis is helpful are described here.

1. This is useful in establishing the pathogenesis and pathology of any disease caused by bacteria, virus, chlamydia, rickettsia, mycoplasma, parasite, toxin, poisons, etc.
2. There are certain diseases in which histopathological examination of tissue is the only alternative to diagnose the disease, e.g. bovine spongiform encephalopathy; the agent of this disease takes a very long incubation period and it is very difficult to isolate and there is no immune response in animal. Therefore, the histopathology remains the only alternative for confirmatory diagnosis.
3. In some cases, the tissues from dead animals are the only available material for laboratory diagnosis. This may occur either due to lack of time or due to negligence in not collecting the material for serological tests or isolation studies. Sometimes the transportation of material from remote areas destroys the other material and the tissues fixed in formalin

only remains for making diagnosis. In all such cases the histopathological examination has a pivotal role.

4. The histopathological procedures produce permanent slides, which can be stored for a long period and one cannot manipulate the findings. Therefore, it is considered the most reliable technique.
5. The histopathological techniques are useful in carrying out retrospective studies. The unstained slides and blocks can be stored for indefinite period, which can be examined even after years for further studies.
6. The presence of causative agents can also be demonstrated in tissue sections using routine histopathological techniques or special staining. In this, Gram's staining procedures are used for demonstration of bacteria while viral inclusions are demonstrated using hematoxylin and eosin or other staining techniques like Macchiavello's stain of Mann's methylene blue-eosin method. The Negri bodies are demonstrated by Seller's stain in case of rabies in animals. In such cases, the isolation of causative agent or their serological examination does not require; since the presence of causal agent in infected tissues gives a confirmatory diagnosis.
7. The detection of chemicals in tissues like enzymes, lipids, etc., is included in histochemical examination, which not only describes the structural changes but also gives an idea about the functional status of the organ.

Microscopic Examination Techniques

The microscopic examination of tissues or organs can be achieved by their smears or by sectioning, the latter being more commonly used in histopathological laboratories.

Smears

The microscopic examination using smears of any organ/tissue/cells is very rapid method which gives the result within hours. In this, the tissue pieces from organs are cut using a sharp knife and the cut surface is soft touched with clean glass slides with some gentle pressure, which gives an impression on the slide. This is also known a impression smears. Generally, 2-5 smears are prepared on a slide. If the collected tissue is too less than it is pressed between two slides and the impressions thus obtained on both the slides are used for study. The wet smears are fixed with ethanol and can be stored or transported to laboratory for examination (Fig. 14.1).

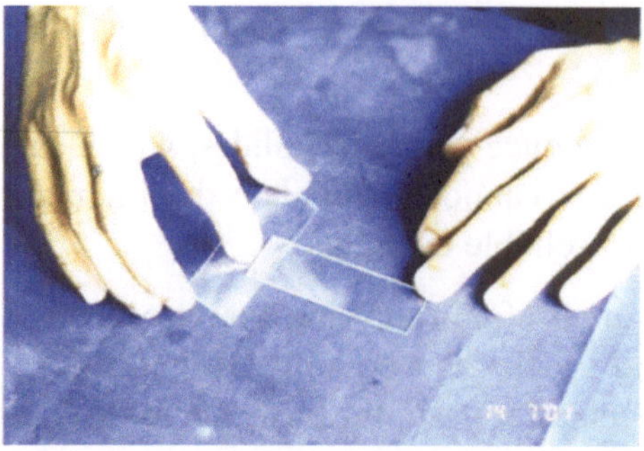

Fig. 14.1: Smear preparation

The impression smears of hippocampus, cerebellum and cerebrum of brain are very useful for demonstration of Negri bodies in rabid animals for diagnosis of rabies. The impression smears are stained with Seller's stain for a few seconds, washed and air dried and examined under oil immersion microscope for the presence of inclusion bodies also known as Negri bodies. These inclusions are characterized by intracytoplasmic, eosinophilic appearance with basophilic granules and are round to oval in shape with clear hollow.

In case of pox infection in animals, the impression smears are prepared from scab or pustule for demonstration of intracytoplasmic inclusions. Sometimes the viral inoculum is inoculated on chorio-allantoic membrane (CAM) of embryonated eggs; the impression smears of CAM yield the viral inclusions in the cytoplasm of the cells. In certain bacterial diseases like hemorrhagic septicemia and enterotoxemia, sometimes it becomes very difficult to demonstrate the organism in blood or tissues. For confirmatory diagnosis the material is inoculated in laboratory animals like mice, guinea pigs, etc. The impression smears (Fig 14.2 & 14.3) are then prepared from liver, spleen and other relevant organs for demonstration of the organism using special stains like Gram's stain.

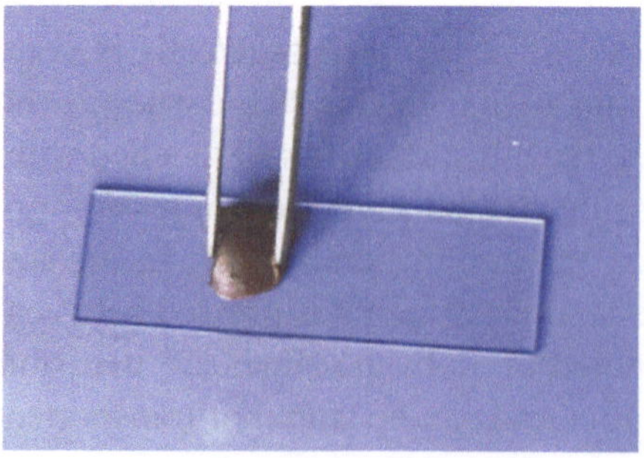

Fig. 14.2: Photograph showing preparation of impression smear

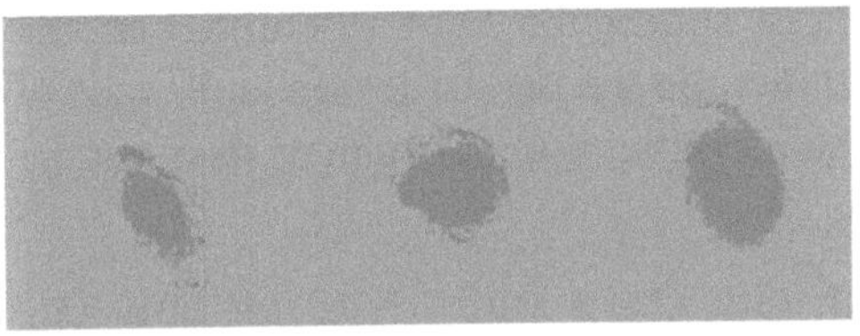

Fig. 14.3: Photograph of impression smear

Vital Staining

Vital staining procedures are not much in use directly in diagnosis. However, for detection of phagocytic cells in body, the vital stains are used. In the living animals when vital staining procedures are used for localization of phagocytic cells, these are known as intravital. *In vitro* use of vital stains known as supravital, e.g. leucocyte migration inhibition test (LMIT), lymphocyte stimulation test (LST), macrophage migration inhibition test (MMIT) and macrophage function tests (MFT).

Routine Histopathological Techniques of Sectioning

The tissue pieces from morbid animals should be collected properly and fixed in a suitable fixative. Then these are processed and sections of 4-5 microns are cut and taken on slides. These sections are stained and mounted to make the permanent preparation of slides. The different steps required for making the tissue slides are being described, briefly.

Collection of Tissues

The collection of tissues is an important step which is many times not properly looked. The whole diagnosis process depends upon the collected tissue pieces. A representative tissue should have been collected carefully and should have the normal as well as abnormal (lesion) part. The tissue must be collected by qualified person after a thorough examination of each organ or system. Sometimes it has been observed that the collection of tissues is performed by attendants or hurriedly by the qualified persons and proper attention is not paid. It should be kept in mind that a representative tissue sample will give the reliable diagnosis. Any mistake in collection of a representative tissue cannot be remedied afterwards. At the time of tissue collection, following points must be kept in mind which will be beneficial for making a correct diagnosis.

1. The tissue pieces from morbid animal should be collected as early as possible after the death of animal. Once the autolytic changes start in the dead body; it will not give a true picture of microscopic lesions due to autolysis.

2. At the time of tissue collection, it should be kept in mind that the representative tissue piece should include the part of lesion and a part of normal tissue, which facilitates the identification of organ or tissue at the time of microscopic examination.

3. The tissue pieces should be cut with sharp knife by using only one stroke. Blunt edged knife may require many attempts for cutting, which destroys the normal architecture of tissues.

4. Tissue pieces for histopathological examination should be collected from all the organs. Sometimes it has been noticed that the tissue sample is taken from that part of body which shows gross lesions; mere absence of gross lesion does not mean that there will not be microscopic alteration. In many disease conditions only microscopic changes occur which are not exhibited grossly. Such selective collection of tissue gives a biased interpretation, so it is better to have tissues from all the organs for proper interpretation and unbiased conclusion of histopathological studies.

5. Tissues should be collected directly in the fixative (Fig. 14.4) and not in any other pot or water. Sometimes it has been observed that at the time of post mortem examination, the tissue samples are collected in petri dishes or in bottle and brought to the laboratory and then fixative is added. This seems to be a wrong practice. The tissue bottle filled with 2/3 fixative must be available at the time of necropsy and tissue pieces should be collected directly in the fixative.

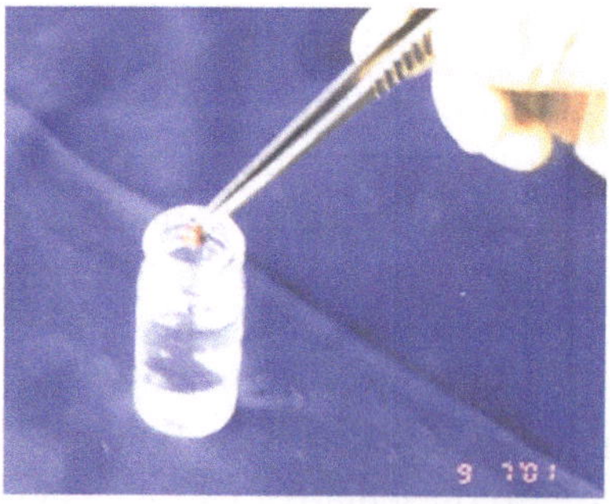

Fig. 14.4: Photograph showing collection of tissue in fixative

6. The size of tissue piece should not be more than 5 mm; it facilitates homogeneous and smooth fixation. The large size tissues do not get fixed properly and in the middle, the tissue gets autolyzed.

7. The tissue pieces from hollow organs like intestines, oviduct, etc. should be cut transversely and placed on a hard paper, then it should be cut longitudinally in such a way that the serosal layer sticks to paper and mucosal layer remains free (Fig. 14.5). After this it should be placed in fixative along with paper. This allows a good fixation and avoids the shrinkage and folding of tissue.

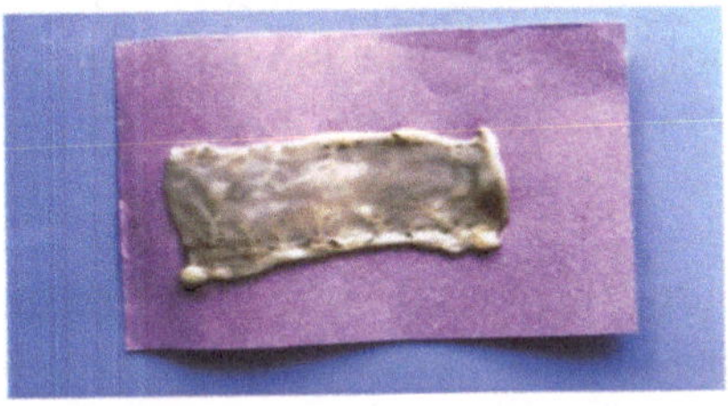

Fig. 14.5: Photograph showing the collection of intestine on a piece of paper for fixation.

8. At the time of post mortem examination, it has been noticed that the fecal matter is removed from the intestines by pressing or squeezing them or after opening the lumen by sharp objects like knife, slides, etc., which causes damage to the mucosal layer. The representative tissue should not be collected from such a damaged portions.
9. The tissues from encapsulated organs should be collected along with capsule or covering. Like, brain should be collected along with meninges; kidneys and liver should be with their capsules. The coverings of such organs also yield useful information on histopathological examination.

Fixation

The fixation of tissues is required for preventing post mortem changes like autolysis and putrefaction by saprophytes, preservation of cellular constituent in life like manner and for hardening of tissues by way of conversion of semisolids to solid material. For proper histopathological preparation and their interpretation, the role of fixative is very crucial. Any faulty fixation cannot be remedied at later stage. An ideal fixative should be one that fixes the tissues quickly and does not interfere with the refractive index of the tissue components.

The choice of fixative depends on the type of investigation required, the formol saline (10% formaldehyde in 0.85% sodium chloride solution)is considered best fixative for routine histopathological studies. The buffered formalin has certain advantage over formol saline and now a days it is recommended for routine use in histopathological laboratories. The buffered formalin can also be used for immunopathological studies. Buffered formalin is widely used and preferred because of its tolerance; tissues can be left for longer periods without excessive hardening or damage and sectioned easily. Since it has neutral pH, the formalin pigment is also not formed in the tissues. However, for immunopathological studies like immunoperoxidase staining techniques, the fixative of choice is formol sublimate. But in the absence of that buffered formalin may also be used. The time required for proper fixation is 6-12 hours for 5 mm thick block of tissue.

Washing

The tissue pieces after 6-12 hours fixation, are taken out from fixative and cut into 2 or 3 small pieces of 2-3 mm size blocks. These blocks are then kept in tissue capsules (Fig. 14.6) or in a gauze tide off with the help of thread and identification marks are kept along with the tissues. The identification number should be written on a small piece of paper with copying pencil. These capsules or gauze containing tissues should be kept in running tap water overnight for at least 12 hours to remove the formalin from tissues.

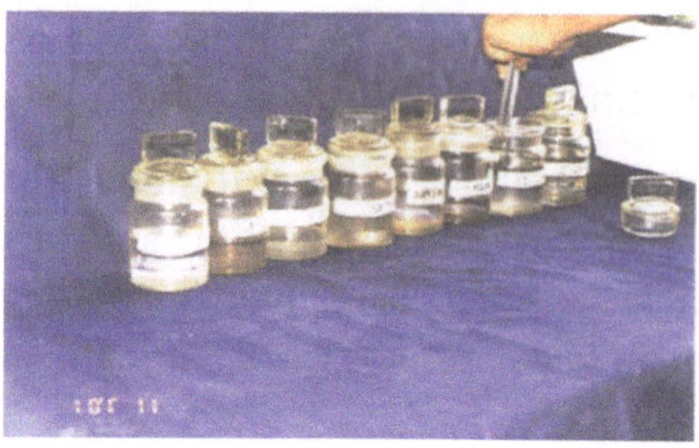

Fig. 14.6: Photograph showing the dehydration of blocks in ascending series of ethanol

Dehydration

In routine practice, the dehydration is done in ascending series of graded ethanol. These tissue blocks are kept in 50% ethanol and then in 70%, 80%, 90%, 95%, absolute ethanol I and absolute ethanol II for one hour each. These ethanol graded series should be kept in tight glass stoppered bottle or in screw cap jars to prevent the evaporation. In last bottle of ethanol II, sometimes copper sulfate is layered in the bottom and covered with filter paper which increases the life of ethanol as it absorbs the water from alcohol. But care should be taken, as soon as the copper sulfate becomes bluish due to absorption of water, the ethanol should be changed (Fig. 14.7).

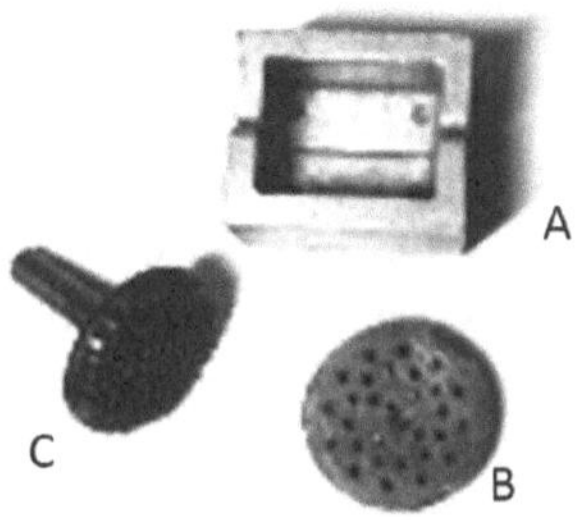

Fig. 14.7: Photograph showing (A) Mould (B) Tissue capsule and (C) Block holder.

To increase the process of dehydration, the tissue blocks should be agitated either mechanically in an automatic tissue processor or by shaking the container periodically. The volume of alcohol should be at least 50 times more than the tissue placed for dehydration.

Clearing

Usually the clearing of tissue blocks is done in xylene (Fig.14.7). Like ethanol, xylene should also be kept in tightly stoppered bottle to prevent evaporation. After dehydration the tissue blocks should be kept in ethanol and xylene (1:1) mixture for one hour, then the blocks are transferred to xylene I and xylene II for one hour each. If xylene is not available then benzene or toluene may be used for 3 hours as their action of clearing is slower than that of xylene. On complete clearing the tissue becomes transparent; then they should be transferred in paraffin wax for impregnation.

Impregnation

For the impregnation of tissue blocks, the paraffin wax is used either in paraffin embedding bath or in oven fixed at 60-62^{0}C temperature. Both the oven and embedding bath are electrically operated with thermostat to adjust the desired temperature. At the time of transfer of tissue blocks from xylene II, the paraffin bath must be kept at 60-62^{0}C so that the paraffin wax is available in liquid form for impregnation. Three changes are given in paraffin wax each of one hour. The paraffin wax should be free from dust or other gross impurities; which can be removed by filtration through muslin cloth.

Casting of Blocks

After 3 hours impregnation of tissue blocks in paraffin wax, the blocks are formed in moulds using molten wax. The tissues are place in moulds (Fig.14.8) in such a way that desired surface should be downward on the base of mould. The sections are cut from this surface, so care must be taken to keep the tissue in a proper manner, which should be cut into sections homogeneously. The mould is then filled with molten paraffin wax and then the blocks are cooled either at room temperature or in cold water. Various types of moulds like 'L' shaped or ring shaped can be used. If the moulds are not available, the blocks can be prepared in glass petri dishes or in empty slide boxes. But care should be taken to lubricate the surface of such petri dishes and other moulds with liquid paraffin or glycerin which facilitates the easy removal of blocks after cooling and hardening of paraffin wax.

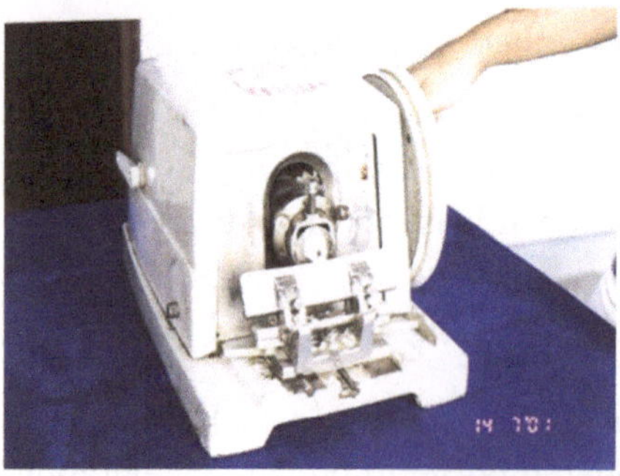

Fig. 14.8: Photograph showing section cutting on microtome

Trimming

The blocks are removed from the moulds and are cut so as to give one tissue per block and the wax is trimmed by knife or by rubbing on a hot plate in order to remove the extra wax on either side of the tissue. The tissue is exposed, which facilitates the side determination on which the section is to be cut. The identification of tissue should be fixed on one side of the block by touching the block with the small paper kept on it, which bears the number, with hot forceps of knife; then the blocks are fixed on block holder (Fig. 14.7C). Care should be taken that the number of marking of block should be kept on dorsal side at the time of trimming of the block on microtome to remove the extra wax and expose the whole surface of tissue. The trimming of blocks is done at 10-15 μm and a separate knife should be used for trimming and section cutting.

Section Cutting

Before the sectioning, the tissue blocks are cooled on ice or by keeping them in refrigerator. The tissue floatation bath should be cleaned and filled with water having a temperature of about 60-62^{0}C. The blocks along with block holders are fixed in the microtome in such a way that the marking number is on dorsal side, giving similar position to the blocks as was during trimming. Usually the sections are cut at 4-6 μm thickness on rotary microtome using a plain edge knife (Fig. 14.9). The knife should be sharp enough so that it cuts the desired thickness sections in the form of a ribbon and does not cause damage to the tissue. By using a brush and forceps, the tissue sections will spread here due to melting of paraffin wax and will take the shape similar to the tissue of that block. One can make out the selection here; the best looking sections 1-5 can be lifted (Fig. 14.10) on a sticky glass slide, which should be kept in a tray at an angle so that the water is removed. The glass slides are made sticky by applying a sticky material on clean and dry glass slides such as egg white and glycerin in 1:1 (V/V) ratio. The sticky material facilitates the sticking of sections on slides, which will not be damaged or removed during further process of staining. Generally 4-5 slides are made from each block and air dried in incubator or at room temperature. Precautions which should be taken into consideration at the time of section cutting are as follows:

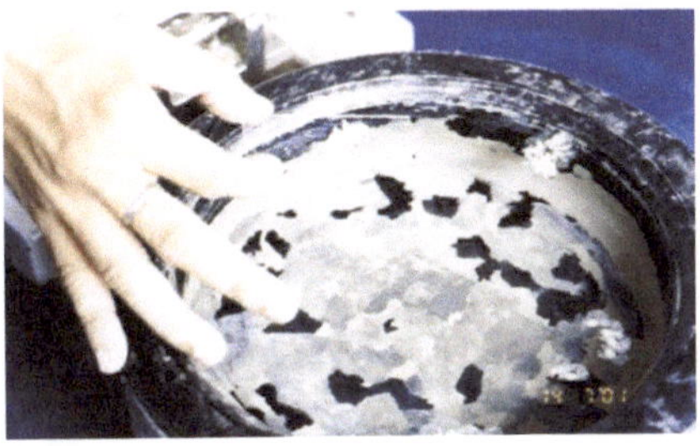

Fig. 14.9: Photograph showing lifting of tissue section from floatation bath

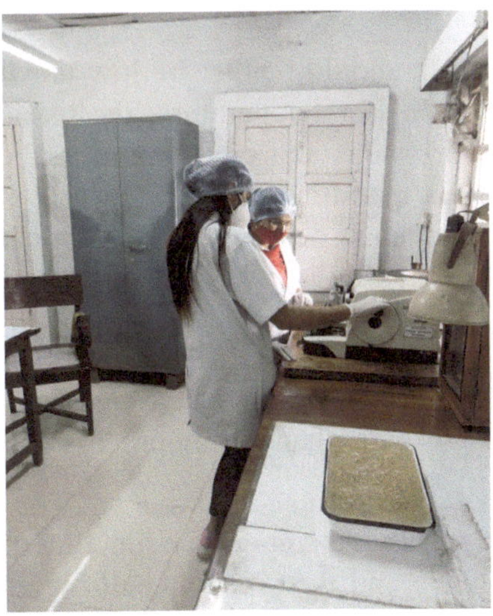

Fig. 14.10: Section cutting on microtome

1. Adjust the microtome gauge at right place, generally it is adjusted at 4-5 μ for routine histopathological examinations.
2. Knife should be properly fixed with the help of screws at an angle of about 45^{0}C. Ensure that all the fittings are tightly fixed.
3. The knife should be sharp enough to cut sections free from nicks (Fig. 14.11). If the nicks are present on section, the position of knife should be changed or the knife should be properly stopped.

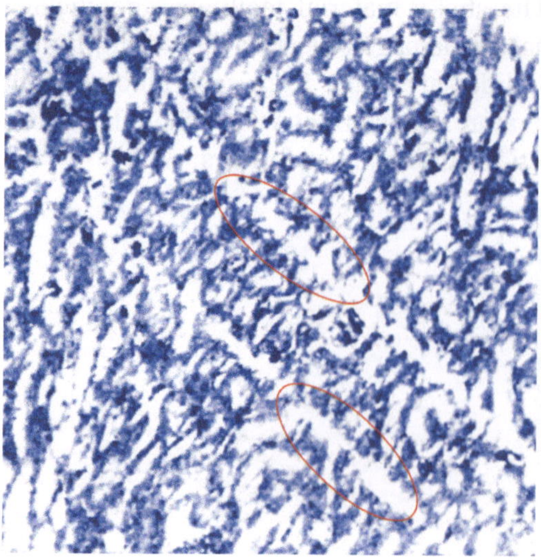

Fig. 14.11: Nicks (lining) in tissue section

4. The temperature of tissue floatation bath should neither be low nor it should be higher than that prescribed. In low temperature, the tissue will not spread properly and its compressions and crease will not be removed, while at high temperature, the paraffin wax of tissue melts quickly making the tissue section fragments, destroying the original shape of the section.
5. Leave the tissue sections on slide making an angle of slide so that air bubble does not appear in between the slide and section.
6. Place little sticky material on slide, if it is more than drying process will take more time.
7. If the ribbon of sections is large then it should be cut at the junction of two sections with a sharp knife or blade and then make small pieces from it.

8. During summer when temperature is above 40^{0}C, the tissue sections should be cut either in a room or laboratory having air-conditioner or desert cooler. If such facilities are not available then make moisture in the environment by sprinkling water on ground. This is necessary because at high environmental temperature, the tissue sections stick to the knife and the ribbon is not properly formed.
9. Drive the microtome smoothly at a regular speed; jerks should not be given.
10. For marking the slides, use a diamond pencil. The marking should be done at the time of section cutting itself.

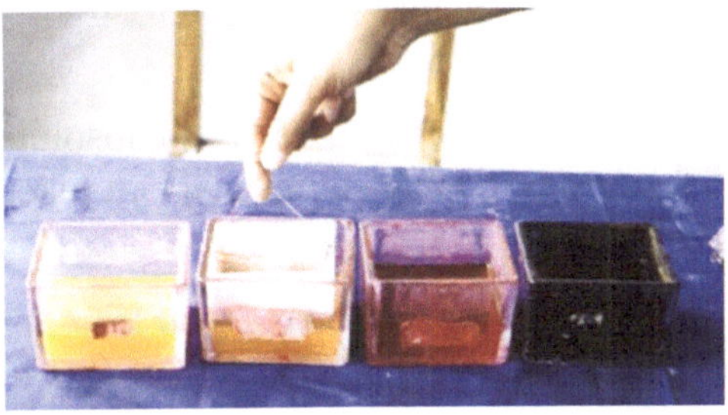

Fig. 14.12: Staining of tissue sections

Staining

Routine Procedures

After drying, the slides are kept in slide cabinets. One slide of each block is selected for staining using the following procedures.

1. *Removal of paraffin:* The slides are slightly warmed either in incubator or on the flame of a spirit lamp and placed in a jar having xylene. Replace the xylene after 10-15 min with fresh xylene for another 10-15 min. This removes the paraffin wax from the tissue sections.
2. *Rehydration:* After removal of paraffin the slides are kept in descending series of alcohol. For this, first they should be kept in absolute ethanol and xylene mixture for 5 min; then in absolute ethanol, 95%, 90%, 80%, 70%, 60% ethanol for 5-6 min in each dilutions. After that the slides are taken in water.
3. *Cleaning of slides:* With the help of muslin cloth, clean the slides from both the sides. Leave only 1 or 2 section on a slide and remove the extra

sections and remnants of paraffin wax. Wash the slides in running tap water.

4. *Staining in hematoxylin* Place the slides in Harris hematoxylin or Meyer's hematoxylin for 10-15 min; shake the slides 2-3 times for proper staining. Remove the hematoxylin solution and wash the slides in running tap water, then dip in acid alcohol for a few seconds, which helps in differentiation. Wash in tap water and place the slides in ammonia water for a few seconds for bluing and place in running tap water in order to remove the ammonia.
5. *Staining in eosin:* Place the slides in 2% aqueous eosin or alcoholic eosin for 2-5 min. After staining in eosin, quickly proceed for dehydration (Figs.14.12 and 14.13).
6. *Dehydration* The slides are placed in 70%, 80%, 90%, 95% and absolute ethanol for dehydration, at least for 5 min in each solution. Then place them in absolute ethanol: xylene mixture (1:1) for 5 min.
7. *Clearing:* Clear the sections in xylene and give two changes at least for 10-15 min each. The clearing in xylene II can be extended for even up to one hour.
8. *Mounting:* Mount the slides with coverslips using Canada balsam or DPX mountant. For this, coverslips of desired size and shape are kept on filter paper and one or two drops of mountant is placed on coverslip. Take out the slides from xylene and place on coverslip in such a way that the section touches the mountant. Press gently and lift the slide (Fig. 30.14). Remove air bubble, if any, by pressing the coverslip with forceps and keep the slides in horizontal position in a tray for drying.
9. *Cleaning and labelling:* After drying, clean the slides with muslin cloth and xylene. Remove the extra mountant using a blade. label the slide with a piece of paper and stick it on one corner of the slide using gum or other adhesive. At the time of examination, the histopathologist should put the name of organ, main changes in sections or disease condition with other remarks on this label.
10. *Examination:* On hematoxylin and eosin staining the nuclei of the cells take blue stain while the cytoplasm becomes pink or red. Examine the tissue section using 10 x objective and if required then in high power or oil immersion (Fig.14.15).

Flow diagram of staining process in routine histopathology

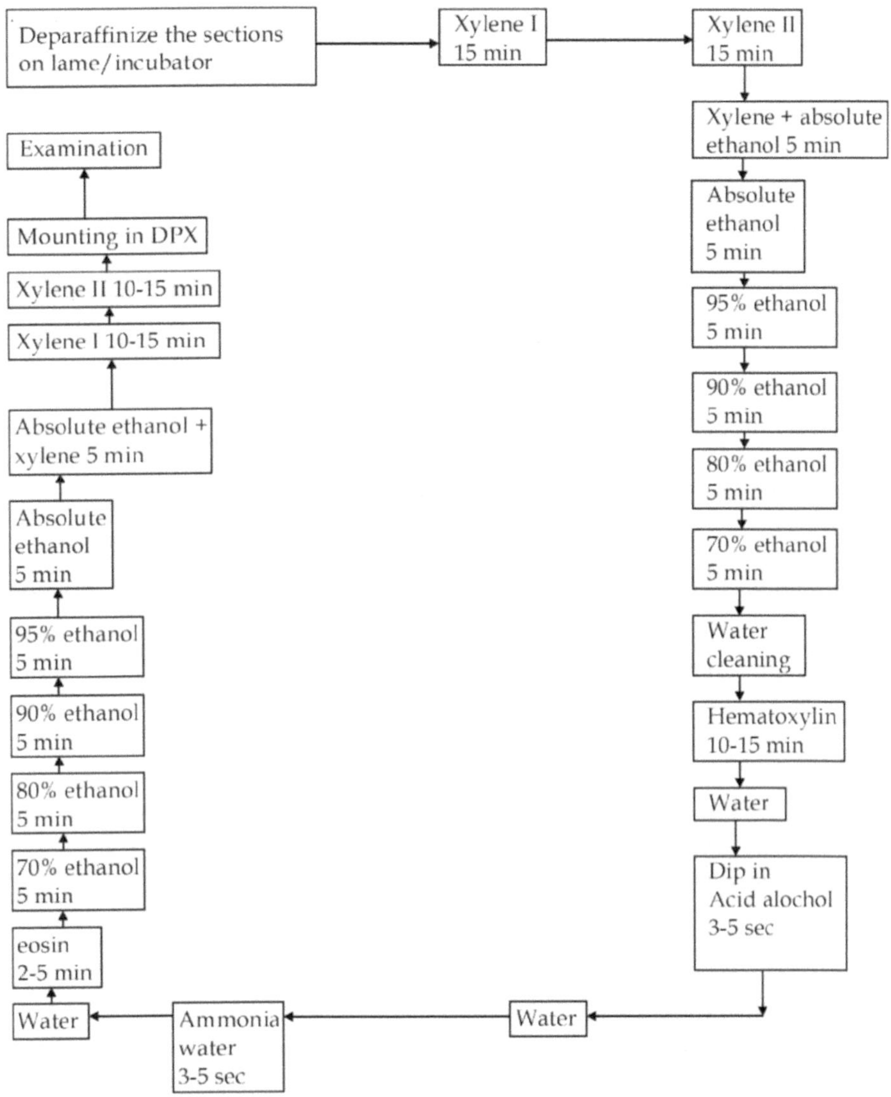

Precautions

Precautions and important tips which should be considered at the time of staining.

1. Check the sections for staining after bluing in ammonia water for hematoxylin stain and after dehydration for eosin stain. If under

staining then repeat the process in case of overstained, the sections can be differentiated for more time in acid alcohol to remove the excess hematoxylin and in ethanol and for removing the excess eosin.

2. Clean the slides thoroughly in water and remove all patches or spots of paraffin; which gives a good look to slides.
3. If on clearing in xylene cloudiness appears then repeat the dehydration process in absolute ethanol for 10-15 min. The cloudiness appears due to presence of water in the sections which reacts with xylene.
4. At the time of mounting, ensure that the tissue section does not get dried. So to eliminate the chance of drying, proceed fast. Ensure the proper mounting of the section on slides. Sometimes the opposite side of the section is mounted and section becomes dry. To ensure proper mounting, one should touch the diamond pencil marking present on the same surface and then mount the section. This can also be checked by touching the slide on reverse side for the presence or absence of tissue section.
5. Cleaning of slides should be performed in such a way that it does not damage the coverslip.
6. Labelling with paper should be done on same side on which the section is present; which will be helpful at the time of examination.

Special Procedures

In routine histopathological techniques, one can demonstrate bacteria, fungus, chlamydia, rickettsia or viral inclusions in the tissue sections by using special staining procedures. These special staining techniques, however, require specific expertise but can be used in a diagnostic laboratory as routine methods. Some important special and useful staining techniques are described below.

Demonstration of Acid Fast Bacilli

The acid fast bacilli are demonstrated in tuberculosis or Johne's disease in animals. The tissues are collected in formol saline or buffer formalin and processed in same manner as for routine histopathological techniques. For special staining of acid fast bacilli following procedures are followed.

Kinyoun's Method

1. Deparaffinize the sections and hydrate in descending series of ethanol as described earlier.

2. Clean the slides in water and give a wash in distilled water for 5 min.
3. Place the slides in carbol fuchsin solution and keep the chamber of slides in a water bath at 56^0C for 1 hour.
4. Thereafter, remove the slides from water bath and keep at room temperature for a few minutes; wash in running tap water.
5. Dip in acid alcohol for differentiation till the colour of tissue becomes pale pink.
6. Wash in running tap water.
7. Place the slides in methylene blue solution for a few seconds, wash in tap water till the colour of sections becomes pale blue.
8. Dehydrate in ascending series of ethanol; clear in xylene and mount in DPX as described earlier in histopathological procedures.
9. Examine the slides under oil immersion. The acid fast bacilli will be bright red in colour with a light blue background.

Precautions

1. Care should be taken as at 56^0C for 1 hour, the stain may get dry. So it is always advisable to keep it in a covered jar in water bath to prevent drying.
2. Differentiation with acid alcohol is a very crucial step and should be controlled carefully; it depends on experience of the histopathologist.

Ziehl Nielsen Method

1. Deparaffinize and hydrate the sections.
2. Clean in water and place in carbol fuchsin for 30 min.
3. Wash in running tap water.
4. Differentiate in acid alcohol for a few seconds or till the sections become pale pink in colour.
5. Wash in running tap water for 5-10 min.
6. Place the slides in methylene blue for a few seconds.
7. Wash in water.
8. Dehydrate in ascending series of alcohol, clear in xylene and mount in DPX.

9. Examine under oil immersion; the acid fast bacilli will be bright red in colour, erythrocytes yellowish orange and other tissue will take a pale blue colour.

Demonstration of Gram Positive/Gram Negative Bacteria

Brown-Hopps Method

1. Deparaffinize and hydrate the sections in water, clean them.
2. Stain the slides with crystal violet for 2 min.
3. Wash in distilled water.
4. Keep the slides in Gram's iodine solution for 5 min.
5. Wash in distilled water.
6. Differentiate in Cellosolve until blue colour no longer comes out from sections.
7. Wash in distilled water.
8. Place in basic fuchsin for 5 min and wash in distilled water.
9. Place the slides in differentiating solution for 5 min.
10. Wash in distilled water and blot dry.
11. Dip the slides in tetrazine for a few seconds.
12. Place the slides in cellosolve 3 changes of 6 dips in each.
13. Clear in xylene I and II for 15 min each.
14. Mount in DPX.
15. Examine the slides under oil immersion. The Gram positive bacteria will be of blue colour while Gram negative will take a red colour against a yellow background.

Taylor's Method

1. Deparaffinize and hydrate the tissue sections to water.
2. Stain in hematoxylin solution for 5-10 min, wash in running tap water for 2-5 min.
3. Dip in ammonia water for a few seconds and wash in running tap water.
4. Place the slides in Hucker's solution for 2 min and wash quickly in water.

5. Place in Gram's iodine for 1 min, wash in water and blot dry.
6. Decolourize in ethyl ether-acetone unit the blue colour comes out, blot with filter paper.
7. Place in basic fuchsin solution for 3 min.
8. Dip in acetone for a few seconds.
9. Place in picric acid acetone solution to differentiate until sections become reddish brown to yellow, which takes about 10-15 seconds.
10. Dip in acetone.
11. Clear in xylene I and xylene II, two changes of 10 min each.
12. Mount with DPX.

Demonstration of Spirochetes

1. During post mortem examination, cut about 1 mm thick slice of tissue from several sites of an organ and fix them in 10% buffered formalin for 24 hrs. Wash in running tap water overnight and place in 95% alcohol for 24 hrs.
2. Transfer the tissues in distilled water and keep till the tissues sink to bottom.
3. Stain in silver nitrate at 37^{0}C in dark for 3-5 days and change the solution daily.
4. Wash in distilled water and place the tissues in reducing solutions for 1-3 days.
5. Rinse in distilled water and dehydrate in ascending series of ethanol.
6. Clear in cedar wood oil for 2 hours.
7. Impregnation or embedding is done in paraffin wax as in case of routine histopathology, cut sections at 4-5 μ, dry and deparaffinize in xylene (3 changes of 5 min each).
8. Clean the slides, remove artefacts and spots of paraffin wax.
9. Mount 1-2 sections per slide with DPX.
10. Examination is done under microscope, the spirochete will be of black colour with yellow to light brown background.

Demonstration of Fungi

Grocott's Method

1. Collect the tissues in formol saline or buffered formalin and process the samples in the same way as in routine histopathology and cut the section at 4-5 μ, deparaffinize and hydrate to water.
2. Place the slides in 4% chromic acid for 1 hour.
3. Wash in running tap water and keep the slides in 1% sodium bisulfite solution for 3-5 min.
4. Wash in running tap water and then in distilled water.
5. Stain with methanamine-silver nitrate working solution at 600C in water bath till section becomes yellowish brown.
6. Wash in distilled water and place in gold chloride solution for 5 min.
7. Wash in distilled water and place in sodium thiosulfate solution for 5 min and wash in running tap water.
8. Stain with light green for 1 min, wash in water, dehydrate in ascending series of ethanol, clear in xylene and mount in DPX.
9. Examine the sections under microscope, the fungi will take a black colour, mycelia and hyphae will be of rose colour with a pale green back ground.

Demonstration of Rickettsia

Pinkerton's Method

1. Tissues are fixed in formol saline or buffered formalin and processed in the same manner, sections of 4-5 μ thick are cut, dried, deparaffinize and hydrated to water.
2. Place in methylene blue solution for overnight and decolourize in 95% ethanol for a few seconds or till blue colour is lost.
3. Wash in distilled water and place the slides in basic fuchsin solution for 30 min.
4. Decolourize in citric acid solution for 1-2 sec.
5. Differentiate in absolute ethanol for a few min, clear in xylene and mount in DPX.
6. Examine the slides, the rickettsia will be of bright red colour and nucleus of the cell will take blue colour.

Demonstration of Inclusion Bodies

Lendrum's Method

1. Tissues should be fixed in buffered formalin or formol saline, processed and sections of 4-5 μ thickness should be cut. Deparaffinize the sections and hydrate to water, clean the slides.
2. Stain with hematoxylin for 5-10 min and wash in running tap water for 15 min.
3. Place the slides in phloxine solution for 30 min and wash in distilled water.
4. Place the slides in tetrazine solution for 5-10 min; dehydrate in ascending series of ethanol, clear in xylene and mount in DPX.
5. Examine the slides under high power or oil immersion and look for inclusion bodies which will take red colour and nuclei will be of blue colour with yellow background.

Modified Macchiavellos' Technique

1. Tissues are fixed in 10% formol saline or buffered formalin, processed and sections of 4-5 μ are cut, dried, hydrated to water and clean the slides.
2. Stain with 0.25% aqueous basic fuchsin for 30 min.
3. Differentiate in 0.5% citric acid rapidly for 1-2 sec and wash in running tap water.
4. Stain in 1% methylene blue for 15-30 sec and wash in water, dehydrate in ascending series of ethanol, clear in xylene and mount in DPX.
5. Examine the slides; the inclusions will take red colour with a blue background.

Mann's Methylene Blue Eosin Method

1. Fix the tissues in formol saline of buffered formalin; process and cut 4-5 μ thick sections; dry and hydrate to water and clean the slides.
2. Stain the slides with methylene-blue eosin for 24 hours in a jar and wash in water.
3. Differentiate in absolute ethanol containing 2-3 drops of 1 N sodium hydroxide.
4. Examine under light microscope, the inclusions will be of red in colour while erythrocytes and other tissues will take blue colour

Histochemistry

Component of tissue	Stain	Interpretation
1. Amyloid	Congo red Toluidine blue	Green Orthochromatic blue
2. Carbohydrate (a) Glycogen (b) Acidic mucin (c) Neutral mucin	PAS (Basic Fuchsin) Bests' carmine Alcian blue Alcian blue	Magenta Nuclei blueMucin-red Neuclei-blue Mucin-blue Nuclei-red Nutral mucin-Magenta Acid mucin-blue Nuclei-pale blue
3. Connective tissue (a) Extracellular collagen (b) Elastic fibres (c) Reticular fibres	Masson's trichrome Van Gieson's Verhoff's elastic Gordon and Sweet's stain (silvernitrate)	Nuclei-blue / black cytoplasm, muscles and RBC-red Collagen-blue. Nuclei-blue / black Collagen-red Other tissue-yellow Elastic fibre-black Reticular fibre-black
4. Lipids Fat	Oil red Sudan black B Osmium tetraoxide	Mineral oil-red Unsaturated fats-Pink Phospholipids-Pink Unsaturated fats-blue/ black Unsaturated lipids-brown black Saturated lipids-unstained
5. Microrganisms (a) Simple Bacteria (b) Acid fast bacteria (c) Fungi (d) Protozoan parasites (e) Viral inclusions (e) Viral inclusions (f) Spirochaete (g) Rickettsia	Grams staining Liehol-neelsen stain Kinyoun's method Gorcott's silver me thanamine Giemsa i. Seller's stain ii. Mann's methylene blue iii. McGrunald iv. Giemsa stain v. Feulgen stain vi. Methylgreen pyronin stain vii. Lendrum's method Mac chia vello's stain Silver stain Pinkerton's method	Gram positive-blue Fibrin, Keratin-blue Gram negative-red Acid fast bacteria-red Background-light blue Fungi-black Red cells-yellow Background-pale green Parasite-dark blue Nuclei-blue Inclusions-pink / magenta Background-pale blue Inclusions-red, Back ground-blue Inclusions-pink Backgroud-blue Inclusions-red/ purple Background-green DNA virus inclusion-green- blue RNA virus inclusion-red Background-light blue. Inclusions-red Nuceli-Blue Background-yellow Inclusions-red Background-Blue Spirochaete-black Background-yellow to light brown Rickettsia-bright red Nucleus & cells-blue.
6. Pigments & Minerals (a) Hemosiderin/ iron (b) Melanin (c) Calcium (d) Copper	Perl's Prussian blue Masson-Fontana Alizarin red Rubeanic acid	Iron-Blue Nuclei-red Melamin-black Nuclei-red Calcium-or agenred Copper-greenish black Nuclei-pale red

Electron Microscopic Procedures

To study the cellular changes at organelles level, the use of electron microscope is evident as these organelles cannot be studied under light microscope because of latter's limited resolution power. In electron microscope one can see the object even after lacs time resolution. Electron microscopic studies are important for the detection of virus, its shape and structure and replication. The cellular changes at ultra-micro level can be demonstrated by electron microscope. In routine, the electron microscope is used for the diagnosis of viral diseases but due to its high cost very sophisticated laboratories can only afford it. In developing countries like India, it is not available in diagnostic laboratories but is only present in research institutions of repute. Therefore, the use of electron microscope in developing countries is for the research purposes rather than to provide diagnosis. However, the basic techniques related to electron microscopy are described for the benefit of readers.

Procedure

1. *Collection of tissue:* For electron microscopic studies, fresh tissues should be collected in fixative. The tissues from dead animals should be collected as early as possible after death using a sharp knife. The size of tissue should not be more than 1 mm. The biopsy material or tissues should be directly collected in the fixative.

2. *Fixation:* Fixation of tissues for electron microscopic studies is done in buffered glutaraldehyde solution, of pH 7.3-7.4. The tissues are fixed for 4 hours at 4^0C and washed in Soreson's phosphate buffer. The tissues are then post fixed in osmium tetraoxide for 1 hour. After fixation in osmium tetraoxide, the tissues can be stored in buffered sucrose solution for longer period in refrigerator.

3. *Dehydration:* The tissue blocks are washed in distilled water and dehydrated in ascending series of ethanol; then the tissues are in propylene dioxide for 1 hour with continuous agitation and then the tissues are embedded in epoxy resins.

4. *Embedding:* Decant the propylene dioxide from vials leaving about 1 ml in bottom with tissues. Add equal amount of embedding media, mix well and keep for 30 min. Discard the mixture and place fresh embedding media and keep in oven at 60^0C for 1 hour with a few agitations. Make the blocks in gelatin capsules, fill the capsule by epoxy resin and place the tissue at the top of capsule and leave in oven at 50-60^0C overnight. The hardened block is then taken out and the excess plastic resin is removed with razor or blade.

5. *Sectioning:* Ultrathin sections are cut on ultramicrotome using glass knife. Glass knives can be prepared in laboratory by breaking a glass sheet either manually or by glass knife maker machine. The surface of glass knife is examined under microscope and the smooth surface free from nicks are selected for sectioning. The sections of less than 0.1 μ are cut and picked up on grids, which are commercially available.

6. *Staining:* The ultrathin sections on grids are stained with lead hydroxide stain. Place a drop of stain on paraffin surface of petri dish containing paraffin wax. Keep grids over the drop of stain, which floats on the drop, with inside contact with solution for 15-20 min. The grid is then washed in distilled water using forceps and dried on a filter paper. The grid is now ready for examination. The viral particles will be of dark colour against light background (Figs. 14.16 and 14.17). The viruses will have central electron dense area with a light outer coat. Tissues from various organs can also be examined by electron microscopy following the same method for ultrastructural alterations. The lymphoid tissue of immunosuppressed animal examined for ultrastructural changes reveal the apoptotic changes in lymphocytes due to pesticide polluted feed consumption (Fig. 14.18)

Flow Cytometry

Flow cytometry is used to study the properties of cells suspended in a single moving stream in flow cytometer with laser light source for fluorescence. Flow cytometer acts as a cell sorter to physically sort out cells from liquid suspension flowing in a single cell stream. It is mainly used to identify and count the CD_4^+ and CD_8^+ molecule bearing lymphocytes in blood. Flow cytometer has a laser light source for fluorescence, cell transportations system in a single stream, monochromatic filters, lenses, mirrors and a computer for data analysis. Various applications of flow cytometry in diagnosis of animal diseases are as under.

1. Immunophenotyping and identification of neoplasms such as bovine leukemia, feline leukemia.
2. Diagnosis of immunodeficiency disorders like bovine immunodeficiency syndrome, immunosuppression in animals.
3. In evaluation of immunomodulator such as effect of Immunopotentiating effect on various cells.

4. Diagnosis of autoantibodies such as autoimmune neutropenia or autoimmune thrombocytopenia.
5. Diagnosis of the cause of allograft rejection through identification and counting of CD_3^+ T cells.

In the identification and counting of CD_4^+ and CD_8^+ cells, lymphocytes are separated from blood and are stained with immunofluorescence method for markers having FITC and rhodamine dyes. Then this cell suspension in passed through laser beam of flow cytometer which counts the cells with green and red fluorescence and records in computer. This system is also known as FACS means Fluorescent Activated Cell Sorter System.

15

Immunological and Serological Techniques

- General considerations
- Agglutination
    - Slide agglutination test
    - Tube agglutination test
    - Capillary tube agglutination test
    - Plate agglutination test
    - Hemagglutination test
    - Hemagglutination-inhibition test
    - Coagglutination test
- Precipitation
    - Agar gel precipitation test
    - Counter immune-electrophoresis test
- Complement fixation test
- Enzyme linked immunosorbent assay
    - Antibody detection
    - Antigen detection
    - Detection of immune complexes in serum
    - Detection of immune complexes in kidneys
    - Optimization of ELISA procedure
- Dot immunobinding assay
    - Detection of antibodies

  - Detection of antigen
- Leucocyte migration inhibition assay
- Lymphocyte stimulation test
- Macrophage function test

General Considerations

Immunological and serological tests are used in the diagnosis of animal diseases since very long. By these methods, one can detect the antibodies specific to a particular infection in serum or antigen in different body tissues or excretions or secretions. The antibodies are produced in animal body as a result of body defence responses against the causative agents. But mere detection of antibodies in serum is not sufficient to conclude the diagnosis as it may happen without apparent illness of the animal. It may occur due to contact of agent and host without clinical disease and it elicits the immune response. The presence of antigen in body tissues or fluids directly correlates with the presence of incriminating agent in the system. It is, therefore, advisable that paired sera should be tested before arriving at any diagnosis. The detection of antigen, however, is considered more specific for diagnosis. Here, many serological and immunological tests are described and the readers may use any of these according to their suitability and availability of materials. Each test has its own advantages and disadvantages and neither of these is fool proof. All care must be taken in order to make the interpretations more reliable and free from bias.

Agglutination

Agglutination is the clumping of particulate antigens, such as bacterial cells, in presence of an immune serum but the particles should have a size of more than 200-250μm to produce a visible reaction. For agglutination, the antigen should be in particulate form of suspension and antigen-antibody reacting sites must be present on the surface of the particles. The homologous antibodies present in serum binds with particulate antigen forming antigen-antibody complexes which settle down leaving a clear supernatant in case of tube agglutination test. Agglutination reactions are more sensitive than immunoprecipitation. The tests are simple and have an added advantage of easy readability.

Applications

1. In diagnosis of bacterial diseases such as brucellosis, salmonellosis, yersiniosis.
2. Blood typing prior to transfusion.

3. Diagnosis of rickettsial diseases like Q-fever.
4. Diagnosis of viral diseases like influenza.

The bacterial cells, which are in suspension form for long periods, are more suitable for agglutination. These cells repel each other in suspension due to electrical charges but when homologous antisera is added, antibodies react with antigens at cell surface. The rate of conduct is increased by agitation or centrifugation of the mixture of cells and antibodies resulting in increased agglutination. The saline solution in which the dilution of serum made will also reduce the electrical charge of the cells and thereby hasten their stick ness. Normal saline solution is found suitable to neutralize the negative potential, however, in case of *Strepotcocci, Corynebcterium* and *Mycobacteria* only 0.3% saline solution is used for optimum agglutination. The bridging between cells by bivalent antibodies and multi-valent antibodies forms aggregates of cells. Serum should be diluted optimally to avoid the pro-zone and post-zone effect in which no agglutination occurs in lower and higher dilutions, respectively (Fig.15.1). Various types of agglutination tests commonly used in the diagnosis of animal diseases are mentioned below.

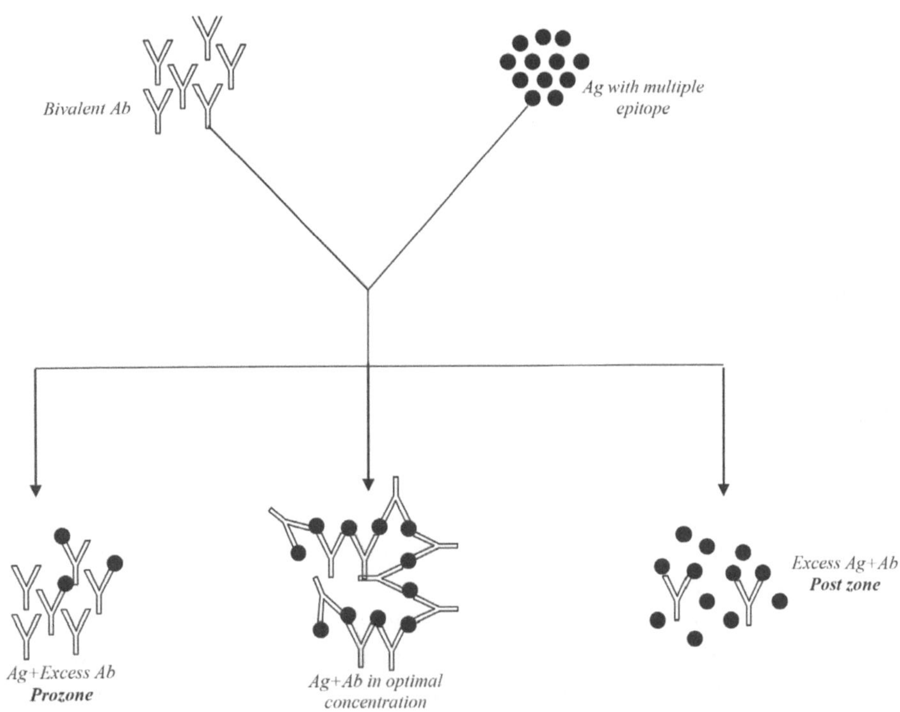

Fig. 15.1: Diagram showing agglutination test

Slide Agglutination Test

This method is quick, simple and requires smaller quantity of reagents. In this test, take a clean, dry glass slide and place a drop of antigen suspension over the middle area of the slide. Add one drop of test serum and mix properly with the help of a clean glass rod or tooth pick. If the homologous antibodies are present, clumps of bacterial cells will occur through agitation. The clumping (Fig. 15.2) can be seen by naked eyes or by using a light microscope. A saline-antigen control should also be used for comparison of the results. The test is mostly used for identification of salmonella organisms or pullorum disease in poultry.

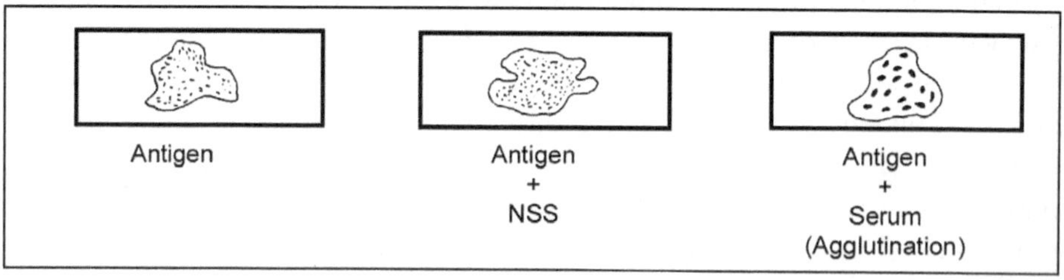

Fig. 15.2: Diagram illustrating slide agglutination test

Tube Agglutination Test

The tube agglutination test is used for the diagnosis and screening of herds for brucellosis in animals. A suspension of brucella organism 0.04% is used an antigen which is commercially available. For diagnosis of brucellosis, a 0.5% carbol saline is used in cattle and buffaloes and 5.0% carbol saline for sheep and goats. To perform this test twofold serum dilutions are made in carbol saline as 1:5, 1:10, 1:20, 1:40.... and so on. An equal amount of brucella antigen is added and mixed properly with agitation of the rack holding tubes. These tubes are then kept at 37°C in incubator for 24 hours. If agglutination occurs, the clumps of antigen and antibody complexes will settle down leaving the clean supernatant (Fig. 15.3). In case of no agglutination, the turbid suspension remains same. The standard tube agglutination is useful in diagnosis of those diseases in which immune carriers are present. There are some sets up to which the test is considered to be negative, e.g. brucellosis positive reactions at 1:20 and 1:40 dilutions are interpreted as negative and doubtful respectively. The titer should be expressed as the highest dilution of antiserum which gives visible agglutination and expressed in IU (International Units). In the brucellosis it is considered 40 IU positive in sheep and goats and 80 IU in man and cattle. To avoid discrepancies in the results, the paired sera should be tested and an increase in fourfold titer of agglutination should be considered as a result of recent infection.

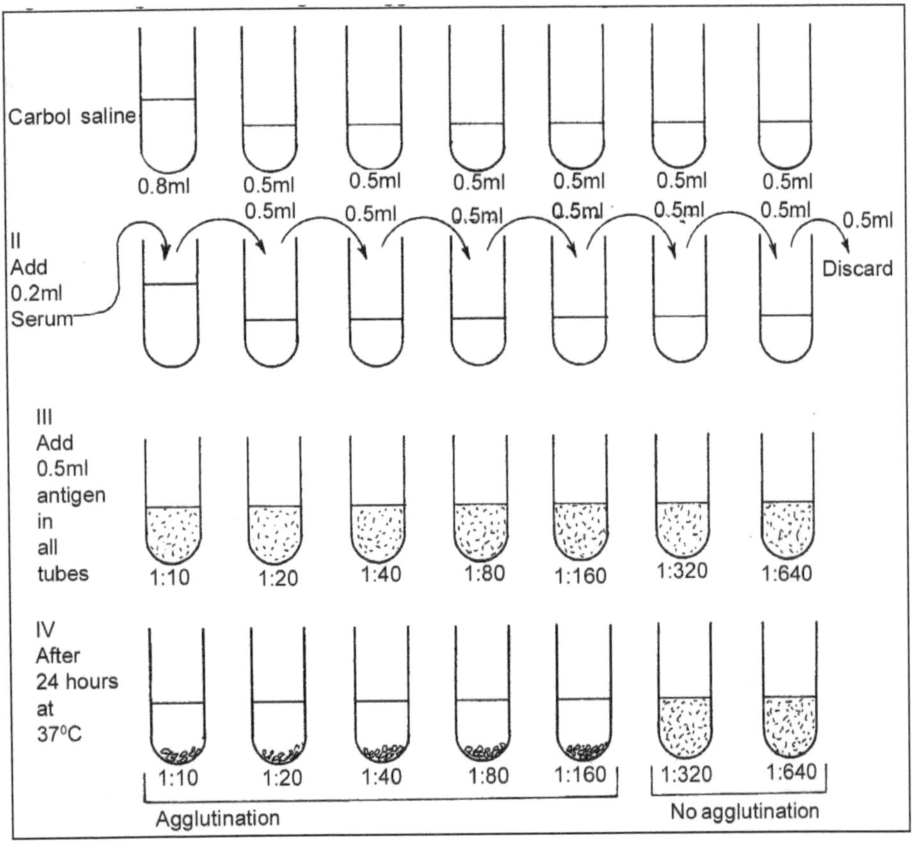

Fig. 15.3: Diagram illustrating tube agglutination test

Capillary Tube Agglutination

Routinely this is used for the diagnosis of Q-fever using particulate coloured antigen. Capillaries are filled half with antigen and half with serum and sealed at one end using clay or plasticin. The capillaries are kept in incubator at 37°C for a few hours; in case of positive sera, there is clumping of antigen at the interphase of serum and antigen which looks like a ring (Fig. 15.4). Positive and negative controls of serum should be run simultaneously.

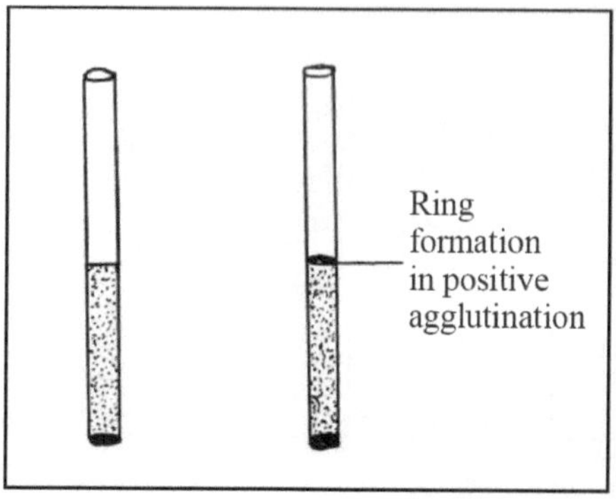

Fig. 15.4: Diagram illustrating capillary tube agglutination test

Plate Agglutination Test

Plate agglutination test is used for rapid agglutination reaction. In this test, a concentrated antigen is used, e.g. in brucella, rose Bengal plate agglutination test, the antigen is having 12% bacterial cells instead of 0.04% in standard tube agglutination test. The dye is also added in antigen to stain the bacterial cells which facilitates the visual reading. The most often used dyes are methyl violet, crystal violet, rose Bengal or malachite green. In this test , 0.03 ml of serum (2-3 drops) is placed in wells of hemagglutination perplex plate and equal amount of coloured antigen is added and this is mixed with a bacteriological loop or needle. For thorough mixing, the plate should be rotated by keeping on a flat surface in clockwise and anti-clockwise direction and incubated it for 3 min at 37°C. In case of a positive test, large clumps of cells will form, which can be seen by naked eyes, e.g.:

1. Diagnosis of brucellosis by rose Bengal plate agglutination test
2. Pullorum testing by plate agglutination test. In pullorum testing, a few drops of antigen are placed on a slide or plate and a drop of blood is added. The antigen will get agglutinated and the clumps can be seen among the erythrocytes, which can be interpreted as under.

Slight agglutination: + weak positive

Moderate agglutination: + + positive

Severe agglutination: + + + highly positive

Hemagglutination Test (HA test)

Hemagglutination test does not depend on formation of antigen-antibody complexes and is used for the diagnosis of certain viral diseases and identification of viruses possessing hemagglutinin. Certain animal and avian viruses belonging to myxovirus, paramyxovirus, togavirus, reovirus, adenovirus, enterovirus and poxvirus groups agglutinate the erythrocytes of chicken, sheep and human 'O' blood. This test can be performed in test tubes (3" tubes, sugar tube) or in 'U' shaped bottom of microtiter plates. If serial dilution of virus and a standard concentration of erythrocytes are added and left for a few hours in incubation at 37^{0}C, the agglutination of red blood cells forms a thin layer covering whole of bottom of tube or plate while in negative, the erythrocytes settle down in bottom and form a button. The highest dilution at which the agglutination of erythrocytes occurs is considered as one hemagglutination unit (HA unit).

To perform hemagglutination test, take a microtiter plate 'U' shaped bottom or 3" sugar tubes in a rack. These should be properly washed, and dried. Place 50 Cl phosphate buffer saline in all columns of the microtiter plate. Take 50 μl virus antigen and place in wells of first column, mix it and transfer from it 50 μl to next and this make the two-fold dilution of virus antigen like 1:2. 1:4. 1:8. 1:16, 1:32 and so on. From the 11th well discard 50 μl mixture and leave the 12 column. Prepare 1% chicken erythrocyte suspension in PBS. For this, collect chicken blood in Alsever's solution, centrifuge it and wash with PBS three times finally the packed red cells are adjusted as 1% in PBS. Place 0.1 ml of the 1% RBC suspension in each column from 1-12, mix it by rotating the plate clockwise and anti-clockwise and leave it in incubator 37^{0}C for one hour and examine it 15 min interval to note the results. 50 μl of 1% chicken RBC in each well and incubate the plate for 30 min. Read the plate for agglutination of RBCs.

In HI positive, there will not be any agglutination of RBC and the highest dilution of serum, inhibiting agglutination of erythrocytes will be the HI titer. An HI titer of 2^5 or more is considered as positive for viral antibodies (Fig.15.5).

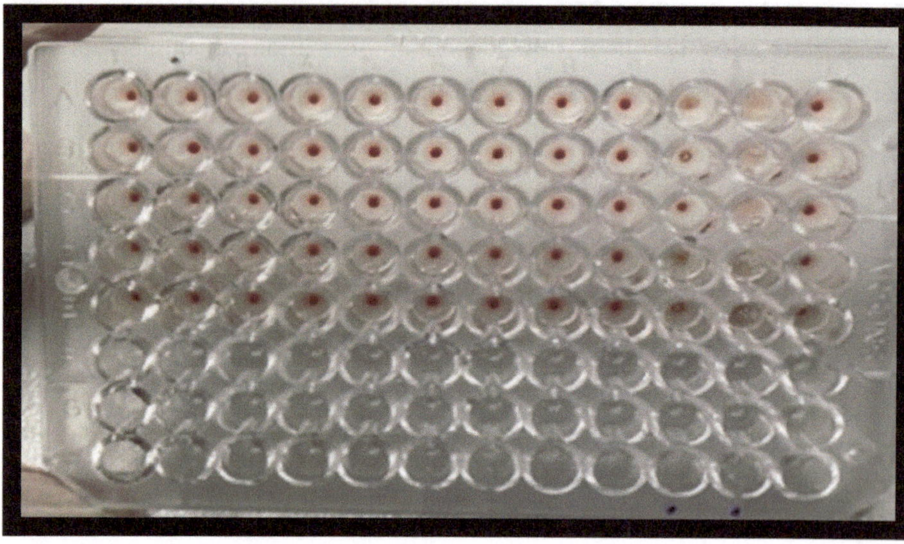

Fig. 15.5: Hemagglutination inhibition test

Coagglutination Test

It includes the stained *Staphylococcus aureus* coated with specific antibodies which detects the antigens in the clinical specimens. The agglutination of *Staphylococcus aureus* occurs in positive test which can be observed by naked eyes. This test has been successfully employed in the diagnosis of brucellosis in bovines and *Hemophilus pleuropneumoniae* infection in pigs.

The coloured *Staphylococcus aureus* are prepared coated with specific antibodies. The growth of *Staphylococcus aureus* cowan I strain (12 hours in trypticase soya broth) is taken and centrifuged. The media trypticase soya broth is supplemented with 1.0% peptone and 0.5% yeast extract. The organisms are pelleted by centrifugation at 3000 g for 30 min and washed three times in 0.01 M PBS (pH 7.2) and finally pellet is suspended in PBS finally pellet is suspended in PBS to 5%. The organisms are killed by 2% formalin and kept at 4^{0}C overnight. The organisms are washed three times in PBS and again suspended in PBS as 5%. This is then heated at 80^{0}C in water bath for 5 min followed by rapid cooling. The suspension of organisms is stained with Giemsa stain at 1:20 dilution for 6-8 hours at 4^{0}C. The stained organisms are washed five times to remove the excess stain and again adjusted to 5% in PBS.

For coating of antibodies, 10 µl of rabbit hyperimmune serum of *Br. abortus* is added with per ml of bacterial suspension and kept for 2 hours at 37^{0}C with intermittent shaking. After 2 hours, this is washed to remove the unbound antibodies and the suspension is finally adjusted to 5% in PBS. For control equivalent volume of normal rabbit serum is coated on *Staphylococcus aureus* suspension. The test sample is prepared from the stomach contents of the aborted fetus. A 1:2 or 1:5 suspension of fetal stomach contents is prepared in PBS containing 1% phenol. On a glass slide or plastic plate, take a drop of coloured suspension of *Staphylococcus aureus* cells and one drop of treated fetal stomach contents. Mix well with a glass rod or toothpick. In case of positive, blue coloured aggregates will be formed within 5 min in the mixture; while the control will remain same and will not show any agglutination. This test has several advantages due to its simplicity, rapidity and usefulness in field diagnosis. The antibody coated *Staphylococcus aureus* is stable for three months at 4^{0}C.

Precipitation

Precipitation tests are employed where the antigen is not particulate but homogenous and soluble in normal saline solution or phosphate buffered saline, e.g. most of the viruses make such solution in PBS. The antigen and antibody complex is not visible by naked eyes so these are provided such a medium in which they combine and produce a visible reaction which can be detected by naked eyes; the test medium used for precipitation reactions is agarose or noble agar. There are many methods which can be employed for the diagnosis of animal diseases.

Agar Gel Precipitation Test

The agar gel precipitation test (AGPT) is based on the ability of antibodies that can form precipitin lines with antigen in gel system. In this test, the antigen and antibodies are allowed to migrate towards each other in gel and a line of precipitation is formed at the zone the equivalence, where the antigen-antibody complexes are formed, which is visible with naked eyes. The test is used for the detection of antibodies in serum or antigen in tissues and excretions or secretions. Microscopic glass slides (25 X 75 mm) or rectangular slides (70 X 100 mm) or even small petri dishes may be used to carry out the test. These slides are precoated with either 0.3% agarose or impregnated in the agar. Agarose (1%) is prepared in normal saline solution or in 0.01 M PBS (pH 7.2). However, in case of poultry, 8% sodium chloride is used. The plates must be uniform in size and should be thoroughly cleaned before use so that any grease on it completely removed. Agarose is poured on the clean slide; 4-5 ml on microscopic slide or 8-10 ml on lantern slide to have a 2 mm thickness of agar on the slide. The slides should be left for 15-20 min to solidify the gel and should be transferred to the humid chamber and placed at 4^{0}C for 15-30 min. Thereafter, wells are cut using a gel cutter; there should be a central well and 4-6 outer wells. Before cutting wells, prepare a diagram on a piece of graph paper for equal distance of wells. The optimum size of wells is 5 mm diameter and distance from central well to outer well should be not more than 5 mm. The gels of wells are removed using suction or needles. The bottom of gels is filled with one drop of 0.1% agarose. If antibodies are to be detected then place the antigen in central well and serum or test samples in peripheral wells using separate pipettes for each sample. If antigen is to be detected then place the known serum or antibodies in central well and test sample in peripheral wells. It is always desirable to have a positive control invariably along with test samples. Place the slide in humid chamber large petri dishes with wet filter paper or cotton inside and keep it at 37^{0}C in incubator. After an incubation of 24 hours, examine the slide for precipitin lines in between the central and peripheral wells. In some cases, it may take long incubation period even up to 7 days or 24 hours at 37^{0}C and 24 hours at 4^{0}C in refrigerator. However, the slides should be examined in morning and evening daily for the development of precipitin lines because over incubation may also lead to the loss of sharpness of bands.

For an increased sensitivity and visibility, the gels are stained with amido black or coomassie brilliant blue. The plates are kept in 0.15M sodium chloride solution for at least overnight to remove the non-precipitating proteins. The plates are then kept in distilled water for 2 hours. Dry the gels in incubator at 370C or at room temperature. Before drying takes place, a drop of agar is placed in the wells in order to prevent the cracking of wells on drying. Stain in 1% amido black prepared in 7% acetic acid for 5 min and de-stain the slides in a 45:10:45 solution of methanol: glacial acetic acid: distilled water. The precipitin lines or bands will take the dark blue colour.

Coomassie brilliant blue is prepared in ethanol, acetic acid and distilled water (45:10:45) solution as 1% and stain gels in this stain for 15-30 min. De-stain with ethanol: acetic acid and distilled water (25:10:65). The precipitin lines will take blue colour, it is three times more sensitive than amido black (Fig.15.6).

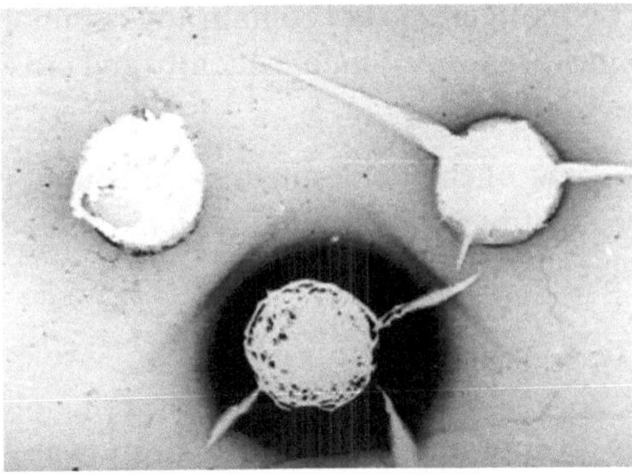

Fig. 15.6: AGPT

A view box should be used to examine the slides for the presence of the well-marked precipitin lines between antigen and antibody wells. It is comparatively a less specific and sensitive test because of its certain inherexnt problems. However, it is preferred because it does not require any sophisticated equipment and is easy to perform. It can be used in the diagnosis of viral, bacterial and parasitic diseases and to monitor the immune response in animals. It is used in differentiation of meat from different species of animals, standardization of toxins and antitoxins and for identification of closely related antigens.

Interpretation

Three basic patterns of result are observed in agar gel precipitation test (Fig. 15.7).

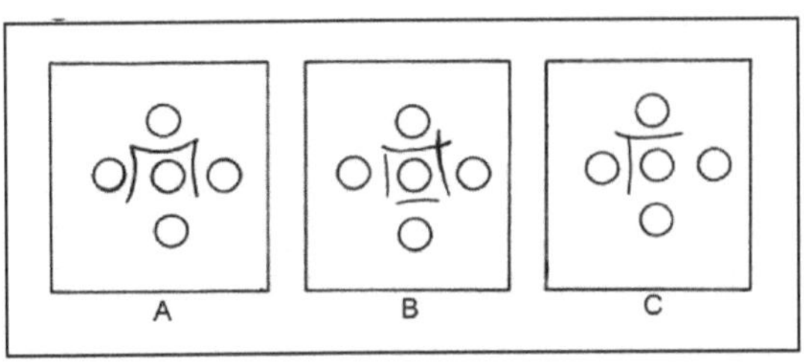

Fig. 15.7: Diagrammatic illustration of agar gel precipitation (A) Reaction of identify, (B) Reaction of non-identify and (C) Reaction of partial identity

1. *Reaction of identity:* It occurs between the identical antigenic determinants. The line of precipitation fuse to form one continuous line in the area.

2. *Reaction of non-identity*: When two antigens do not contain any common antigenic determinant, the two lines are formed independently and cross without any interaction.
3. *Reaction of partial identity:* If some of the determinants are common they give a continuous line of identity whereas unique determinants recognize on one of the antigen; so the spur is formed.

Counter Immuno-electrophoresis Test

The counter immune-electrophoresis is performed using the basic principle that at a particular pH, antigen moves towards anode and antibodies towards cathode under electrophoretic conditions. When these two fractions meet, a line of precipitation is formed similar to the precipitation line obtained in agar gel precipitation test. In this method, lantern slide of 70 X 100 mm size is taken and cleaned well. This is impregnated in 0.3% agarose prepared in veronal buffer pH 8.6. There after 8-10 ml of 1% agarose prepared in veronal buffer is poured on the slide and allowed to solidify. Keep this for 15-30 min in refrigerator at 4^{0}C. Then the wells are cut in parallel with a distance of 5 mm. On one slide there should be 5-6 wells. The gels are removed from the wells and the wells are sealed by one drop of 0.1% agarose. The wells are filled with antigen in one row and antibodies or serum in another row. The slides are then kept in an electrophoresis apparatus in such a way that the antigen wells are towards cathode and anode side wells contain antibodies. The slide is adjusted with filter paper strips which make the connection of veronal buffer to agarose of the slide. The filter strips are properly wet with veronal buffer and both chambers of anode and cathode are filled with freshly prepared veronal buffer (0.05 M, pH 8.6) up to a desirable quantity. The electrophoresis apparatus is now run using an anodic current of 7.5 mA/slide for 1-2 hours. After electrophoresis, the slides are taken away and examined for the presence of precipitin lines present in between the antigen and antibody wells using a view box. These slides can also be stained like AGPT slides as described earlier. This test is considered to be comparatively quick and more sensitive than AGPT. This is being used extensively in diagnostic laboratories; however, it requires a costly power pack which should be efficient enough to control the current and only desired current is achieved during operation. Further, the counter immune-electrophoresis requires trained and experienced staff, who can prepare the chemicals and run the instrument. Care must be taken that pH of the veronal buffer is not be less than 8.6 and it does not leak from the chamber. Like, AGPT, this test can also be used for detection of antigen or antibody (Fig.15.8).

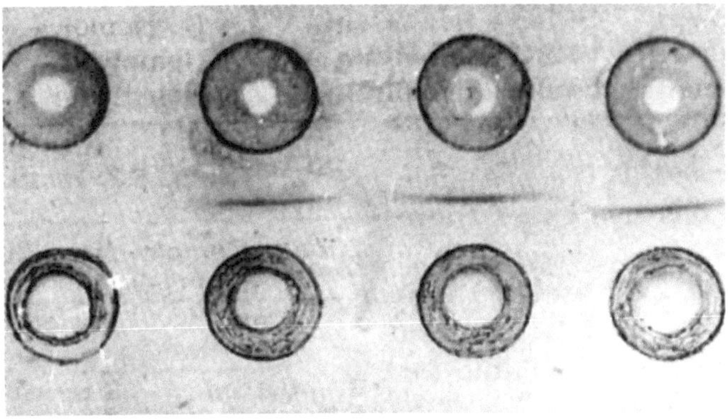

Fig. 15.8: Counterimmunoelectrophoresis test. Note the presence of precipitin lines in between the wells

Complement Fixation Test

The complement is a normal component of serum of animals; the highest concentration being present in guinea pig serum. The complement combines with antigen antibody complex to cause the lysis of bacterial cells. The complement fixation test is considered to be time consuming and cumbersome, even then it is used for the detection of foot and mouth disease virus antigen in vesicular fluid for diagnosis and typing of the virus. In brucellosis even after development of other diagnostic tests, complement fixation test is considered quite specific and other tests are compared with CFT. For the detection of antibodies by complement fixation test, the test serum is heated at 56^{0}C for 30 min for destruction of complement and a known amount of complement is added in the form of guinea pig serum. Then the test serum mixed with complement is added to a known antigen and incubated with 2% sheep red blood cells as indicator. If the antigen is detected by complement fixation test, the known sera and test sample are mixed in the presence of complement and in positive cases there is no lysis of sheep red blood cells (SRBC); while if antigen and antibody are not specific, the complement will not be utilized (not fixed) and it will remain available for hemolysis of SRBC (Table 15.1).

Table 15.1: The complement fixation reactions

No.	Step I	Step II	Results	Interpretations
1.	Agl + Abi + Complement	SRBC + Hemolysin	No Hemolysis	+
2.	Agl + Ab2 + Complement	SRBC + Hemolysin	Hemolysis	-
3.	Ag2 + Abi + Complement	SRBC + Hemolysin	Hemolysis	-

Procedure

A general procedure of complement fixation test is as under applied in the diagnosis of bacterial and viral diseases.

Materials Required

1. *Bacterial or viral antigen.*
2. *Test serum samples:* These samples should be heated in a water bath at 56^{0}C for 30 min to destroy the complement present in serum.
3. *Guinea pig serum:* The guinea pig serum is used as source of complement; the potency of complement should be determined before use by the following method. For titration of complement, 0.1 to 0.5 ml of diluted (1:30) complement is taken with 2 units of hemolysis and 0.5 ml SRBC. The final volume is adjusted as 3 ml using normal saline solution. The unit of the complement will be minimum amount of complement that causes hemolysis. Incubate at 37^{0}C for few hours. The minimum amount of complement causes hemolysis is the complement unit.
4. *2% sheep RBC:* The blood of sheep is collected under sterilized conditions in Alsever's solution and centrifuged at 2000 rpm for 10 min, the supernatant is discarded and the RBCs are washed with normal saline solution to get the RBC free from complement and fibrin. The final volume of RBC is prepared as 2% in NSS.
5. *Hemolysin:* Hemolysin is prepared in rabbits using 10% sheep red blood cells suspension in NSS. The intramuscular injections (4-5) are given in rabbits to raise hyperimmune serum against SRBC. Four days after the last injection, the rabbits are bled and the serum is collected and preserved by adding an equal amount of neutral glycerin. The stock solution of hemolysin in prepared as under.

Glycerinized serum	- 2.0 ml
5% phenol in NSS	- 4.0 ml
NSS	- 94.0 ml

   The titration of hemolysin should be done using complement and SRBC in the following manner as detailed in Table 15.2.

   Each tube, after mixing, is kept in incubator at 37^{0}C for a few hours. The hemolysin unit will be the highest dilution which gives complete hemolysis of SRBC.

5. *Complement fixation test:* After the optimization of hemolysin

Table 15.2: Complement fixation test

Tube	Hemolysin (0.5 ml)	Complement (1:30)	SRBC (2%)	NSS
1	1:1000	0.3 ml	0.5 ml	1.7 ml
2	1:2000	0.3 ml	0.5 ml	1.7 ml
3	1:3000	0.3 ml	0.5 ml	1.7 ml
4	1:4000	0.3 ml	0.5 ml	1.7 ml
5	1:5000	0.3 ml	0.5 ml	1.7 ml
6	1:6000	0.3 ml	0.5 ml	1.7 ml
7	1:7000	0.3 ml	0.5 ml	1.7 ml
8	1:8000	0.3 ml	0.5 ml	1.7 ml
9	1:9000	0.3 ml	0.5 ml	1.7 ml
10	1:10000	0.3 ml	0.5 ml	1.7 ml

Incubate the tubes at 37^{0}C for 1 hour. If the serum is having antibodies against known antigen, the complement will be fixed with antigen and antibody complex. Then 0.5 ml of 2% SRBC and 2 units of hemolysin is added in each tube. Make the final volume 3 ml by adding NSS. Incubate for 1 hour. If the test is positive then no hemolysis will occur but in case of negative sera (serum not having homologous antibodies) hemolysis of SRBC will occur. It is always advisable to use positive and negative controls of the test. Before start of the test serum samples should be heat inactivated at 56^{0}C for 30 min. The results of complement fixation test are expressed in concentration of antibody titer in serum. In brucellosis 1:40 is considered positive for the disease.

Enzyme Linked Immunosorbent Assay

Enzyme linked immunosorbent assay (ELISA) is a widely applicable and accepted test routinely used now-a-days for diagnosis and confirmation of infectious disease. It has the same principle and sensitivity as radioimmunoassay (RIA) and replaced the later being less expensive and safe in handling during procedure. In radioimmunoassays, the use of radioisotope labelled antibodies or antigen are hazardous to the health and it requires the costly gamma or beta counter to interpret the results. The basic principle of ELISA is same as RIA but in place of radioisotope labelled antibodies, in ELISA an enzyme is used. This assay is also used for the detection of antigen as well as antibodies.

For detection of antibodies, the known antigen is coated on the surface of wells of polystyrene plate (96 wells) and then test serum samples, properly diluted, is added. After incubation, the plates are washed and conjugate enzyme labelled species specific antibody is added which binds with the antibodies present in test serum and can be detected by adding substrate which gives a coloured reaction that can be seen by naked eyes or read in spectrophotometer. For detection of antigen, the sandwich assay is preferred. In sandwich assay, antibody is bound to the solid phase (polystyrene plate). This antibody is known as capture antibody. Then the specimen suspected for presence of antigen is added. After appropriate incubation, the plate is washed and second antibody specific to antigen is applied, which is conjugated with enzyme in direct method while in indirect method this antibody is plain and anti-antibody conjugated with enzyme is applied which is known as indicator antibody. In indirect method the secondary antibody should be raised in a different animal species with that of capture antibody. The reaction is detected by applying enzyme substrate, which gives coloured reaction. The coloured reaction can be seen by naked eyes or is read by spectrophotometer.

Advantages

1. ELISA can be used for the diagnosis of bacterial, viral and parasitic diseases.
2. A large number of samples can be tested at a time simultaneously.
3. It is widely used as it is most sensitive and specific.
4. In this assay, the use of monoclonal antibody increases specificity.
5. The use of automated dispensing, washing and photometric methods reduce the time. Many different ELISA systems are reported in literature but for diagnostic purpose in a veterinary diagnostic laboratory, the most commonly used assays with widely used chemicals and procedures are described.

Requirements

The requirement for chemicals and other material along with their preparation are given as under:

1. *Solid phase system:* The polystyrene is very popular solid phase system which is generally used in ELISA. It has less background staining effect. The polystyrene is used as microtiter plates having 96 wells including 12 lines and 8 rows, which may be round or flat bottomed. The strips of single row of wells are also found detachable which can be used in case the number of samples is less. The antigen or antibody binds with the solid phase but its nature is not fully understood; it may have a hydrophobic binding.
2. *Coating buffer:* For coating, 0.05 M carbonate and bicarbonate buffer of pH 9.6 is used for immobilization of antigen or antibody on the polystyrene plate. Although buffers have little or no effect on the immobilization of antibody or antigen, yet the coating is satisfactory

in the buffer. A low pH buffer like 0.01 M PBS or 0.01 M Tris buffer can also be used as coating buffer. Partial denaturation of proteins may increase the sensitivity of ELISA system as it increases the coating on polystyrene. The antibodies can be partially denatured by 0.05 M glycine HCl buffer of pH 2.5 containing 0.1 M NaCl for 10 min at room temperature and neutralizing with 0.05 M Tris buffer. The lipid antigens or viral envelops can be denatured by sodium deoxycholate (1 mg/ml).

3. *Washing solution:* The most commonly used washing solution is PBS-tween; which constitutes 0.2 M PBS (pH 7.2)containing 0.05% tween-20.

4. *Enzyme conjugates:* The following enzyme conjugated with antibodies are used:

   a. Horse raddish peroxidase-Commonly used in ELISA procedures.

   b. Alkaline phosphatase.

   c. Beta-galactosidase

   d. Urease.

   The anti IgG conjugated with enzymes having highly purified grades are available from many private concerns like Sigma Chemical Co., Hi media etc. Each of the conjugates has some advantages or disadvantages but the most widely used conjugates are peroxidase and alkaline phosphatase.

5. *Substrates:* The substrates are specific to the enzyme used as conjugate.

A. *For peroxidase conjugate:* There are many substrate which are used for detection of the peroxidase conjugated antibodies.

   i. *Orthophenylene diamine dihydrochloride:* Orthophenylene diamine dihydrochloride (OPD) is used as 8 mg in 15 ml of 0.1 M citric acid-phosphate buffer (pH 5.0) containing 5 µl 30% H_2O_2. This reagent is prepared just before use. To stop the reaction of this enzyme, 100 µl of 1 M H_2SO_4 is used in each well. The absorbance can be read at 492 nm in spectrophotometer.

   ii. *Tetramethyl benzidine dihydrochloride:* $3,3^1,5,5^1$- Tetramethyl benzidine dihydrochloride 10 mg and dimethyl sulphoxide 1.0 ml is added in 100 µl of 0.1 M sodium acetate-citric acid buffer (pH 6.0). Mix 30 µl of 30% H_2O_2 and use this substrate immediately after preparation. A pale blue colour will develop. Stop the reaction with 100 µl of 2 M H_2SO_4 which changes colour as bright yellow from a pale blue colour. The absorbance can be read at 450nm.

iii. *ABTS:* 10mg 2,2'-Azino-bis (3-ethyl-benzthiazoline-6-sulfonic acid) in 100 ml citric acid phosphate buffer is mixed and 20µl of 30% H_2O_2 is added just before the use. It produces green colour with peroxidase enzyme; the absorbance of which is read at 405 nm.

iv. *5-Amino salicylic acid:* 100 mg of 5-amino-salicylic acid is mixed in 100 ml of 0.01 M sodium phosphate buffer containing 1 mM EDTA and adjusted to pH 6.0. Add 20 µl of 30% H_2O_2 immediately before use. The reaction can be stopped with 1 M NaOH. It gives brown colour with peroxidase and its absorbance can be read at 450 nm.

B. *For Alkaline phosphatase conjugate:* Alkaline phosphatase is a good substitute of horse raddish peroxidase and is being used where inherent peroxidase activity is suspected. For alkaline phosphatase, P- nitrophenyl phosphate (PNP) substrate is used. 5 mg of nitrophenyl phosphate is mixed in 5 ml diethanolamine buffer (pH 9.8). It gives a yellow colour, which can be stopped by adding 3 M NaOH in the wells. The absorbance of the reaction can be read at 405 nm.

C. *For Beta-galactosidase conjugate:* For beta-galactosidase conjugate, ortho-nitrophenly beta-D- galactosidase (ONPG) substrate is used. 90 mg of ONPG is dissolved in 10 ml PBS containing 10 mM $Mgcl_2$ and 0.1 M 2-mercapto-ethanol. Heat the solution at 50°C to dissolve the contents and store at room temperature in dark. Dilute this to 1:10 in PBS (pH 7.2) just before use. It gives a yellow colour which can be stopped by 1 M Na_2CO_3 and absorbance can be read at 410 nm.

D. *For urease conjugate:* The following solution is used as substrate for urease conjugate:

(i) Bromocresol purple-8.0 mg

(ii) 0.01M NaOH – 1.48 ml

(iii) Make to 100 ml by adding distilled water

(iv) Urea- 100 mg

(v) EDTA –0.2 mM

The pH of 5.0 should be adjusted with 1 mM HCl. It gives yellow to blue colour which is visible.

Procedure

Antibody Detection (Fig. 15.9 I & II).

1. Coat the wells of polystyrene microplate with 100 μl of known antigen diluted in coating buffer. Keep the plate for overnight at 4°C or 2 hours at 37°C.
2. Wash the plate three times (5 min each) with washing solution. Tap the plate against any soft paper or towel after each washing to get rid of any un-adsorbed material in the well. The washing solution should be according to enzyme conjugates being used in the assay such as:
   a. Use PBS-tween with peroxidase conjugate
   b. Use Tris-tween with alkaline phosphatase conjugate
   c. Use PBS with beta-galactosidase conjugate
3. For immobilization of remaining unsaturated sites of polystyrene plate well, use 5% skimmed milk or 3% bovine serum albumin or 1% gelatin. Keep this suspension for at least 1 hour at 37°C.
4. Wash and tap the plates as described in step 2.
5. Apply 100 μl of appropriately diluted serum in duplicate wells and keep the plate at 37°C for 2 hours.
6. Wash and tap the plate as in step 2.
7. Apply in appropriate dilution 100 μl of anti IgG conjugate in each well and keep the plate for 1 hour at 37°C.
8. Wash and tap the plate as in step 2
9. Apply 100 μl substrate in each well and note the time. Stop the reaction within 30 min by using an appropriate stopping reagent.
10. Read the absorbance from spectrophotometer.

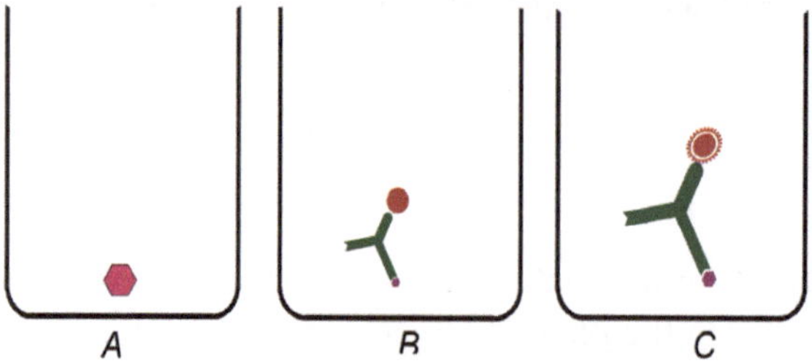

Fig. 15.9(i): Diagram showing direct-ELISA for antibody detection

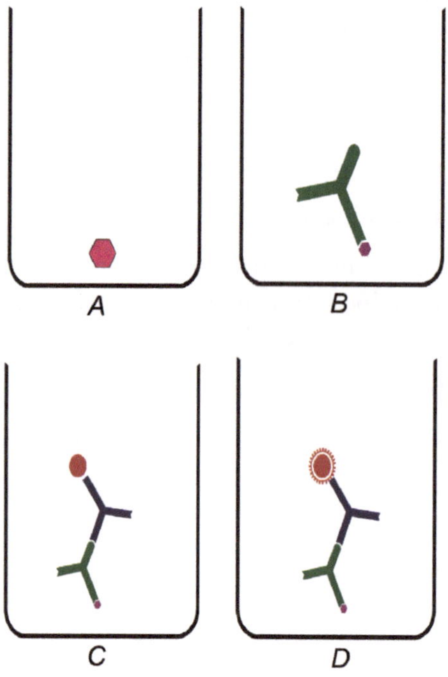

Fig. 15.9(ii): Diagram showing indirect-ELISA for antibody

Antigen Detection (Fig. 15.10 I & II)

For antigen detection, the sandwich ELISA technique is used; procedure of which is as follows.

1. Coat the well of polystyrene plates with primary antibody in optimum dilution in coating buffer and keep it at 4^{0}C for overnight or for 2 hours at 37^{0}C.

2. Wash the plate with washing solution three times of 5 min each and tap against any soft paper or towel etc.
3. Block the remaining unsaturated sites in well by using 3% bovine serum albumin or 5% skimmed milk or 1% gelatin for 1 hour at 37^{0}C.
4. Wash tap the plate as in step 2.
5. Apply 100 µl of specimen in which antigen is to be detected. Keep the plate at 37^{0}C for 2 hours.
6. Wash and tap the plate as in step 2.
7. Apply the second antibody (detector antibody) 100 µl per well raised in different animal species than that of primary capture antibody. Keep the plate for 2 hours at 37^{0}C.
8. Wash and tap the plate as in step 2.
9. Add 100 µl of anti-IgG-conjugate for 2 hours at 37^{0}C. (This is anti-antibody conjugated with enzyme).
10. Wash and tap the plate as in step 2.
11. Apply 100 µl of appropriate substrate to each well and keep the plate for 30 min at 37^{0}C.
12. Stop the reaction with appropriate stopping reagent.
13. Read the absorbance by spectrophotometer or take visual reading (Fig.15.11).

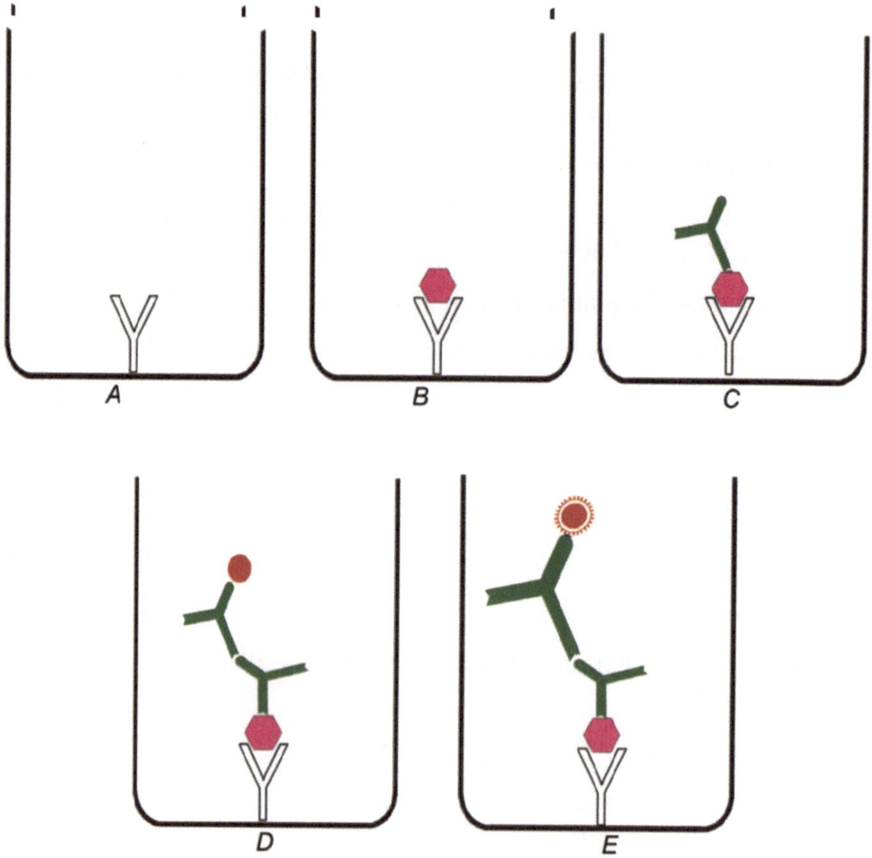

Fig. 15.10(ii): Diagram showing indirect-ELISA for antigen detection (sandwitch-ELISA)

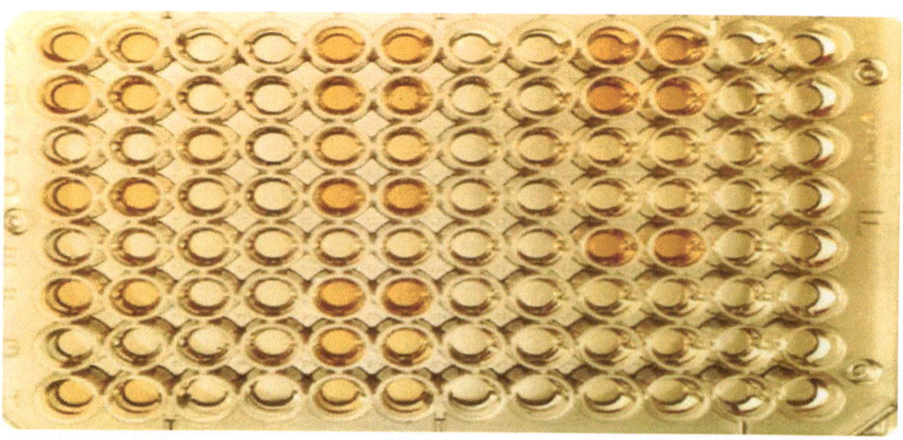

Fig. 15.11: ELISA

Detection of Immune Complexes in Serum (Fig. 15.12).

1. *Test serum:* One ml 8% polyethylene glycol (PEG-6000) MW 6000 in PBS pH 7.2 is mixed drop by drop in 1 ml serum with constant stirring. Leave the tube for 1 hr at room temperature and then centrifuge it at 1500g for 1 hr at 4^{0}C. Discard the supernatant and suspend the pellet in 2 ml of 4% PEG-6000 and centrifuge again. Discard the supernatant and finally dissolve the pellet in 0.5 ml PBS (pH 7.2).
2. Coat the plate with antibodies against the agent for which immune complexes are detected. (e.g. if immune complexes are detected in bovines due to trypanosomes, then the plate is coated with antibodies of trypanosomes raised in mice or rabbits or any other species other than bovines). Keep the plate at 4^{0}C for overnight.
3. Wash the plate three times with washing solution for 5 min each; tap the plate after each washing.
4. Apply the diluted precipitate of serum in PBS as prepared in Step 1 (dilutions can be made twofold like 1:2, 1:4, 1:8, 1:16 and so on) and keep the plate for 1 hour at room temperature for 37^{0}C.
5. Wash the plate as in step 3.
6. Add anti-bovine IgG-enzyme conjugate in proper dilution for 1 hour at room temperature.
7. Wash the plate as in step 3.
8. Apply appropriate substrate for 30 min, stop the reaction with stopping reagent.
9. Take the absorbance in spectrophotometer or visually read the plate.

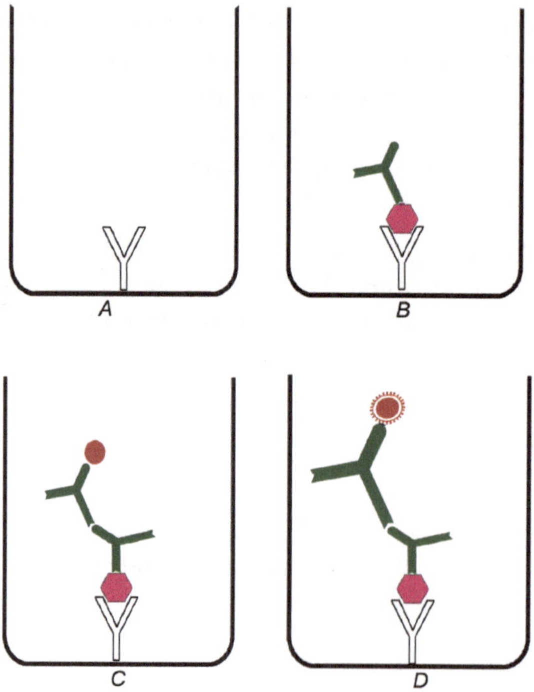

Fig. 15.12: Diagram showing ELISA for the detection of immune complexes

Detection of Immune Complexes in Kidneys

1. Collect the kidneys of animal and store at -20⁰C till use, but freshly collected kidneys are preferred.
2. Cut the kidneys in two parts longitudinally and remove the capsule. Separate out the cortex portion of kidneys and make small pieces of it.
3. Wash in 0.01 M PBS (pH 7.2) two times using centrifugation.
4. Mince and homogenize the kidney tissue in blender or in pestle and mortar.
5. Centrifuge and pass through 80 um membrane of cellulose membrane filter; then pass the fluid through 60 um membrane to isolate the glomeruli. (the glomeruli are trapped in mesh).
6. Wash with 0.01 M PBS.

7. Weight the isolated glomeruli and mix in 10 ml of 02. M glycine - HCl buffer of pH 2.4.
8. Incubate it at room temperature for 2 hours with gentle stirring.
9. Centrifuge at 5000 x g for 20 min.
10. Dialyse the supernatant against PBS at 4°C for 48 hours with frequent changes.
11. Remove the fluid from dialysis and centrifuge at 5000 x g for 20 min.
12. Concentrate it and measure the protein content by Lowery method.
13. Perform ELISA for the presence of immune complexes as in serum.

Dot Immunobinding Assay

The need of rapid and specific diagnostic tool(s) for detecting a wide variety of viral, bacterial, fungal and parasitic diseases of man and animals has always been an area of considerable importance for clinicians. Many infectious diseases are diagnosed by isolating, growing and identifying the infectious agent from clinical specimens. These methods demand well equipped and well trained and skilled staffed microbiology and virology laboratories. Days to weeks are sometimes spent in arriving at an unambiguous diagnosis which lead into failure to meet the need for an early management of the disease by the clinician. Although isolation and identification of the microorganism provides incontrovertible diagnosis of the disease but rate of success is limited. Alternatively, methods detecting seroconversions to particular micro-organisms can be of great diagnostic importance. Laboratory based diagnosis of majority of infectious diseases involving seroconversion has largely been depended on the assays using antigen-antibody reactions. Historically, agglutination tests in various forms have been used for the diagnosis of diseases such as leptospirosis, salmonellosis, brucellosis etc. Some of these agglutination tests still in use indicating their usefulness to prevail despite some inherent problems associated with these assays. Tremendous advancement has been made in the field of immunodiagnostics with a view to develop a technology which should be able to provide rapid and specific diagnosis of infectious diseases. Amongst the various immunodiagnostic tools enzyme immunoassay becomes increasingly popular for the detection of humoral immune response (seroconversion) or microbial antigens for the purpose of diagnosis.

Background

The most popular among the enzyme immunoassays is the Enzyme Linked Immunosorbent Assay commonly termed as ELISA which finds a wide application in studies of infectious diseases. The popularity of ELISA is primarily due to its high sensitivity, excellent specificity and relative simplicity as compared to other immunoassay methods. Although radioisotopes are the most widely used labels for immunoassays, the use of an enzyme as a label has offered an excellent alternative to radioimmunoassay (RIA) procedures. In general, ELISA results can be read or quantitated by readily available and relatively inexpensive spectrophotometers. Minimal training is required to perform ELISA, facility licensing or special handling of reagents and wastes is not required, and there is no radiation hazard. Reagents for ELISA are relatively cheap, stable, and easy to prepare and the technique lends itself well to automation. The time required for preparation of reagents is minimal. In the performance of the assay, the time required for successive incubations may be a limiting factor in applications, although incubation periods can be shortened significantly. Despite several merits of ELISA as outlined above, the assay has some important limitations. Particularly the requirement of an ELISA reader to obtain accurate measurements mainly restricts its application to laboratory settings. The situation in many areas, particularly in developing countries where application of electrical equipment is difficult due to non-availability of electricity, is quite different. For such areas it will be important to have an enzyme immunoassay which should be as excellent as ELISA and should not require any electrical equipment like spectrophotometer. The development of an enzyme immunoassay for screening of monoclonal antibodies which basically required no equipment including ELISA reader, was named as "Dot Immunobinding Assay" because the final outcome of the assay constitute a colour dot against a white background in positive reactions. Later several modification of this assay were developed according to the demand and convenience, and scientists working in the field of diagnostics have demonstrated that the Dot Immunobinding Assay is as good as ELISA for diagnosing infectious and non-infectious diseases. The other commonly used name for this assay is Dot-ELISA.

Principle

The basics of the Dot Immunobinding Assay are similar to that of any solid phase immunoassay such as RIA or ELISA except that nitrocellulose membrane is used as an adsorbent matrix instead of plastic surface. The antigen is dotted on to nitrocellulose membrane and the membrane then first incubated with test antibody, and second with enzyme conjugated antibody directed against the first antibody. Specific antigen-antibody reaction is developed as a coloured dot against the white background at the site of antigen deposition. In case of negative reaction, no colour development takes place at the site of antigen deposition.

Development of Assay

Development of Dot Immunobinding Assay in the laboratory is easy and any laboratory involved in immunodiagnosis of infectious disease could standardize this assay for immunodiagnosis without much cost and effort because basically no equipment is required. Several formats have been evolved for carrying out this assay for the purpose of diagnosis of infectious diseases since its development. The idea of direct deposition of antigen on to nitrocellulose membrane came into mind by looking at solid phase systems of nucleic acid hybridization to nitrocellulose. This is commonly done in dot hybridization method in which, instead of being blotted DNA fragments from a gel, the DNA sample is applied directly to the nitrocellulose membrane as a spot or dot and detected subsequently using radio-labeled probes. Similarly, in Dot Immunobinding Assay the antigen is directly dotted on to nitrocellulose membrane and then exploited for the detection of specific antibody. The steps given below will provide an insight into the protocol of this assay as to how it is developed.

Protocol

Basic requirements to develop Dot Immunobinding Assay include:

- Solid phase matrix.
- Antigen.
- Serum sample in which antigen specific antibody is to be detected (Primary antibody).
- Anti-immunoglobulins conjugated to an enzyme (Tracer antibody).
- Substrate solution according to the tracer antibody enzyme conjugate.
- Chemicals, reagents, glass ware and plastic ware to prepare buffers and solutions required for the assay.

This assay could be developed to detect either antibody in the serum sample or antigen in the clinical sample. Depending on the interest the protocol of the assay could be modified accordingly. However, the basic requirements as given above remain the same. For detection of antibody in the serum sample the indirect method is most popular as with ELISA. But for the detection of antigen the direct method has commonly been used.

Antibody Detection

Solid phase matrix

Nitrocellulose membrane is the solid phase matrix most conveniently employed in the Dot Immunobinding Assays. The membrane of 0.22µm or 0.45µm pore size has been used as such or supported by some kind of plastic surface to facilitate the handling of membrane in subsequent steps. Small squares of nitrocellulose membrane are prepared so that the individual square could be placed into each well of a 96-well microtitre plastic plate. Nitrocellulose based 96-well microtitre plates have been used for the rapid detection of human infection with visceral leishmaniasis. The nitrocellulose membrane cut to fit the top of a 96-well microtitre plate has been employed for the detection of antibodies against *Entamoeba histolytica.* Although nitrocellulose membrane cut into strips have been found useful in detecting antibody against *Trypanosoma cruzi* in human sera but these strips were considered very inconvenient as nitrocellulose is very fragile and tears quickly. This critically limits their use outside the laboratory under field conditions. To overcome this problem nitrocellulose membrane following deposition of antigen is glued to flat, pliable plastic strips. This dipstick format has been found easy to handle and resistant to breakage of nitrocellulose membrane during handling. Later, the dipstick format of this assay became much popular and has been used by several workers in diagnosing several infectious diseases.

Antigen

The antigen preparation in solution, preferably in neutral buffer or in normal saline or in distilled water, can be used. Whole cells, either viable, killed or formalin fixed such as protozoa, bacteria, viruses and fungal agents or their sonicated extracts, are all reported to bind to the nitrocellulose membrane. The extracts obtained from microbial agents by treating them with some chemicals such as ethanol or detergents like NP-40, excretory-secretory antigen extracts from cestode, hydatid cyst fluid antigen, tick salivary gland antigens and rat brain synaptosomal membranes bind to the nitrocellulose membrane.

Dotting of antigen

The antigen preparation is dotted or deposited on to nitrocellulose membrane with the help of a micro-capillary or some other device like Hamilton micro syringe. Glass Hamilton syringe calibrated in 0.1µl increments up to 10µl is very convenient for this purpose and produces dots of uniform size. While dotting, the antigen solution forms a small circular dot on to the membrane at the site of deposition which quickly disappears on air drying the membrane.

At this stage the protein molecules or any other bio-molecules in the antigen preparation bind with the nitrocellulose membrane. The nature of binding or interaction between antigen and nitrocellulose membrane is still not clear but the binding appears to be very strong and irreversible as it is not disturbed even if treated with some detergent. However, incubation of the nitrocellulose membrane dotted with antigen at 80°C for 30 minutes has been advocated to improve the binding particularly if whole bacterial cells are used as antigen. If the incubation of antigen dotted membrane at somewhat higher temperature is not possible due to non-availability of incubator, drying time at room temperature can be increased or a hair dryer can be used.

The amount of antigen in terms of volume to be deposited on to nitrocellulose membrane is an important step while developing this assay. This primarily depends upon the concentration of proteins or other antigens present in the antigen preparation. If the preparation contains lesser amount of antigen then higher volumes can be dotted on to the membrane to achieve desired concentration of antigen on to the membrane where subsequent antigen-antibody reaction takes place. This can be accomplished by depositing the antigen preparation several times at the same place and drying the membrane between the dotting of antigen. At this stage, drying the dotted antigen on the membrane with the help of a hair dryer will greatly facilitate the step of dotting of antigen. An antigen preparation could be applied on to membrane in volumes ranging between 0.1µl and 3µl conveniently. In case the preparation contains much higher concentration of antigen then smaller volumes of antigen could be dotted on the membrane. The absorptive capacity of nitrocellulose membrane for different kinds of proteins and other antigens is approximately 100 µg/cm2. The nitrocellulose membranes with small pore sizes are optimal when solubilized antigen preparation are used, because protein is bound at or near surface. The pore size of nitrocellulose does not seem to adversely affect the reactivity of the assay when antigen preparation containing whole protozoa of 5-10µm diameter is applied to the membrane.

In practice, approximately 0.5µl to 1µl volume of antigen preparation is dotted on to the nitrocellulose membrane. This volume of solution produces a dot of antigen on the nitrocellulose membrane which is easily appreciable. A 0.1µl volume of antigen preparation produces a 0.3 mm diameter dot on the nitrocellulose membrane which is well above the resolution limit. The antigen dotted nitrocellulose membrane can be stored for a few months between 4 to 8°C without an appreciable loss in antigen activity.

Blocking

Subsequent to dotting of antigen, blocking of unsaturated sites on the nitrocellulose membrane is an essential step in Dot Immunobinding Assay to prevent non-specific adsorption of the immunological reagents. The nitrocellulose membrane is incubated with a blocking reagent for a 1 hour period at room temperature or 37°C. Blocking of all unsaturated sites on the membrane can be achieved with a range of protein or detergent solutions as given below:

Blotto

It is a 5 per cent w/v solution of non-fat dry milk powder dissolved in phosphate buffer saline (PBS) containing 0.02 per cent sodium azide. It is cheap and gives clear background but it deteriorates rapidly. It is to be prepared fresh before use.

Blotto/Tween

It consists of 5 percent w/v non-fat dry milk powder dissolved in PBS containing 0.02 percent sodium azide as above but also contains 0.1 to 0.2 percent Tween-20. It is similar to Blotto as it is also cheap and gives clear background but deteriorates rapidly. It is also to be prepared fresh before use.

Tween

Tween-20 alone has also been found to be an effective blocking agent. It works well between 0.1 and 0.2 per cent in PBS. It is cheap but sometimes it gives residual background.

Gelatin

Gelatin is prepared as 1.0% in washing solution PBS Tween which provides good blocking of unsaturated sites of nitrocellulose strips.

Bovine Serum Albumin (BSA)

Majority of the initial reports regarding ELISA indicate use of BSA as a blocking reagent. It is also very effective between 2 and 3 per cent solution prepared in PBS in Dot Immunobinding Assay when good signal strength is required. The main disadvantage of this is that it is relatively more expensive.

Horse Serum

Horse serum diluted between 8 and 10 percent in PBS containing 0.02 percent sodium azide gives very clear background. The main disadvantage is its cost and its incompatibility with anti- horse immunoglobulin conjugates.

Above mentioned blocking agents work satisfactorily in some circumstances, hence a careful choice is necessary to ensure compatibility with the detection reagent. For example, use of whole serum for blocking is inappropriate if enzyme conjugated Protein A is used as a detection reagent. The compatibility of the blocking reagent with the detection system can be tested by taking a fresh piece of nitrocellulose membrane, blocking it and then treating with the detection system.

Two blocking solutions that are compatible with nearly all detection systems are non-fat dried milk and BSA. If protein blocking solutions cause problems with excessive background, then blocking in Tween-20 or gelatin should be tried. It should be noted that both milk and BSA contain phosphotyrosine, and will confuse the interpretation of certain tests with antibodies specific for anti-phosphotyrosine antibodies. Some preparations of milk contain inhibitors of alkaline phosphatase enzyme. In such cases if no signal or high background is detected then some other blocking agent should be tried. The nitrocellulose membrane following dotting of antigen and blocking step can be processed further immediately or can be stored at -20°C for a few weeks. For storing, it is essential to wash the membrane thoroughly with distilled water, dry it at room temperature and pack in an airtight plastic cover.

Incubation with Serum Sample

Serum sample obtained from an individual is incubated with the antigen dotted nitrocellulose membrane for specific antigen-antibody reactions to take place. If specific antibodies are present in the serum sample of the individual they will interact with the antigen dotted on to nitrocellulose membrane and bind firmly. It is important to provide a favourable environment for an optimal reaction between antibody in serum and the antigen on the nitrocellulose membrane. For this, serum sample is diluted in some kind of buffer solution like PBS or Tris buffer saline (TBS) at physiological pH (pH 7 to 8) and incubated with the nitrocellulose membrane containing antigen. The incubation is carried out for 2 hours at room temperature or 1 hour in an incubator at 37°C. It is always appreciated if the serum dilutions are prepared in the blocking solution. Inclusion of blocking solution will help in lowering the background reaction because it will inhibit or interfere in non-specific binding of antibody to the solid phase matrix. Some workers prefer overnight incubation of nitrocellulose membrane with diluted serum at 4°C. Although incubation overnight increases the sensitivity of the assay but an increase in background is also commonly observed.

Washing of Nitrocellulose Membrane

An important step in all solid phase immune assays, including Dot Immunobinding Assay, is washing because this step allows separation of bound antigen or antibody from that of free antigen or non-reactive antibody as the case may be. The solid phases initially used to immobilize antigen or antibody include particles of cellulose, agarose and polyacrylamide. Separation of unbound antigen or antibody in washing step was to be achieved by centrifugation. The procedure tended to be labour intensive where large number of samples were to be processed. With the development of ELISA in tubes for antibodies and subsequent 96-well ELISA plate format simplified the step of separation of non-reactive antigen or antibody to a great extent. Similarly, washing step in Dot Immunobinding Assay, particularly of dipstick format, is very simple because following incubation of nitrocellulose membrane with the diluted serum the dipsticks are washed in washing solution. The dipsticks are immersed in washing solution in a container by holding them in hand from the opposite end to membrane and then washing them by quick backward and forward movements for one minute. The process is repeated three times using 3 different containers. The washing solution commonly used for this purpose is PBS containing 0.1 per cent Tween-20. In this way many dipsticks can be washed in a short period of time and the procedure is very suitable to be carried in all laboratory settings. Washing of nitrocellulose membrane not in the dipstick format is comparatively labour intensive and requires more time because it cannot be handled as vigorously as done in dipstick format. This could lead to more background. Use of nitrocellulose membrane strips or a bigger piece increases the chances of tearing off of membrane during washing steps.

Incubation with Conjugate

Following washing after first incubation in diluted serum sample the nitrocellulose membrane is incubated with the anti-species specific immunoglobulin conjugated to an enzyme, commonly termed as conjugate, for a period of 1-2 hour. If specific antigen-antibody interaction had taken place at the stage of incubation with serum sample then antigen bound immunoglobulins at this step will bind with anti-species immunoglobulin conjugate during incubation. The incubation in diluted conjugate is usually carried out for 2 hours at room temperature or 1 hour at 37°C to obtain optimum reaction. Dilution of conjugate is normally prepared in some physiological buffer like PBS or TBS. It is again preferred that blocking agent should be included in conjugate diluting solution as given above to suppress the background reaction.

The anti-species specific immunoglobulin enzyme conjugates can be prepared in the laboratory by raising high titred antiserum in a heterologous host and then conjugating the anti-immunoglobulins with an appropriate enzyme. Although conjugates can be prepared in the laboratory but they are commercially available in the market at a very competitive cost. However, conjugates against every animal species are not available commercially, hence it is advisable to prepare those conjugates in the laboratory which are not available commercially in the market.

Determination of optimum dilution of the conjugate to be used in the assay is very important step because an inappropriate dilution could result in higher background reaction or reduce the sensitivity of the test. The working dilution of most commercially available conjugates is predetermined by the manufacturers and provided with the product information. In majority of the cases the recommended dilution works well in the hands of clinicians, However, sometimes it needs to be determined in the laboratory if problems like higher background arise. In addition, it is imperative to find out the working dilution of a conjugate which is prepared in the laboratory. To determine the optimum dilution to be used in the assay, appropriate serial dilutions of the conjugate are checked with the immunoglobulin of the species against which the conjugate has been prepared.

Most common enzymes which have been used to chemically link anti-immunoglobulins to prepare conjugate are horse radish peroxidase and alkaline phosphatase. Both the enzymes have merits and demerits. In general, an enzyme should have the following properties:

- Possess a high specific activity at physiological pH
- Be readily available and also relatively inexpensive in a purified form
- Be stable enough to allow conjugation, purification, and storage without significant loss of activity
- Catalyze a reaction in which the product can be easily quantitated
- Not occur naturally in the solution to be assayed

The conjugates possessing horse radish peroxidase or alkaline phosphatase enzymes have been used in Dot Immunobinding Assay and found equally good. However, horse radish peroxidase conjugate appears to be comparatively more popular.

Washing of Nitrocellulose Membrane

Subsequent to incubation in conjugate the nitrocellulose membrane needs thorough washing as described above. At least 3 washing each of 5 minutes should be done prior to incubation with substrate solution. By thorough washing at this stage much better results which are free from any background, can be obtained. The dipstick format of Dot Immunobinding Assay provides a very convenient way by which the nitrocellulose membrane could be handled manually for washing thoroughly at this step and also after incubation with serum sample.

Incubation with Substrate Solution

This is the final step in which specific antigen-antibody reaction is visualized. The nitrocellulose membrane is incubated with the substrate solution at room temperature and development of a coloured dot is observed. The incubation time could vary from few minutes to 30 minutes depending on the substrate employed. A wide range of substrates are available which on reaction with the conjugate i.e. enzyme linked to anti-immunoglobulins, yield insoluble products of different colours. This detection method is simple and requires no special equipment. The development of coloured dot at the site of antigen deposition can be seen with unaided eyes. This also provides an immediate result. Many substrates have been used to detect the presence of horse radish peroxidase conjugate in Dot Immunobinding Assay. Satisfactory results can be obtained with diaminobenzidine (DAB), 4-chloro-1-naphthol, or 3-amino-9-ethylcarbazole. Details about two substrates are given below.

Diaminobenzidine

It is an exceptionally sensitive substrate, yielding a brown colour product at the site of antigen deposition in the form of a dot. The substrate solution is always prepared fresh by dissolving 10 mg of DAB in 50 ml of 50 mM Tirs-buffer (pH 7.6) and adding 20µl of 30 percent (v/v) H_2O_2. The nitrocellulose membrane is immersed in the substrate solution and assessed for the development of a brown colour reaction at the site of antigen deposition which takes only a few minutes to develop. To stop the reaction, the membrane is washed with distilled water. The developed nitrocellulose membranes, after thorough washing, are air-dried and can be stored indefinitely in a sealed container. The drawback of this substrate is its over sensitiveness as it reacts fast so that it is very easy to over develop resulting in high background.

Chloronaphthol

The 4-choloro-1-naphthol is relatively insensitive substrate but gives an intense blue-black colour product in an easily controlled reaction. Background binding of the product to the nitrocellulose membrane is very low.

- Prepare the stock solution of chloronaphthol by dissolving 0.3 gm in 10 ml of absolute ethanol. The stock is stable at -20°C for at least one year.
- Just prior to development add 0.1 ml of stock solution to 10 ml of 50 mM Tris buffer (pH 7.6). A copious white precipitate could form which is removed by filtration.
- Add 10 µl of 30 percent H_2O_2 solution per 10 ml of working chloronaphthol solution.
- Make sufficient substrate solution as needed.
- Immerse nitrocellulose membrane in the above prepared substrate solution and allow to develop colour reaction at room temperature. Approximately 30 minutes are required for incubation to complete the reaction.
- Remove the nitrocellulose membrane from substrate solution after 30 minutes to stop the reaction, wash with distilled water and air-dry.
- The membrane can be stored in a sealed container though the colour fades noticeably on long storage.

The most popular substrate which precipitates on reacting with alkaline phosphatase conjugate and has been used in immunoblotting and Dot Immunobinding Assay is a mixture of bromochloroindolyl phosphate (BCIP) and nitro blue tetrazolium (NBT). This substrate generates an intense black-purple coloured product at the site of enzyme binding. The substrate solution is stable in the absence of enzyme. The reaction proceeds at a steady rate, thus allowing accurate control of the development of the reaction. The BCIP/NBT substrate characteristically produces sharp reaction with very little background colouring of the membrane.

- Prepare stock solutions of NBT, BCIP and alkaline phosphatase buffer. These are stable at 4°C for at least one year.
- ***NBT***: Dissolve 0.5 gm of NBT in 10 ml of 70 percent dimethylformamide.
- ***BCIP***: Dissolve 0.5 gm BCIP (disodium salt) in 10 ml of 100 percent dimethylformamide.

- ***Alkaline phosphatase buffer***: 10 mM sodium chloride, 5 mM magnesium chloride, 100 mM Tris-buffer (pH 9.5).
- Just prior to use, prepare fresh substrate solution by adding 66 ml of NBT stock to 10 µl of alkaline phosphatase buffer. After proper mixing add 33 µl of BCIP stock and use within 1hour. Make sufficient substrate solution as needed.
- Immerse nitrocellulose membrane into substrate solution and allow reaction to proceed for 30 minutes.
- To stop the reaction, rinse the membrane with PBS containing 20 mM EDTA which chelates the Mg++ ions.
- The membrane can be stored for a long period in sealed containers.

Antigen Detection

When the assay is needed for detection of antigen in the clinical material both direct and indirect methods could be used. In direct method, the clinical material is dotted directly on to the nitrocellulose membrane with the help of a micro-capillary or Hamilton syringe. The remaining sites of the nitrocellulose membrane are saturated with some blocking reagent as above. The antigen specific antibody conjugated to an enzyme (conjugate) is allowed to react with the antigen dotted on to the nitrocellulose membrane and then developed with a suitable substrate solution. The main disadvantage of direct method of Dot Immunobinding Assay is that the conjugation of antibody is to be done against each and every microbial agent of interest. In addition, some compromise has to be made with sensitivity despite excellent specificity. Alternatively, nitrocellulose membrane bound antigen is first allowed to react with some high titered antiserum and then bound antibody is detected with a conjugate against the bound antibody. Using this approach scientists have successfully demonstrated rotavirus antigen in fecal material from diarrhoeic calves and claimed that the method could be used for rapid diagnosis of rotavirus infection in animals (Fig.15.13). In addition, they have also advocated that the Dot Immunobinding Assay is as sensitive as ELISA or polyacrylamide gel electrophoresis (PAGE) but much rapid and simple to perform.

Similarly, detection of human immunodeficiency virus (HIV)-associated antigens has been simplified by the application of direct method of this assay. Antigens were detected by dotting the polyethylene glycol precipitated supernatants from infected cultures directly on to nitrocellulose membrane and sequentially incubating with an anti-HIV rabbit or human antiserum and then in an alkaline phosphatase conjugated anti-rabbit or anti-human antibody conjugate. The colour reaction was developed using NBT/BCIP substrate solution. They showed that the assay was nearly as sensitive as the reverse transcriptase (RT) assay in detecting HIV antigens in experimentally infected peripheral blood mononuclear cells, as well as in a T-cell line and is useful in detection of HIV antigens in studies of viral pathogenesis.

A two-site Dot Immunobinding Assay for antigen detection could also be designed. In this method the antibody prepared against antigen of interest is dotted on to nitrocellulose membrane. Following blocking step the dotted membrane is incubated with the clinical sample in which the antigen is to be detected. The antigen in the sample is trapped by the antibodies. The trapped antigen then could be detected by second antibody conjugated with an enzyme.

Standardization

It is important to standardize several variables of an enzyme immunoassay, including Dot Immunobinding Assay, prior to its application for immunodiagnostic purposes. The most important variable which needs to be standardized is determination of optimal concentration of antigen to be used in the assay. Other critical variable is dilution of serum producing positive reaction considered to be indicative of infection. Standardization of conjugate is seldom required as most manufacturers provide information regarding optimal working dilution to be used in the assay. As far as standardization of time required for incubation and incubation temperature is concerned, the antigen-antibody reaction effectively takes place at room temperature within a period of 1-2 hours.

For determining optimal concentration of antigen and antibody dilution to be used in the assay, the most acceptable procedure is the checker board analysis in which variables like conjugate concentration, incubation period and time and other factors are kept constant and various concentration of antigen are analysed against various dilution of pooled positive and pooled negative sera. The pooled positive sera should comprise serum samples from at least five positive animals or individuals exhibiting moderate to high antibody titres against the antigen in question. It is always better to include more number of positive individuals to prepare a pool of positive sera. Similarly, pooled negative sera is prepared from negative individuals preferably from an area that is free from that particular disease. When antigen is in soluble form the criterion of antigen concentration could be determined in terms of protein concentration whereas if particulate antigen such as whole cell bacteria or whole protozoan-parasites are used in the assay, then number of particulate microorganisms is taken into consideration. Both soluble and particulate antigens have been used to standardized Dot Immunobinding Assay for the serological diagnosis of brucellosis in animals. The particulate antigen in the form of heat killed whole cell *Brucella abortus* organisms and sonic extract of these organisms were dotted in various concentration on to nitrocellulose membrane of dipstick format of Dot Immunobinding Assay. In case of particulate antigen the number of *B. abortus* cells vary between $1x10^{10}$ and $1x10^{6}$ micro-organisms per ml of PBS. One microliter (1µl) of each dilution was dotted on to nitrocellulose membrane of required number of dipsticks indicating that the number of bacterial cells deposited varied between $1x10^{7}$ and $1x10^{3}$ per dot. These dipsticks were checked with various dilutions (1:50 to 1: 25600) of pooled positive and pooled negative sera in checker board analysis. It was observed that $1x10^{7}$ to $3x10^{7}$ bacterial cells per ml (i.e. $1x10^{4}$ to $3x10^{4}$ cells per dot) produce optimal reaction. A cell concentration above 1′108 cells per ml gave slight background reaction with low dilution (1:50) of pooled negative sera. The analysis also indicated that 1:200 dilution of serum is optimal to be tested because below this dilution of serum a background reaction could develop. Hence, optimum concentration of bacterial cells should be determined independently in each case. Interestingly very parallel results were obtained in a study of antibody response to formalin fixed *Leishmania donovanii* in which $2.5x10^{4}$ protozoan parasite were dotted on to nitrocellulose membrane. Similarly, optimum concentration of any soluble antigen preparation should be determined. In case of *B. abortus*, soluble antigen prepared by sonication and centrifugation the optimum concentration of antigen was reported to be 300 ng (based on protein content) protein per dot whereas 500 ng protein per dot was shown to produce optimum results in assaying antibodies against *Entamoeba histolytica* in human patients.

Sensitivity and Specificity

The sensitivity of any immunoassay depends on its ability to detect minimum amount, of antibody in a given sample. In other terms the lower limit of detection is the sensitivity of an assay. It should always be kept in mind that as the sensitivity of an assay increases the specificity of the assay decreases. In a study on diagnosis of brucellosis in cattle it has been found that the sensitivity of Dot Immunobinding Assay is comparable to that of ELISA as both the methods produce positive reaction up to the equal titres of antibody and none of the assay gives positive reaction with negative serum samples. The lower limit of detection if determined using purified immunoglobulins directly dotted on to nitrocellulose membrane as an antigen then it ranges between 0.1 ng and 1 ng. However, this lower limit of detection is difficult to establish while performing the assay for detection of antibody by indirect method.

Flow Diagram of Dot Immunobinding Assay Procedure

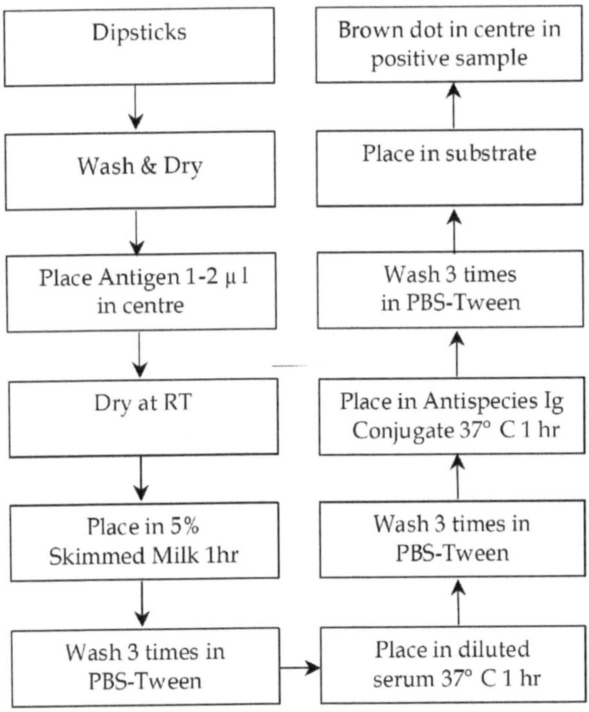

Reproducibility

The assay reproducibility is an important criterion which is always considered by a clinician. In a study carried out on 167 serum samples it was observed that 90 per cent samples produced same reciprocal titres on repeated testing but 10 per cent displayed variability of one titre dilution. Besides, pooled positive and negative control sera were assayed 20 times. The pooled positive sera reacted at the same titre 18 times while the negative control was uniformly unreactive. Assay reproducibility for detecting visceral Leishmaniasis was also found to be slightly higher in the Dot Immunobinding Assay compared to ELISA and much better than the complement fixation test. Twenty five coded sera from cases of amoebiasis at four different occasions were checked for antibody titres to assess the reproducibility of the assay. It has been found that 23 (92 per cent) sera did not show any variation in titres whereas titres of two sera varied on two occasions, but the variation was not more than ±1 titre dilution. None of the negative control sera showed any reactivity at any occasion.

Cross Reactivity

The problem of serological cross-reactivity due to existence of cross-reactive antigens could be seen with some microbial agents. For example, the lipopolysaccharide, an immunodominating antigen of *B. abortus,* shows complete serological cross-reactivity with the lipopolysaccharide of *Yersinia enterocolitica* O9. Similarly, the capripox virus serologically cross-reacts with contagious pustular dermatitis virus. In such cases any serological assay, including Dot Immunobinding Assay, will be unable to detect specific antibody responses. However, use of an etiological agent specific antigen in an immunoassay could provide specific diagnosis of a disease as shown in diagnosing capripox virus infections in sheep by Western blotting and by ELISA in cattle.

Comparison with ELISA

Both the assays are based on the same principle that the antigen is allowed to bind to a solid phase and then exploited for all antigen-antibody reactions to take place at the site of antigen deposition. In case of ELISA the final outcome is the appearance of development of a coloured solution in a well of a 96-well microtitre plate whereas in Dot Immunobinding Assay, a coloured dot is developed at the site of antigen deposition. Some important characteristics of both assays are summarized in Table 15.5.

Table 15.5: Showing comparison of DIA and ELISA

Assay Characteristic	**DIA**	**ELISA**
Technical expertise required	No	Yes
Electrical equipment required	No	Yes
Field application	Yes	No
Cost per test	Low	Comparatively high
Sensitivity	Comparable	High (pg-to ng)
		(up to ng)
Specificity	Same	Same
Test time	3-4 hour	5-6 hours
No. of incubations	3	4
No. of washes	3	3-4
Colour reaction	Easy to photo- graph	Difficult to photo-graph

Comparison with RIA

Dot Immunobinding Assay is a solid phase enzyme immunoassay and in principle, analogous to radioimmunoassay (RIA) and immunofluorescence. The only major difference is in the use of an enzyme rather than an isotope or fluorescent dye as the label on one of the immunological reactants. Scientifically this may seem be a small difference, but it can result in quite marked differences in the development, production and availability of the tests. Radioimmunoassays of clinical importance commonly used 125I as the label. The 125I has a short half life necessiating frequent quality control of reagents, thereby limiting use in remote areas. In addition, there are legal restrictions on the use and disposal of such isotopes which result in these assays being limited to highly sophisticated centres. The necessity for highly trained personnel and expensive instrumentation further restricts the wider use of radioimmunoassays. In contrast, Dot Immunobinding Assay reagents are stable, having long shelf life and consequently reducing costs of quality control. The non-hazardous nature of the reagents means that they can be used by any laboratory, and requirement of no equipment to assess the results encourages the use of Dot Immunobinding Assay by smaller laboratories, even those located in remote areas.

Application in Diagnosis of Diseases

Dot Immunobinding Assay is an efficient method for diagnosing infectious diseases of man and animals either by detecting the presence of antibody produced against infectious agent or by detecting the presence of etiological agent or its components in clinical samples. In principle, the assay can be used to diagnose any infectious disease of man or animals (Table 15.12). In addition, the assay has been found useful for the diagnosis of many infectious diseases of plants. The assay has been found promising in detecting *Leishmania* antigens in vector sandflies (*Lutzomyai anthophora)* fed on mice or hamsters infected with cutaneous Leishmaniasis agent. The flies were squashed on to nitrocellulose membrane and after drying the membrane processed with high titred anti-*Leishmania* serum and suitable enzyme conjugate and substrate. Positive reaction was observed in 66 percent of infected flies. The uninfected sandflies, with or without blood meals, failed to yield positive results.

Table 15.6: Application of DIA in diagnosis of diseases

Sr.No.	Disease
1.	Trypanosomosis
2.	Potato virus
3.	HIV infection
4.	Capripox virus infection
5.	Brucellosis
6.	Yersiniosis
7.	Contagious pustular dermatitis
8.	Rotavirus infection
9.	Blue tongue

Sr.No.	Disease
10.	Amoebiasis
11.	Cytomegalovirus
12.	Salmonellosis
13.	Leishmaniasis
14.	Leptospirosis
15.	Hydatid disease
16.	Aflatoxicosis
17.	Reovirus infection

Leucocyte Migration Inhibition Assay

Leucocyte migration inhibition assay (LMI) is performed to assess the cell mediated immune response in animals and poultry. About 5 ml blood is collected in heparinized vials from animals. Add equal amount of PBS (pH 7.2) or HBSS and place it was layered on 5 ml histopaque or Ficoll solution in a tube and centrifuge at 400 g for 10 min. After centrifugation clear upper layer is discarded and middle opaque layer is collected in another test tube and mixed with equal amount of PBS (pH 7.2). It is again centrifuged at 250 g for 10 min repeating the process three times in order to wash the lymphocytes. Lymphocytes can also be prepared from spleen and lymph nodes and in poultry from thymus and bursa. For the purpose, collect these tissues separately in HBSS under anesthesia and place them in small beakers; cut into small pieces by using sterile scissors and forceps and filter through muslin cloth sieve. The filtered suspension of lymphocytes is allowed to stand for 15 min, the supernatant containing lymphocytes is taken and washed 3 times with PBS and passed through a millipore support screen and glass wool.

The viability of the lymphocytes is determined with trypan blue dye exclusion method. The dead lymphocytes will stain with trypan blue dye while the live lymphocytes will not take the colour and remain same, therefore the percent viable cells are counted in the lymphocyte population.

The cells are finally suspended in RPMI media containing 5% fetal calf serum with 4 X 106 cell count per ml. The cell suspension is allowed to be aspirated in capillaries. On filling the capillaries are sealed at one end with plasticin and centrifuged at 250 xg for 5 min. The capillaries are cut at cell and fluid interphase with the help of glass cutter and the stubs of capillaries containing packed leucocytes are placed in leucocyte migration inhibition chamber with the help of sterile grease. The chambers are filled with RPMI 1640 media containing 5% fetal calf serum, antibiotics and antifungal agents. Duplicate chambers of control and antigen are prepared for each sample. In test wells, 0.2 ml sonicated or killed antigen is also added. Grease is applied on the rim of the chamber and it is sealed with coverslip. Care must be taken that there should not be any air bubble in the chamber. These chambers are placed in large petri dishes moistened by wet filter paper and incubated for 2 hours at 37^{0}C (Fig.15.14). The area of migration of leucocytes in each chamber is measured with the help of camera lucida and planimeter or by using overhead projector and planimeter and the pre cent migration inhibition is calculated with following equation.

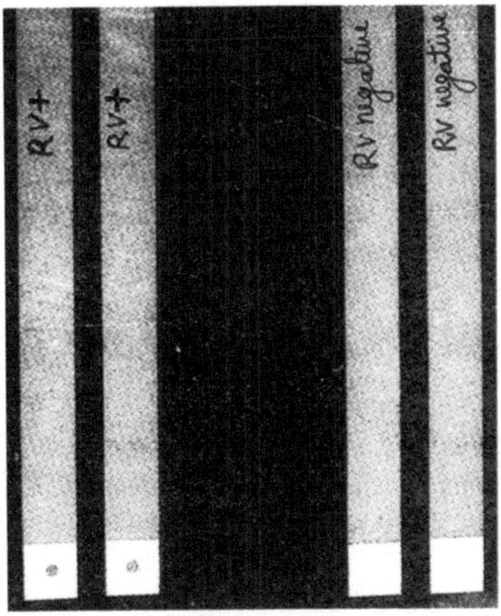

Fig. 15.13: Dot immunobinding assay. Note the presence of brown/black dot in positive nitro cellulose strips Control Migration inhibition

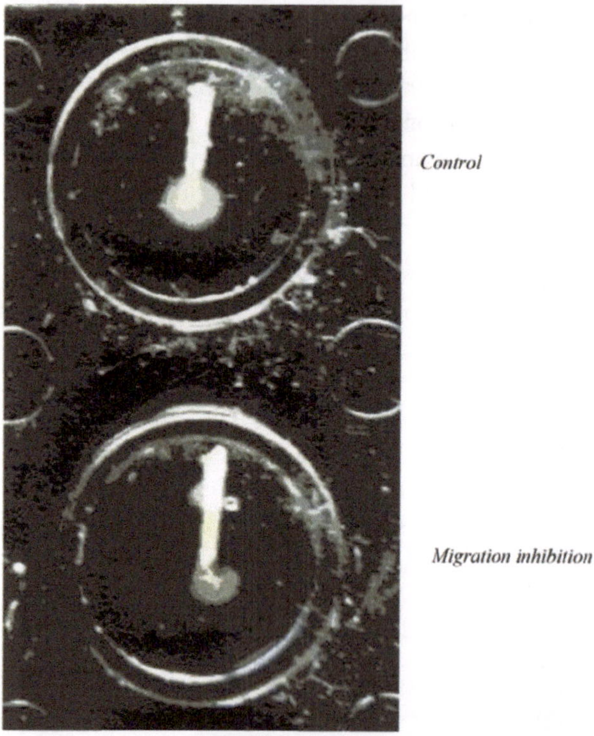

Fig. 15.14: Leucocyte migration inhibition test

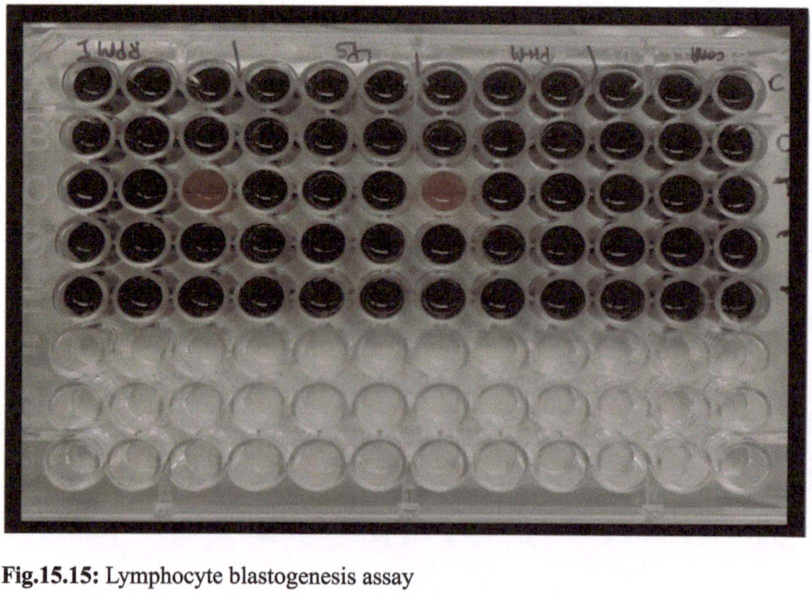

Fig.15.15: Lymphocyte blastogenesis assay

Lymphocyte Stimulation Assay

[3H] thymidine Method

The lymphocytes are separated as described in LMI assay and their viability is assessed by trypan blue dry exclusion test and 95% viability of cells should be assured. A differential count is also carried out in order to see that the lymphocytes should be approximately 90% in the cells. These cells are allowed to grow in a 96-well flat bottom sterile microtiter plate. 100 μl of lymphocyte suspension in RPMI-1640 medium with 10% fetal calf serum and 100 μl of mitogen (PHA or Con A) is placed in triplicate wells. The control wells receive only 100 μl RPMI-1640 medium and 100 μl of lymphocyte suspension. Besides, one can also use antigen for lymphocyte stimulation which will provide the information about specific cell mediated immune response. The plates are covered with cover provided with the plate and are sealed with the help of cello-tape and are incubated at 37^{0}C for at least three days under 5% carbon dioxide pressure. Thereafter add 0.5 μl Ci/well of tritium labeled thymidine ([3H] thymidine) into the plate and incubate the plate for 6 hours. Harvest the cells with multiple automated sample harvestor onto filter paper, dry the filter paper at room temperature and place the cells in scintillation vials with 1 ml of scintillation fluid and count the radioactivity by using beta scintillation counter.

MTT Dye Method

The lymphocytes are separated as described earlier and their viability is assessed by trypan blue dye exclusion test. The lymphocytes having more than 95% viability should be used. On differential count, one should see that the lymphocyte population must be more than 90%. Now a flat bottom 96-well sterile microtitier plate is taken and the triplicate wells are prepared for mitogen (PHA or ConA), antigen and control. The plates are charged with 100 μl of lymphocytic cells in RPMI-1640 medium, and 50 μl of mitogen; equal amount of cells and 50 μl of antigen and in control wells 100 μl cells and 50 μl of RPMI-1640 medium. The plate is sealed with cello tape and is incubated at 37^{0}C under 5% CO_2 pressure for three days . The pipette 50 μl of MTT (4 mg/ml) dye to all wells before the 4 hours of the end of culture i.e. at 68 hours of incubation. Keep the plate for incubation at 37^{0}C in CO_2 incubator. After 4 hours, the contents of the plates are discarded, and washed with PBS. Thereafter, 100 μl of acid isopropanol (0.04 N HCl in isopropanol) is added to each well and mixed properly. The development of blue purple colour is measured by spectrophotometer or ELISA reader at wave length of 570 nm. The triplicate wells averaged and mean OD of antigen stimulated, mitogen stimulated and control wells is calculated. The mean control OD is subtracted from mean antigen stimulated and mitogen stimulated OD to get delta OD, which is plotted on a graph to make out further conclusions (Fig.15.15).

Macrophage Function Test

For macrophage function test, the peritoneal macrophages or peripheral blood neutrophils are collected. The functions of macrophages are assessed generally by following methods; macrophage migration inhibition assay, nitro blue tetrazolium test and bactericidal activity test. The peritoneal macrophages are collected by inoculating paraffin oil intraperitoneally 2-3 days before the start of experiment. The animals or poultry are sacrificed or the peritoneal exudate through syringe and needle or pipette after laparotomy. The exudate is centrifuged with HBSS and the macrophages are collected. One should give at least three washings with HBSS. Then finally suspend the cells in HBSS/ RPMI-1640. Count the live and dead cells.

For peripheral blood neutrophils, collect 5 ml heparinized blood in sterile culture tubes and add equal amount of PBS or HBSS. Centrifuge the blood at 1200 rpm for 5 min and collect the supernatant plasma in other tube. Centrifuge it at 2000 rpm for 20 min and discard the supernatant, resuspend the cells sediment and wash at least three times with HBSS and finally suspend in RPMI-1640 complete medium. Determine the viability of cells.

Macrophage Migration Inhibition Assay

The assay is carried out in the same way as LMI assay

Nitroblue Tetrazolium Test

The cells are incubated in a mixture of solution containing 0.3 ml (0.2% NBT in PBS), 0.2 ml cell suspension and 0.1 ml endotoxin activated plasma (15µl of endotoxin in 1 ml of normal animal plasma incubated at 37°C for 30 min) for 30 min at 370C preferably in water bath. This reaction is stopped with addition of cold PBS. Centrifuge the cell suspension at 500 xg for 5 min. Discard the supernatant and resuspend the cells in 0.5 ml PBS. Put a drop on clean and dry glass slide and make smear. Dry in air and fix in methanol for 2 min. Counter stain the cells with 0.5% safranin solution for 2 min, wash the cells, dry and mount in DPX mountant. The NBT positive cells are counted in percent, these are the cells which contain black/blue granules of stain in the cytoplasm of the cells. In place of endotoxin, one can also use the killed bacterial suspension.

Bactericidal Activity Assay

The bactericidal activity is determined by mixing 3.0 ml macrophage cell suspension (10^7 cell/ ml), 1.0 ml *Staphylococcus aureus* or *E. coli* (2 X 107/ ml) and 0.4 ml normal animal serum and incubating it at 37^{0}C for 30 min in shaker to enhance the phagocytosis. The reaction can be stopped by adding cold HBSS or PBS. Centrifuge the cell suspension at 400 x g for 2-3 min and discard the supernatant. Wash the sediment for at least three times with HBSS and finally resuspend the cells in 4.0 ml HBSS and 37^{0}C. The cells are collected (0.1 ml) at the start of incubation and then at hourly interval for 2 hours. These cells are washed and 1 ml distilled water is added and the cells are disrupted by vigorous pipetting. The ten fold dilutions are prepared from this suspension and 0.1 ml of each dilution is plated on nutrient agar/tryptose soya agar plate and incubated overnight at 37^{0}C. The discrete colonies are counted and the count of bacteria per ml is calculated and compared with the counts at 0,1 and 2 hour. Normally at one hour, neutrophils or macrophages kill 50-70% organism after phagocytosis. But this capacity of macrophages reduces and the bacterial count is not much affected in case of macrophage dysfunction.

16

Immunopathological Techniques

- Allergic Tests
- Single intradermal test
  - Tuberculin test
  - Johnin test
  - Double intradermal test
  - Comparative test
  - Mallein test
- Immunofluorescence Techniques
  - Direct method
  - Indirect method
- Immunoperoxidase Techniques
  - Detection of antigen
  - Demonstration of antibody producing cells
  - Detection of immune complexes
  - Peroxidase-antiperoxidase method
- Avidin-Biotin Methods
  - Enzyme labelled avidin-biotin method
  - Bridged avidin-biotin method
  - Avidin-Biotin-complex assay
- *In situ* hybridization

Allergic Tests

The administration of an allergen into the skin of a previously sensitized animal results in hot and painful swelling at the site, 2-3 days after injection. Histologically, the area is heavily infiltrated with mononuclear cells comprising mainly of macrophages and lymphocytes. Such allergic tests are being used in the diagnosis of chronic diseases particularly tuberculosis, paratuberculosis (Johne's disease) and glanders and are based on type IV hypersensitivity reactions which are the manifestation of 'T' cell response. The cells involved in allergic tests are T-lymphocytes, macrophages, regulatory B-lymphocytes and basophils.

The allergens are prepared by killing the causative organisms of disease and filtering them from culture media. These allergens are named after their principal organisms like tuberculin for *Mycobacterium tuberculosis*. Special purified protein derivative (PPD) is used now a days for eliciting delayed type of hypersensitivity reactions and detection of reactors. The allergens viz. tuberculin, Johnin and mallein are commercially available from Indian Veterinary Research Institute, Izatnagar (India) and Central Veterinary Laboratory, Webridge (U.K.).

In literature, many types of allergic reactions are described for detection of tuberculosis, Johne's disease and glanders reactors. Single intradermal (SID) and comparative intradermal (CID) tests are recommended for routine screening of animals to detect the reactor of tuberculosis and Johne's disease. However, double intradermal (DID) test can also be employed for screening of animals but it is considered expensive and sometimes impracticable.

Single Intradermal (SID) Test

Tuberculin Test

Tuberculin testing is done for the diagnosis of tuberculosis in animals and birds. In bovines, the tuberculin is injected in the skin of neck; in pigs, in ear and in birds, in wattle. In single intradermal test, 0.1 ml of tuberculin or PPD is injected intradermally in the middle portion of neck of bovines, a site preferred due to maximum sensitivity. Prior to tuberculin injection, the skin should be cleaned, shaved and thickness of skin fold measured using a Vernier calliper. The reaction can be read after 72 hours of the injection; the positive reaction is characterized by a hot, red and painful swelling with an increase of 4 mm or more in skin fold. However, some diagnosticians consider that skin thickness should be double to declare a positive reactor (Fig.16.1).

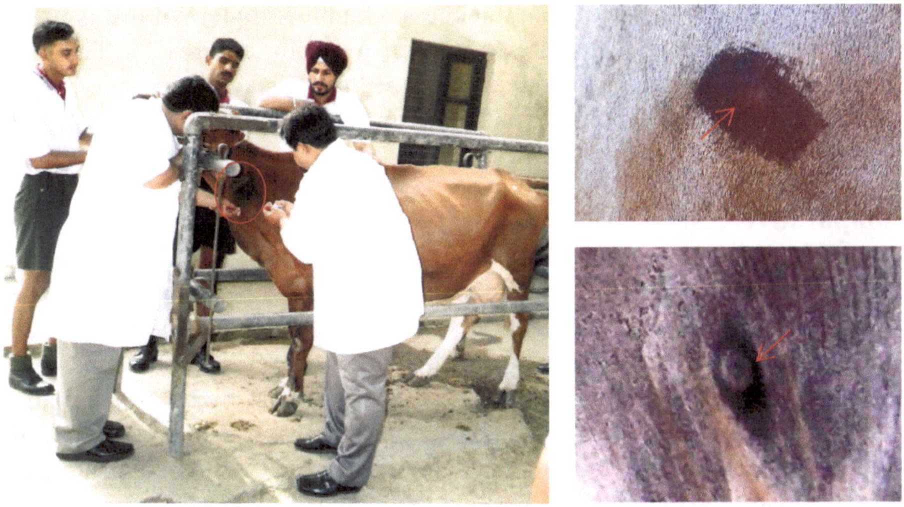

Fig. 16.1: Tuberculin testing in cows (A), Skin after inoculation of tuberculin (B) and after 72 hrs skin thickness in positive case (C).

Johnin Test

Johnin testing is performed in bovines for the detection of reactors of Johne's disease. In this test, instead of tuberculin, Johnin or its PPD fraction is used. An injection of 0.1 ml Johnin is given intradermally in clean and shaved area of cervical region. If the tuberculin and Johnin testing are done simultaneously, Johnin is injected in the skin of the opposite side of neck. An increase of 5 mm or more in thickness of skin fold after 72 hours is considered positive for Johne's disease. The confirmation of the test can be made by performing a comparative test after 2 months.

The main advantage of single intradermal test is its simplicity besides being less expensive in comparison to other tests. However, the disadvantages include lack of its specificity, as the mammalian tuberculin is not specific to differentiate among *Mycobacterium bovi, M.avium, M.tuberculosis* and *M. paratuberculosis*. This test is also not able to detect cases of minimal sensitivity such as may occur in the early or late stages of disease, in old cows and in cows which have recently calved.

Double Intradermal Test (DID)

The double intradermal test is performed in same manner as in single intradermal test, the only difference is that a second injection of tuberculin or Johnin is given 7 days after the first injection at the same site and the skin thickness is measured 24 hrs after the last injection. In positive reactor, there should be an increase of 5 mm or more in skin thickness. Double intradermal test is useful to detect those animals which are poorly sensitized for any reason. The main disadvantage of this test is the requirement of three visits to complete the test which becomes more expensive and sometimes impracticable. However, it is more accurate than the single ID test.

Comparative Test

The comparative test depends on the greater sensitivity to homologous tuberculin. In this test, the mammalian and avian tuberculin are injected simultaneously in the neck region about 10-15 cm apart. The test is read after 72 hours and an increase of skin thickness of either site is considered positive for that particular type of organism. If thickness more at mammalian tuberculin injected site the case is considered positive for tuberculosis while the increased thickness at the site of avian tuberculin is considered positive for Johne's disease/avian tuberculosis/skin tuberculosis.

The test is not meant for primary screening, but is routinely used for confirmation of the results of single intradermal test. However, it can be used as primary test where the presence of Johne's disease or avian tuberculosis is suspected or skin tuberculosis is apparent. A variable degree of desensitization will occur in the skin over the area of injection site so that when retesting is necessary, it is advisable to allow an interval of about two months to elapse, and the skin on the opposite side of the neck should be used.

False positive and false negative reactions may occur in these allergic tests which may also be looked into before making any interpretation.

1. Situations/circumstances in which false negative results may occur:
    a. Early stage of infection. Tuberculin test may become positive only after 6 weeks of infection.
    b. Late stage of infection.
    c. In old animals.
    d. Test carried out just after parturition.
    e. Within 60 days of tuberculin test.
2. Situations or circumstances in which false positive results may occur.
    a. Animals sensitized to other allergens like hydatid disease, bovine farcy, etc.

b. If the animal is infected with nonpathogenic mycobacteria (saprophytic).

Mallein Test

The mallein is a bacteria free filtrate from a fluid culture of *Pseudomonas mallei,* the cause of glanders in equines. In this test, 0.2 ml of mallein is injected intra dermo pelpebrally (IDP) into the skin of lower eyelid using a tuberculin syringe. The test is read after 48 hours and a positive reaction includes marked edema of eyelid, with blepharospasm and a severe purulent conjunctivitis. The mallein test is routinely used to screen the equines for glanders and is considered quite specific. As the glanders is a communicable and notifiable disease, the test has its significance in detecting positive reactors in eradication programme of disease (Fig 16.2).

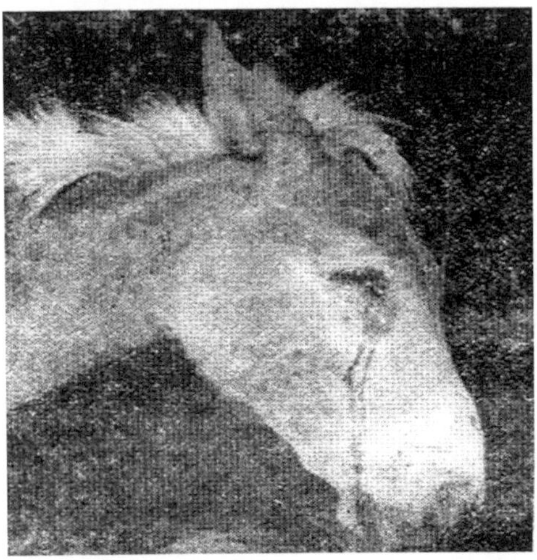

Fig. 16.2: Photograph showing mallein reaction

(1) DNCB/DNFB induced DTH Reaction

Sometimes chemicals (DNCB/DNFB) are used to measure the DTH reaction nonspecific to any disease agent. For the purpose the skin of the area should be cleaned and shaved to remove hair/feather follicles. About 1 cm2 area is marked with marker pen and 0.25 ml of DNCB/DNFB (10 mg/ml) is applied intradermally in the marked area. The vehicle (acetone) is used as control on another side of skin. After 15 days of sensitization, 0.25 ml of DNCB/DNFB (1 mg/ml) is again applied intradermally on same site and vehicle on control area. Measure the skin thickness at 0, 12, 24, 36, 48 and 60 hours of post challenge. Examine the area for erythema, induration, ulceration and scab formation (Fig. 16.3 to 16.5).

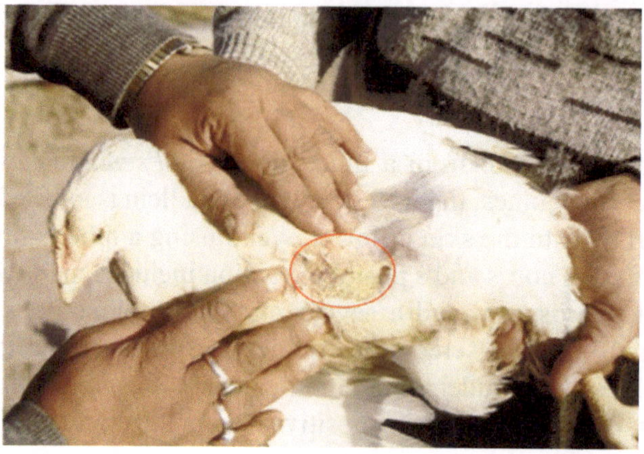

Fig. 16.3: DTH Reaction due to DNFB in poultry

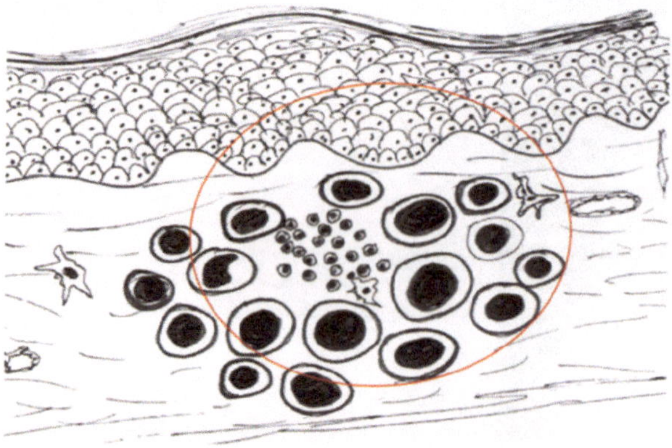

Fig. 16.4: Diagram showing microscopic picture of DTH reaction

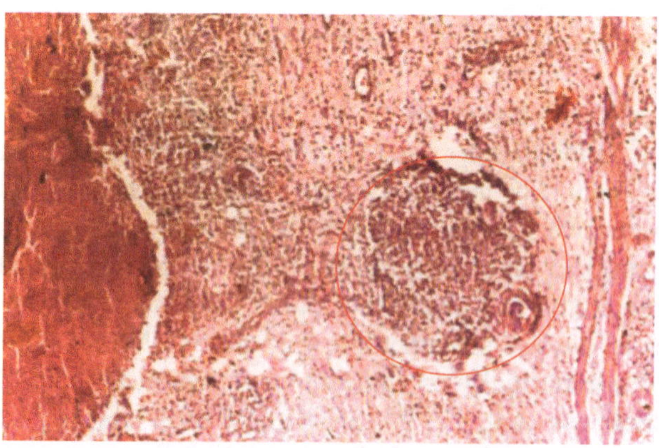

Fig. 16.5: Microscopic picture of DTH Reaction- Lympho-follicular reaction

Immunofluorescence Techniques (IFT)

Immunofluorescence techniques are being used in diagnosis of several viral and bacterial diseases since long and are considered one of the confirmatory tests for the diagnosis of rabies in animals. This provides definitive diagnosis within a few hours and is the simplest way of identifying the new isolates of viruses. The immunofluorescence test involves the detection of antigen in specimen with the help of antibody commonly labelled with dye fluorescein isothiocyanate (FITC) through direct and indirect methods. Using immunofluorescence techniques, antigen can be demonstrated in frozen tissue sections, biopsy materials, exfoliated cells and scrapped cells, Besides, cell cultures can be used for identification of viral antigens. Formalin fixed tissue sections can also be used after digestion with proteolytic enzymes to get better results. This test is simple, rapid and quite sensitive but requires a fluorescent microscope for demonstration of fluorescence. The routine immunofluorescence procedures used are discussed under two heads.

Direct Method

In the direct method, primary antibody is labelled with (FITC) dye and antigen is detected in specimen by applying the FITC labelled antibodies (Fig.16.6). Direct method has the advantage of its rapidity.

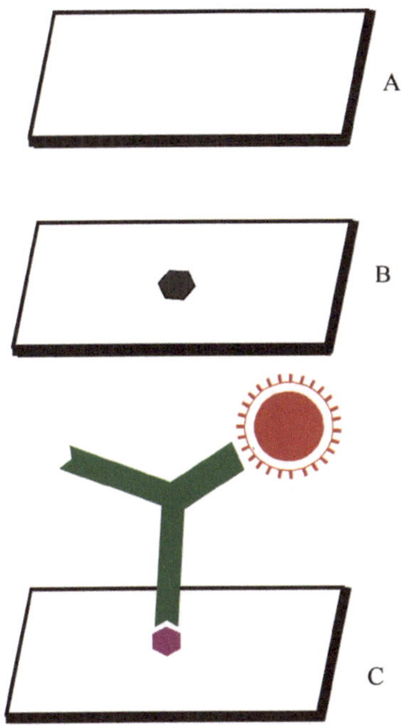

Fig. 16.6: Diagram showing direct immunofluorescence test

Indirect Method

In the indirect method, the primary antibody is not labelled with fluorescein dye but a secondary antibody is labelled; the secondary antibody is raised against the species of origin of primary antibody (Fig.16.7). For example, if the primary antibody is raised in rabbit, the secondary antibody will be antirabbit immunoglobulin tagged with FITC. The primary antibody is specific for antigen while secondary antibody is specific to primary antibody; thus the indirect method has several advantages over direct method of immunofluorescence.

1. The primary antibody against different infectious agents can be prepared in one animal species (e.g. rabbit), which requires only one conjugate, i.e. antirabbit IgG-FITC conjugate for diagnosis of all diseases against which the sera are raised in rabbit.
2. Indirect method is more sensitive due to additional combining sites made available by primary antibody.
3. The indirect method can also be used for detection of antibody in serum using known antigen in the form of smear, tissue section or cell cultures.

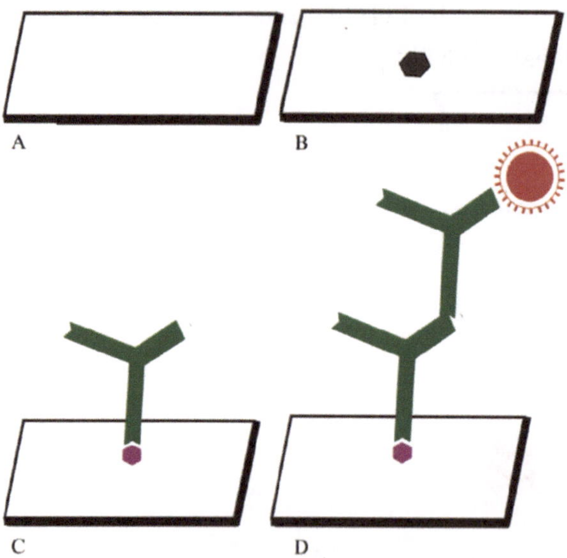

Fig. 16.7: Diagram showing indirect immunofluorescence test (**A.** Glass slide, **B.** Antigen on smear /tissue section **C.** Primary antibody birds with antigen and **D.** Immunofluorescence)

Procedure

Immunofluorescence Test for Diagnosis of Rabies

1. Frozen tissue sections or impression smears are made from medulla, cerebellum and hippocampus of the suspected animal. Tissues are touched on clean glass slides for impression smears. It is always better to have duplicate slides for immunofluorescence test; one for test and another for control.

2. The slides are air dried and fixed in chilled acetone for 30 min to 1 hour.

Flow diagram of Immounofluorescence test.

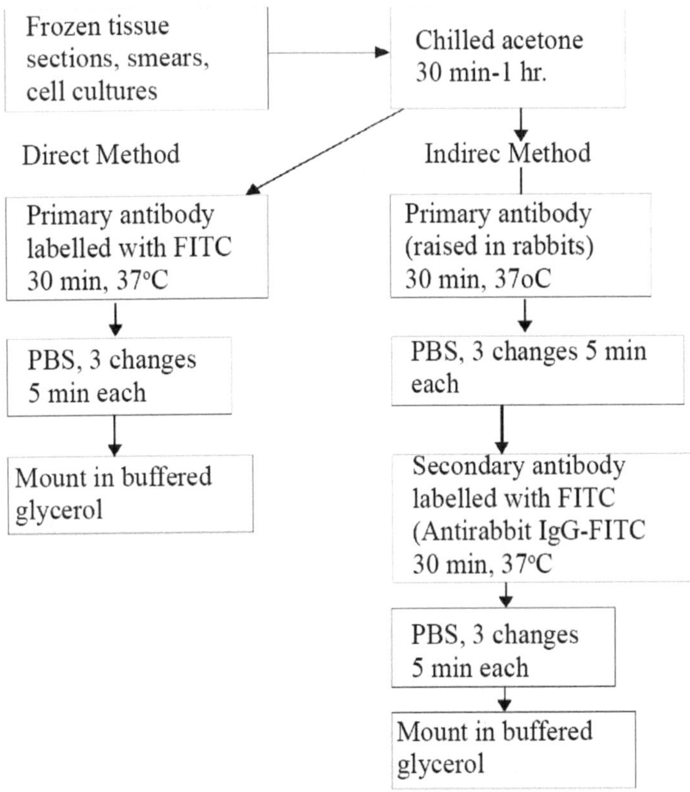

3. The primary antibody directed against rabies virus in rabbits are applied on test slides where as, control slides are treated with normal rabbit serum negative for rabies antibodies for 30 min at 37^{0}C in a humid chamber.

4. Wash the slides three times in 0.1 M PBS (pH 7.2) for 5 min each.

5. Apply antirabbit IgG-FITC conjugate in optimum dilution for 30 min at 37ºC in humid chamber.
6. Wash the slide thrice in PBS for 5 min each.
7. Place a drop of buffered glycerol (glycerol 9 parts: 0.1 M PBS (pH 7.2) 1 part) on section or smear.
8. Mount with coverslip. Keep the mounted slides in humid chambers at 4ºC.
9. Examine the slides under fluorescent microscope. In positive cases, the yellow-green fluorescing cells can be demonstrated.

Immunofluorescence test for diagnosis of rotavirus infection in calves

a. *Fecal smear method:* Make a fecal suspension (1:10) in 0.1M PBS (pH 7.2) and prepare smears on clean glass slides.
b. *Intestinal scrapped cell method:* Take about 5-10 cm long segment of intestine from duodenum, jejunum and ileum, open and remove the contents gently. Scrape the mucosal cells using clean glass slides or knife and prepare smear.

2. Dry the smears in air and fix them in chilled acetone for 30 min.
3. Apply antibovine rotavirus serum raised in rabbits on test slides while normal rabbit serum negative to bovine rotavirus antibodies is applied on control slides. Keep the slides for 30 min at 37ºC in humid chamber.
4. Wash the slides in 0.1 M PBS (pH 7.2) three times for 5 min. each.
5. Apply antirabbit IgG-FITC conjugate in optimum dilution for 30 min at 37ºC in humid chamber.
6. Wash the slides in PBS; three changes of 5 min each.
7. Place a drop of buffered glycerol on smear and mount with coverslip.
8. Examine the slides under fluorescent microscope. Cells containing rotavirus in test slides will show a positive yellow green fluorescence (Fig.16.8).

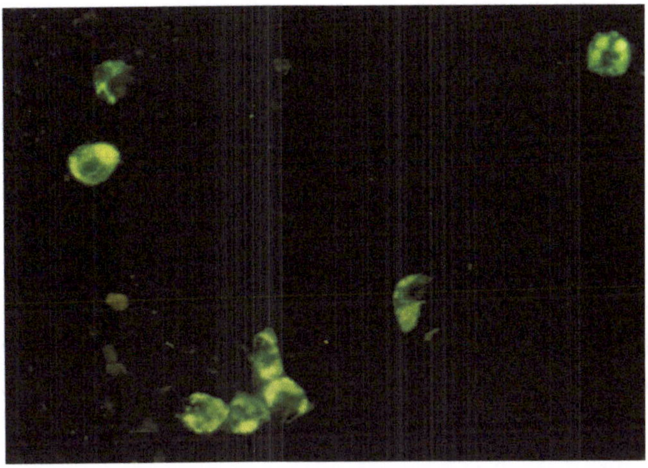

Fig. 16.8: Photomicrograph showing immunofluorescence for demonstration of antigen in cells

Immunoperoxidase Techniques

Immunoperoxidase techniques are being successfully used for the detection of antigen in tissue sections in many diagnostic laboratories. This technique requires the antibody labelled with an enzyme known as horse raddish peroxidase (HRP) instead of fluorescein dye used in immunofluorescence tests and the antigen-antibody complexes are detected using an enzyme substrate, which gives coloured reaction visibile to eyes. It has several advantages over immunofluorescence technique and it does not require the expensive equipment like a fluorescent microscope. In immunoperoxidase technique, clear non-fading permanent preparations are produced which are visualized under ordinary light microscope. The slides stain with immunoperoxidase can be stored for a long period in the same way as other histopathological slides. This technique is also useful in studying the role of dual infections by using a second antibody directed against another antigen. Further, the immunoperoxidase techniques are valuable for retrospective studies using previous paraffin blocks.

The basic principle of immunoperoxidase techniques is similar to that of immunofluorescence for detection of antigen in tissues. As in case of ELISA, primary antibody labelled with horse raddish peroxidase is used in direct method (Fig.16.9) while in indirect method the secondary antibody is labelled with enzyme (Fig.16.10). The presence of antigen-antibody complexes is detected by using diaminobenzidine tetrahydrochloride (DAB) as substrate which gives insoluble brown colour precipitate. The main disadvantage of immunoperoxidase technique is the endogenous peroxidase present in various cells like leucocytes, which may give false positive results. To overcome this problem, before applying primary antibody the endogenous peroxidase activity should be removed and control slides should always be run for comparison. The immunoperoxidase techniques are not only used for detection of antigen in tissues but also for demonstration of specific antibody producing cells. Besides, tissues, cell monolayers, impression smears, exfoliated cells and scrapings can also be used for demonstration of antigen by immunoperoxidase.

In immunoperoxidase method, cryosections or the tissues fixed in formol saline or buffered formalin are used but for a better contrast of staining, tissues and cell monolayers should be preserved in formol sublimate; which constitutes 9 parts saturated mercuric chloride solution and 1 part of formaldehyde. Tissues are fixed in formol sublimate for 24 hours; thereafter, the fixative is replaced by 80% ethanol.

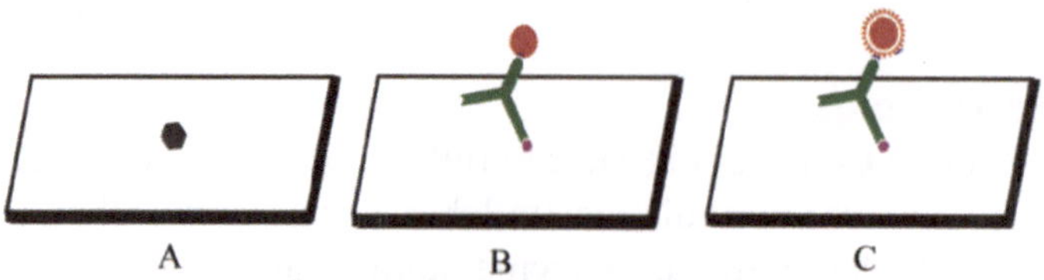

Fig. 16.9: Diagram showing direct immunoperoxidase test (**A.** Antigen in tissue section, **B.** Conjugated antibody binds with antigen, and **C.** peroxidase reaction of substrate.

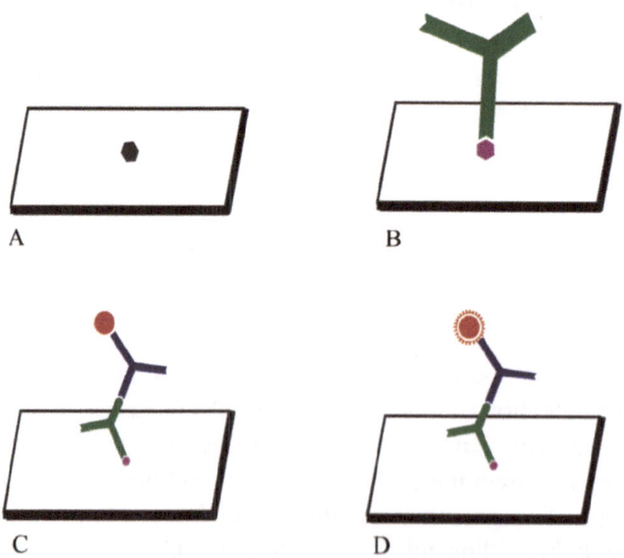

Fig. 16.10: Diagram showing indirect immunoperoxidase test (**A.** Antigen in tissue section, B. Primary antibody binds with Ag **C.** Secondary antibody binds with primary antibody and antigen complex and **D.** peroxidase reaction of substrate.

Detection of Antigen

Procedure

The paraffin embedded tissue sections of 4-5 μ thickness are made using standard istopathological procedures and the slides, after drying, are processed in following ways.

1. *Removal of paraffin and hydration:* After applying gentle heat, the slides are kept in xylene for at least 30 min (two changes of 15 min each), then in xylene absolute ethanol (1:1, V/V) for 5 min and hydrated in descending series of ethanol i.e. absolute, 95%, 90%, 80%, 70%, and 50% ethanol (5 min in each).
2. *Clearing:* Slides are then taken into water and cleaned with muslin cloth. The extra sections are removed here from slides.
3. *Removal of mercuric chloride deposits* : In formol sublimate fixed tissue sections, residual mercuric chloride deposits are present which can be removed by placing the slides in Gram's iodine for 5 min followed by immersion in 5.0% sodium thiosulfate solution for 5 min. Thereafter the slides are washed in 0.2 M PBS (pH 7.2).
4. *Inhibition of endogenous peroxidase:* The endogenous peroxidase activity can be inhibited by using 0.5% hydrogen peroxide in methanol, 10% hydrogen peroxide in methanol, 0.07% hydrochloric acid in ethanol and by periodic acid- sodium borohydride. However, the latter method of removing endogenous peroxidase activity is considered quite satisfactory as it does not permit any false positive reaction. It is done by placing the slides initially in 0.01 M periodic acid solution for 10 min followed by 0.003 M sodium borohydride solution for30 min. Finally, slides are washed in 0.2 M PBS (pH 7.2) thrice for 5 min each.
5. *Application of primary antibody:* (a) For direct method, the primary antibody directed against antigen is labelled with peroxidase conjugate and applied on sections in optimum dilutions for 24 hours at 4^0C. (b) For indirect method, the primary antibody raised in rabbits directed against antigen is applied in optimum dilutions on tissues for 24 hours at 4^0C. For control slides use normal rabbit serum which is negative for specific antibodies; wash the slides in 0.2 M PBS (pH 7.2) three times for 5 min. each.

Flow diagram of Immunoperoxidase techniques for detection of antigen in tissue

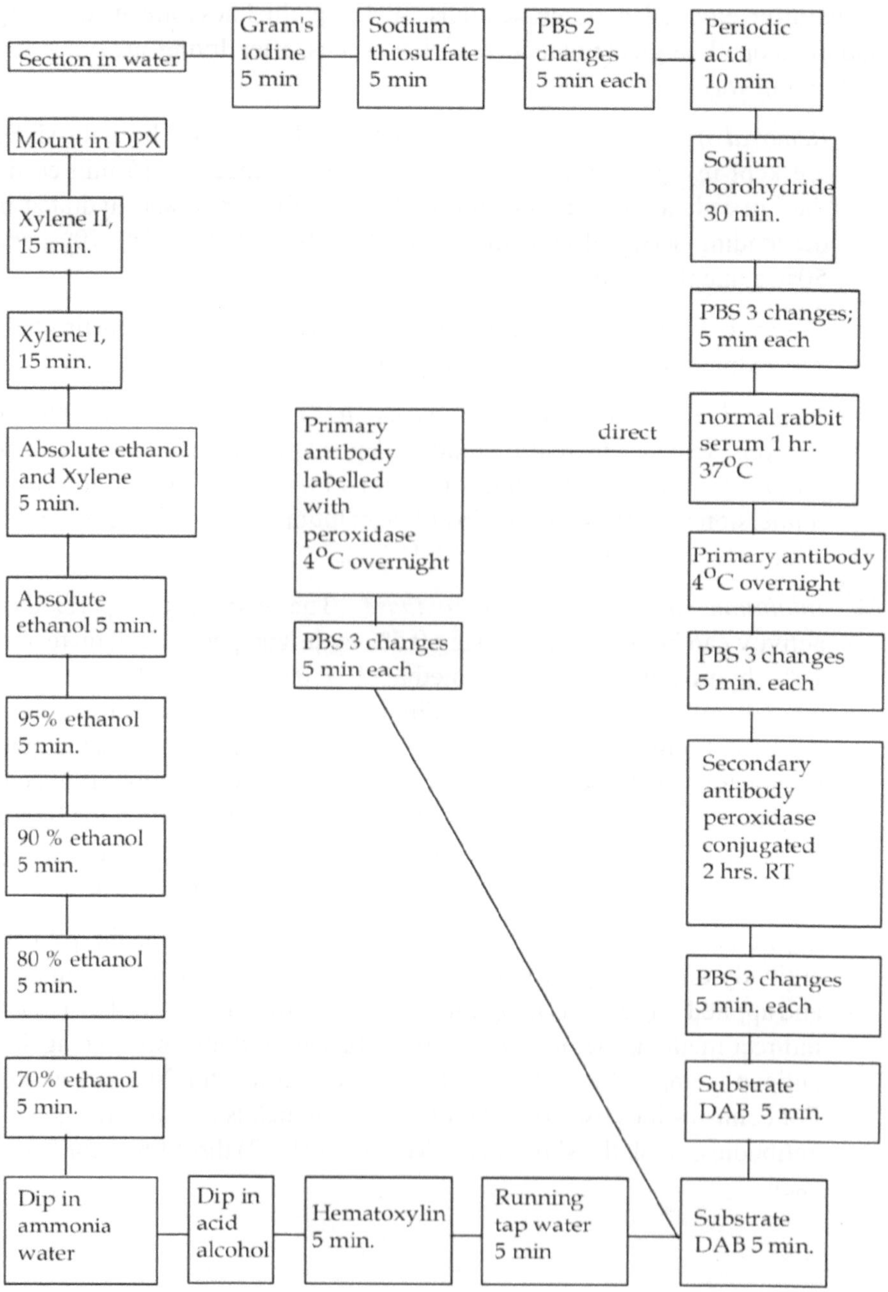

6. *Application of secondary antibody* : This step is not required in direct method. For indirect method, apply antispecies antibody (antirabbit immunoglobulin) peroxidase conjugate in proper dilutions on tissue sections for 2 hours at room temperature. Thereafter wash the slides with 0.2 M PBS (pH 7.2) three times for 5 min each.

7. *Application of substrate:* Apply freshly prepared 0.05% diaminobenzidine tetrahydrochloride in PBS containing 0.01% H_2O_2 for 5 min and wash the slides in running tap water for 5 min to stop the reaction.

8. *Counter staining:* Stain the slides in Meyers or Harris hematoxylin for 5 min, differentiate in acid alcohol and blued in ammonia water or tap water.

9. *Dehydration and clearing:* Dehydrate the slides in ascending series of alcohol, i.e. 50%, 70%, 80%, 90%, 95% and absolute ethanol, by placing the slides for 5 min in each dilution. Thereafter place the slides in absolute ethanol: Xylene (1:1) mixture for 5 min and clear in xylene for 30 min (two changes of 15 min each) and mount in DPX.

10. *Examination/Interpretation:* The stained slides are examined under ordinary light microscope for the presence of antigen which will have a brown red colour against light blue back ground (Fig.16.11). Compare the results with control slides for proper interpretation.

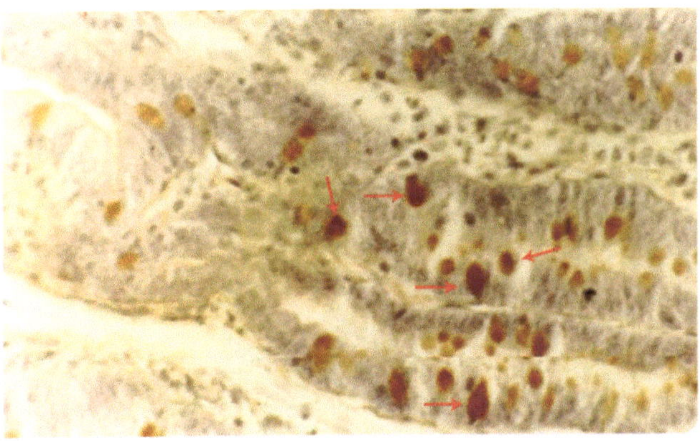

Fig. 16.11: Immunoperoxidase technique for demonstration of rotavirus antigen in intestines

Demonstration of Antibody Producing Cells

For detection of specific antibody producing cells in tissues, the following step is added before application of primary antibody in immunoperoxidase techniques of antigen detection.

Application of antigen: After the inhibition of endogenous peroxidase activity and washing the slides thrice in PBS, the antigen is applied over the sections for 1 hour at 37^{0}C so as to bind it with antibodies present on the surface of lymphocytes in tissues. Thereafter washing is done in PBS (3 changes of 5 min each) and other steps are followed similar to those of immunoperoxidase techniques (with the application of primary antibody).

Examination and Interpretation

The slides are examined under ordinary light microscope. Specific antibody producing cells appear as brown red coloured cells which can be counted in test slides. The control slides are also examined for comparison, which are stained as described for antigen detection. The brown red coloured cells (Fig.16.12) are counted in comparison to controls. Localization of antibody producing cells is useful for diagnosis of those conditions in which the infectious agent is removed quickly from the body, e.g. rotavirus infection. Rotavirus is eliminated from the intestinal tract of calves within 6-7 days: thereafter only antibody producing cells can be demonstrated. Further, this method is useful in enumeration of isotype specific cells in tissues particularly in infections in which local immune response plays a significant role (Fig. 16.13).

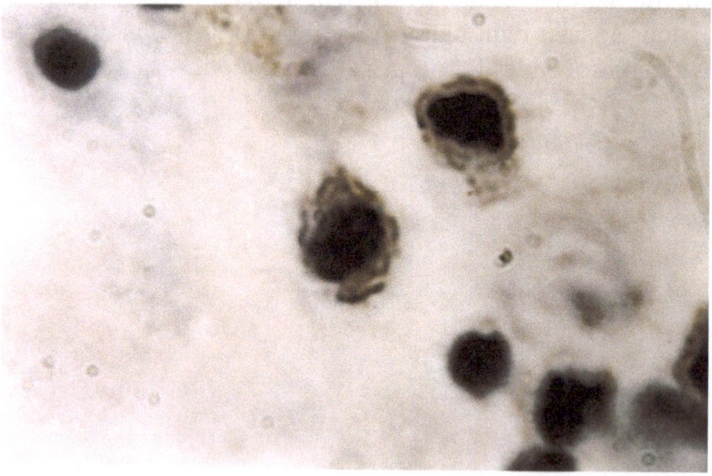

Fig. 16.12: Photomicrograph showing demonstration of T- and B-cell subsets by immunoperoxidase technique

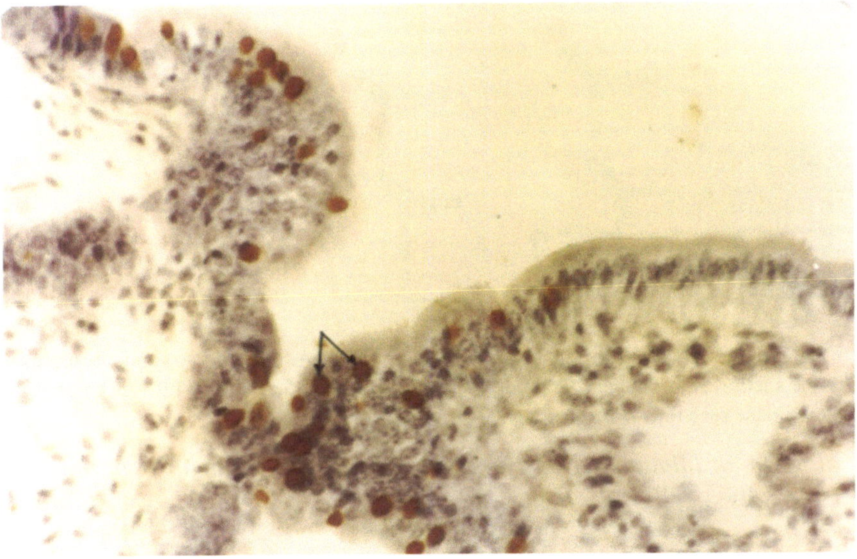

Fig. 16.13: Photomicrograph showing detection of antibody producing cells by immunoperoxidase technique

Detection of Immune Complexes

Immune complexes are localized in kidneys as they are responsible for glomerulonephritis which is an emerging disease condition in animals. Immune complexes are formed as a result of antigen-antibody reaction in the body; normally they are phagocytosed by macrophages and removed from the system. When the quantity of these complexes is pathologically increased, they get deposited in the glomerulus and cause inflammation. Thus the demonstration of immune complexes in the glomeruli has been considered diagnostic in glomerulonephritis and type III hypersensitivity reaction seven if the exact cause is not known. The exact etiology for the formation of immune complexes appears to be difficult to establish. Various techniques are used for localization of immune complexes of which immunoperoxidase (Fig.16.14) and peroxidase-antiperoxidase (PAP) methods are considered sensitive and reliable.

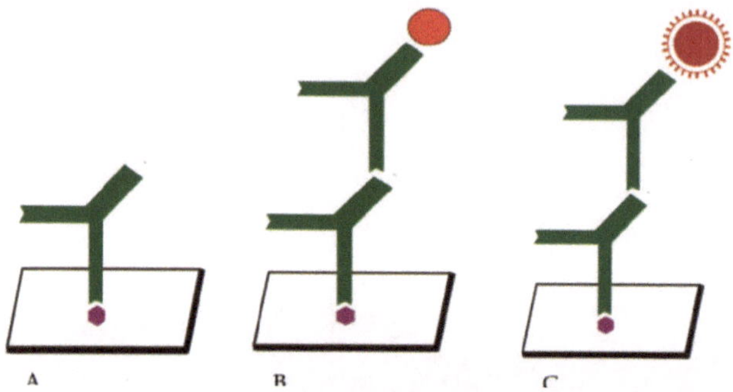

Fig. 16.14: Diagram showing immune complex in kidneys (A. Antigen antibody complex in smear/tissue section B. secondary antibody Peroxidase conjugated binds with Ag-Ab complex and C. Peroxidase reaction with substrate

Flow diagram of Immunoperoxidase technique for demonstration of antibody producing cells.

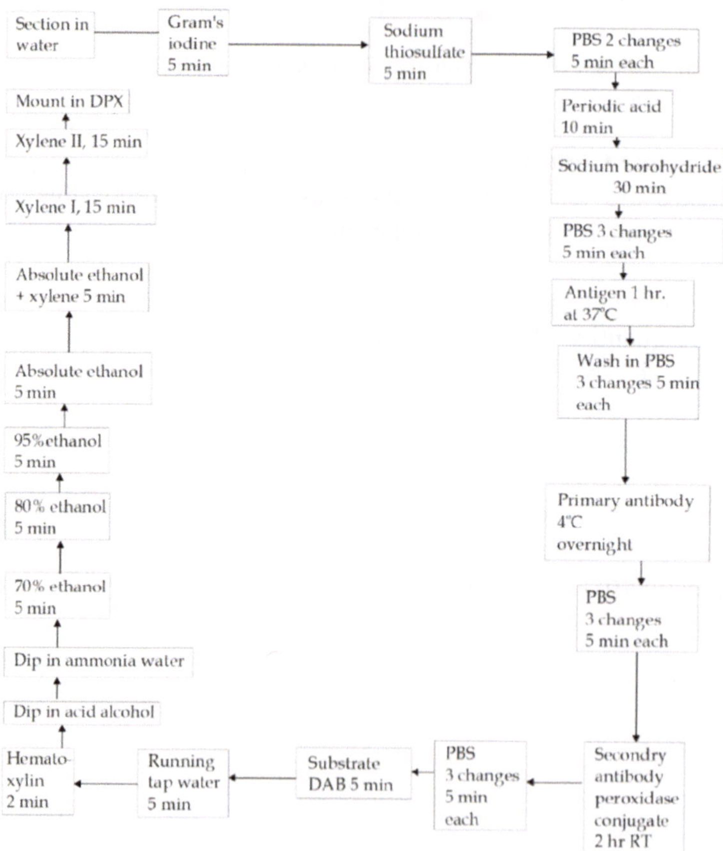

Procedure

For the demonstration of immune complexes, IgM, IgG, IgA and C_3 are localized in the glomeruli of either frozen sections or formalin fixed sections of kidneys. The tissue pieces of kidneys are collected in formol sublimate or neutral buffered formalin; after 24 hours the former is replaced by 80% ethanol. The tissues are processed in same manner as described under immunoperoxidase techniques up to removal of mercuric chloride deposits and thereafter the following steps are carried out.

1. Incubate the sections with 0.1% trypsin and 0.1% calcium chloride solution (pH 7.8) for 1 hour at 37^{0}C.
2. Wash the slides in 0.2 M PBS (pH 7.2) three times for 5 min each.
3. Apply anti IgG, anti IgM, anti IgA and anti C_3 of the species in which the immune complexes are demonstrated, i.e. if immune complexes are demonstrated in kidneys of cattle, use antibovine IgG peroxidase conjugate, antibovine IgM peroxidase conjugate, antibovine IgA peroxidase conjugate and antibovine C3-peroxidase conjugate. Use separate sections or slides for each immunoglobulin isotype (IgG, IgM, IgA) and complement fraction (C_3).
4. Wash the slide in PBS three times for 5 min each.
5. Apply substrate diaminobenzidine tetrahydrochloride (DAB) 0.05% in 0.1 M tris hydrochloride buffer containing 0.01% hydrogen peroxide for 10 min at room temperature.
6. Wash the slide in running tap water for 5 min to stop the reaction.
7. Counterstain with hematoxylin for 5 min; dehydrate in ascending series of alcohol, clear in xylene and mount in DPX as described under immunoperoxidase techniques.

Flow diagram of Immunoperoxidase technique for demonstration of Immune complex in kidneys.

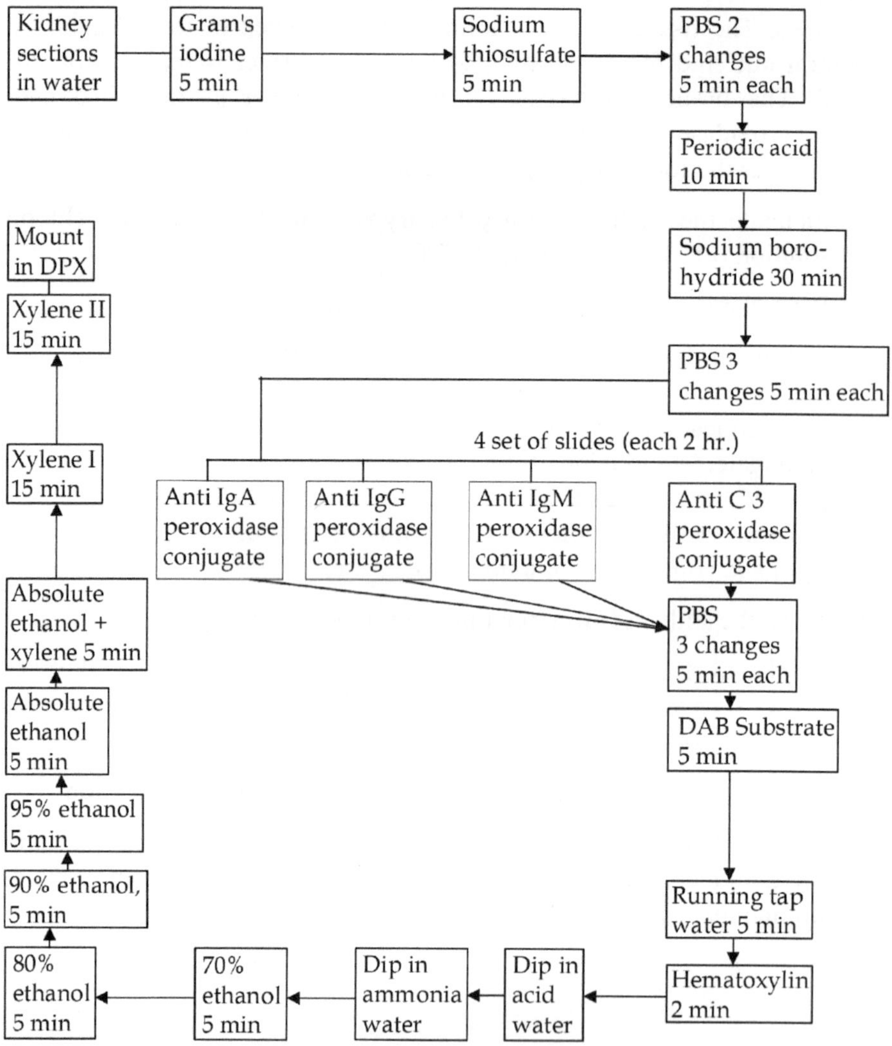

Interpretation

The slides are examined under ordinary light microscope for the presence of immune complexes in glomerulus. The granular brown red coloured immune complexes are observed in glomerular basement membrane in case of immune complex mediated glomerulonephritis. (Fig. 16.15).

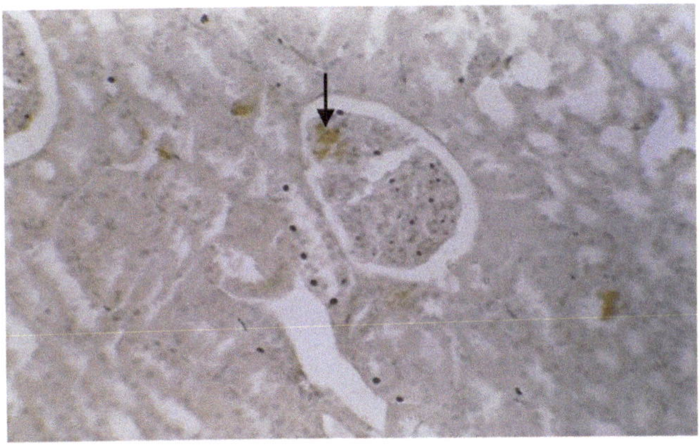

Fig. 16.15: Photomicrograph of kidney showing immune complexes using immunoperoxidase technique

Peroxidase-Antiperoxidase Method

The peroxidase-antiperoxidase (PAP) method has the same principle as indirect immunoperoxidase techniques but involve three reagents, i.e. primary antibody, secondary antibody and peroxidase antiperoxidase complex. The PAP complex includes an enzyme known as horse radish peroxidase and its antibody. The primary antibody is specific to antigen and the secondary antibody is capable of binding with both primary antibody and PAP complex because both are produced in the same animal species. The PAP method is more sensitive than the direct and indirect immunoperoxidase techniques but it has a disadvantage that it is time consuming.

Procedure

The peroxidase-antiperoxidase method is almost similar to the immunoperoxidase (Fig. 16.16) but the following additional steps are required after step 6, i.e. application of secondary antibody.

1. Apply unconjugated secondary antibody, e.g. antirabbit IgG for 30 min at 37^{0}C. Wash the slides in PBS three times (5 min each.).
2. Place a few drops of PAP complex on sections and incubate for 30 min at 37^{0}C. Wash the slides with PBS three times for 5 min each.
3. Continue with step 7 of the immunoperoxidase techniques.

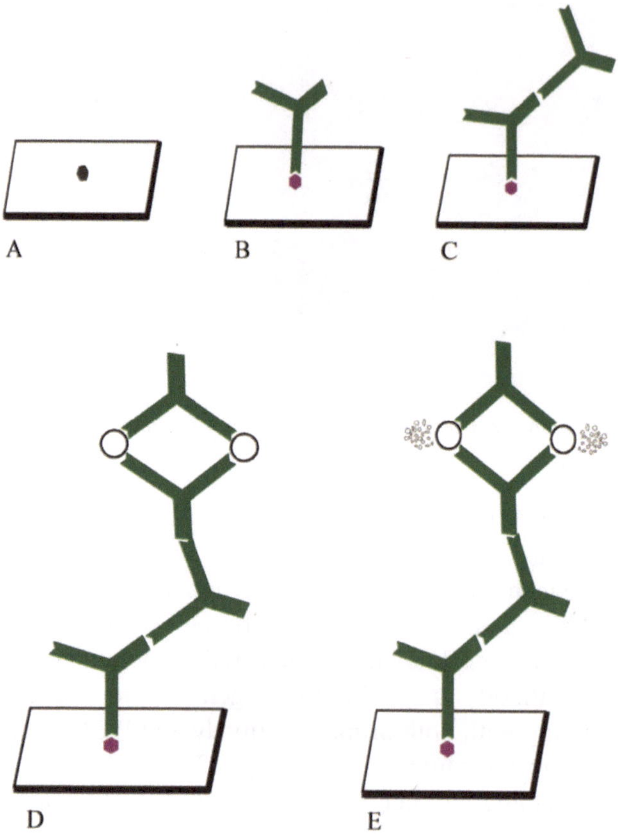

Fig. 16.16: Diagram showing PAP techniques **A.** Antigen in tissue section/ smear, antibody binds with primary antibody +antigen. **D.** PAP complex binds with **C.** and **E.** Peroxidase reaction of substrate on **D.**

Interpretation

Examine the slides under ordinary light microscope and interpret in same manner as described under indirect immunoperoxidase techniques.

Avidin-Biotin Techniques

The avidin-biotin method is considered to be a more sensitive method than other immunoperoxidase techniques. This is based on the ability of egg white glycoprotein "avidin" to bind with four molecules of vitamin "biotin". In avidin-biotin techniques, the secondary antibody is labelled with biotin which is detected by either avidin labelled with peroxidase or bridged avidin-biotin method or by using an avidin-biotin complex. This method, because of its sensitivity, can be used for detection of those antigens which are present in meagre amounts viz. hormones. The avidin-biotin system is performed in three different ways which can be used for detetcion of antigen, immune complexes and antibody producing cells.

Enzyme Labelled Avidin-Biotin Method (Fig.16.17)

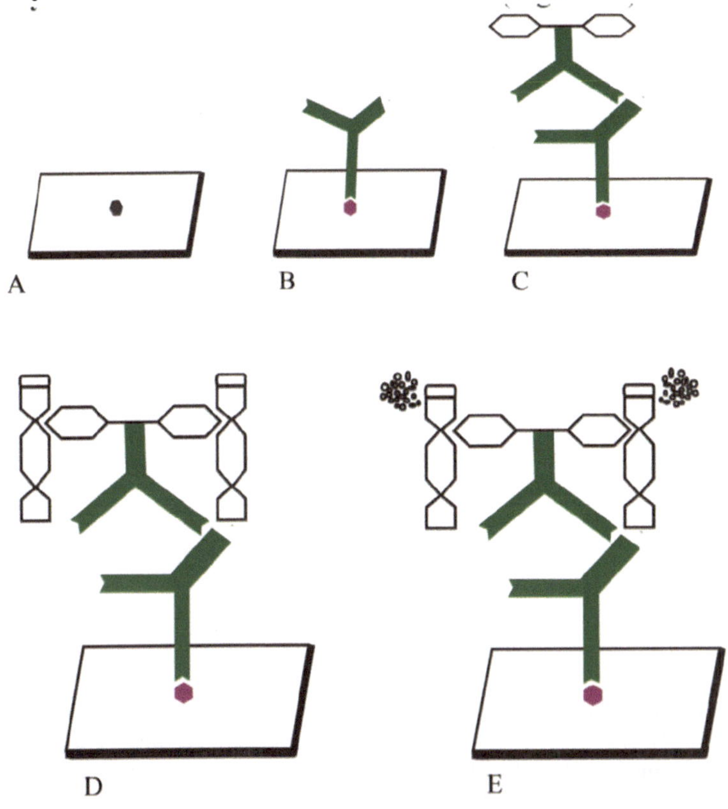

Fig. 16.17: Diagram showing enzyme labeled avidin-biotin techniques (**A.** Antigen in smear/ tissue section **B.** Primary antibody binds with antigen, **C.** Secondary antibody labeled with biotin binds with B, **D.** Avidin conjugated with Peroxidase binds with **D.** and **E.** Peroxidase reaction with substrate)

In this method, the biotinylated secondary antibody and peroxidase conjugated avidin are used. The technique is similar to immunoperoxidase method up to step 5 which is followed as under:

1. Apply biotinylated secondary antibody for 1 hour at 37^{0}C, there after wash the slides with PBS three times for 5 min each.

2. Place the avidin-peroxidase conjugated on sections for 1 hour at 37ºC and wash the slides thrice in PBS (5 min each).
3. Continue with step 7 onward as detailed under imunoperoxidase techniques.

Bridged Avidin-Biotin Method (Fig.16.18)

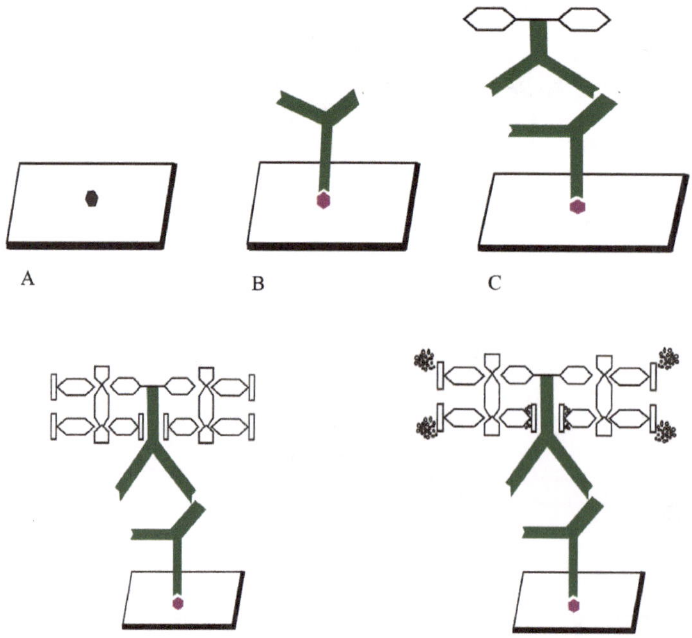

Fig. 16.18: Diagram showing bridged avidin-biotin techniques (**A.** antigen in smear/tissue section **B.** Primary antibody binds with antigen. **C.** Secondary antibody conjugated with biotin binds with **B, D.** Avidin binds with **C, E.** Biotin conjugated with peroxidase binds with Avidin at **D** and **F** Peroxidase reaction of substrate)

1. The biotin labelled secondary antibody is applied as above (1) on slides, wash three times in PBS (5 min each).
2. Apply avidin 10 mg/ml in PBS on the sections for 15 min at 37ºC. Wash three times in PBS (5 min each).
3. Apply biotin labelled with peroxidase on sections for 1 hour at 37ºC. Wash three times in PBS (5 min each).
4. Follow from step 7 onward as described in immunoperoxidase techniques.

Flow diagram of PAP method

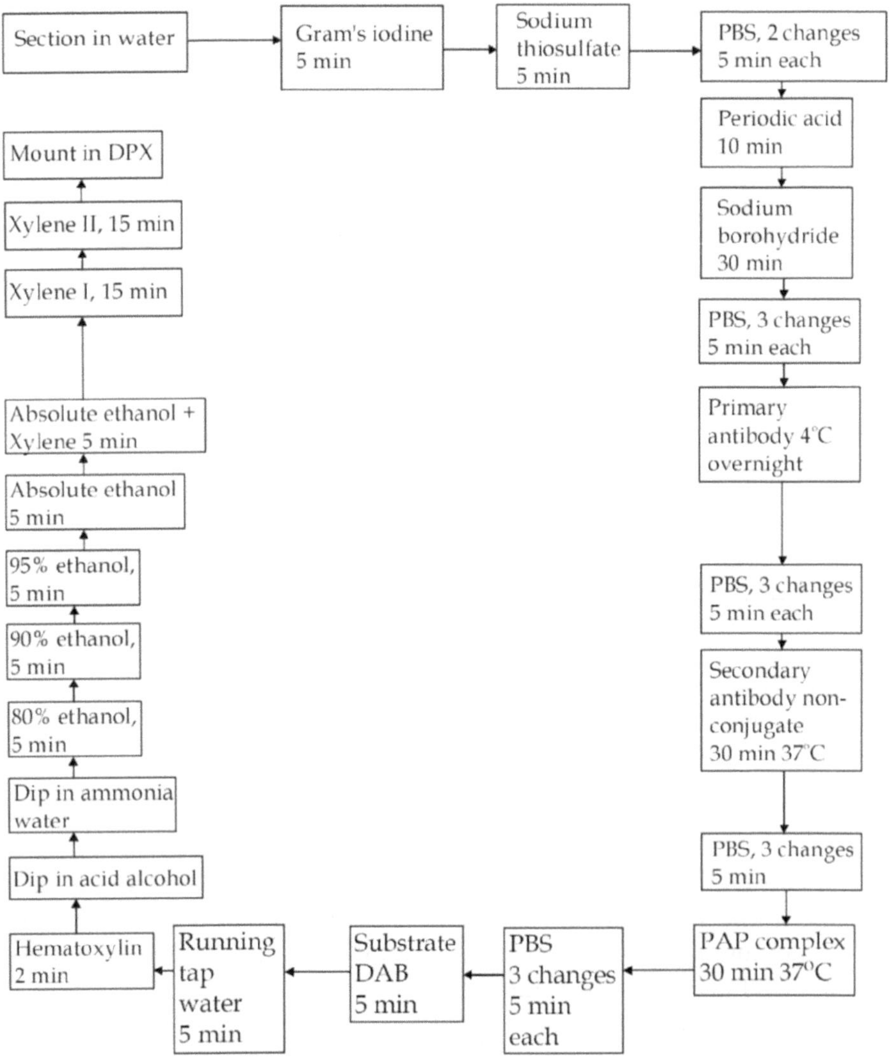

Avidin-Biotin Complex (ABC) Assay (Fig.16.19)

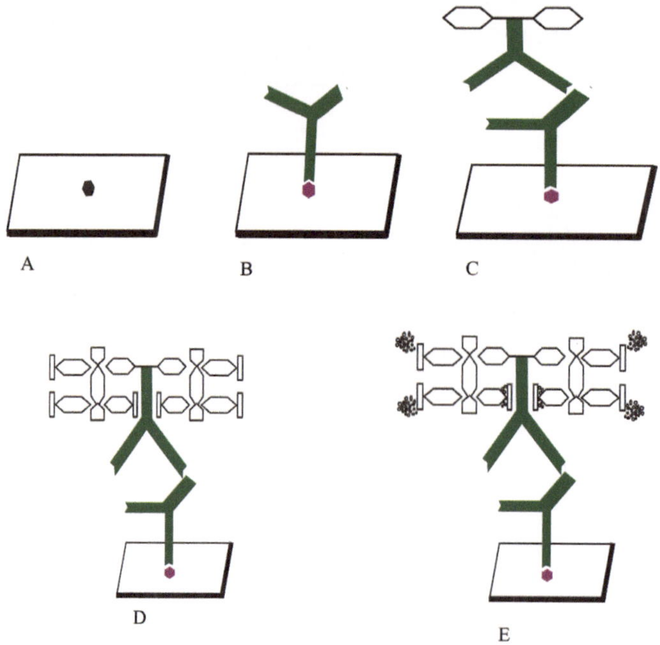

Fig. 16.19: Diagram showing avidin-biotin complex assay (**A.** Antigen in smear/ tissue section **B.** Primary antibody binds with antigen **C.** Secondary antibody labeled with biotin binds with B, **D.** Avidin-Biotin –peroxidase conjugate binds with C and **E.** Peroxidase reaction of substrate)

1. The step (1) of enzyme labelled avidin-biotin method is followed in same manner.
2. Apply avidin-biotin peroxidase complex mixture on slides for 1 hour at 37°C. The avidin-biotin peroxidase mixture contains 5 μg avidin, 2 μg biotin conjugated with peroxidase in 1 ml PBS (pH 7.2). Wash the slides in PBS three times for 5 min each.
3. Follow step 7 of the immunoperoxidase techniques described earlier.

Interpretation

Interpret the slides as described in immunoperoxidase method. The avidin-biotin techniques represent one of the most recent developments in immunoperoxidase staining.

Flow diagram of Avidin-Biotin Techniques

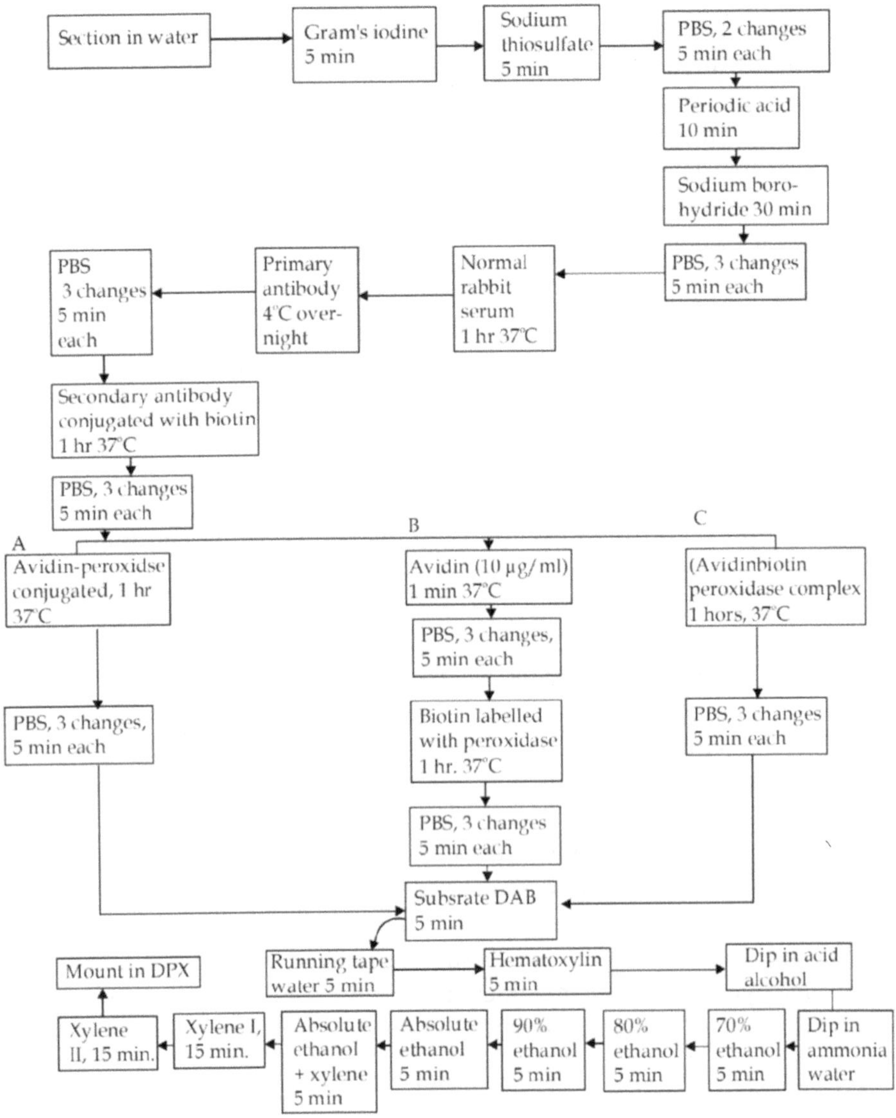

In Situ Hybridization

The *in situ* hybridization of nucleic acid is an extremely useful technique developed recently for diagnosis of infectious diseases, particularly for detection of latent viruses or tumour viruses in cells. This technique utilizes the complementary DNA or RNA probes (c DNA or c RNA probe) for detection of viruses intracellularly. The specific nucleotide sequences complementary to the virus can be synthesized in laboratory and labelled with radioisotope or biotin; this labelled complementary nucleotide sequence is known as "probe". *In situ* hybridization involves the denaturation of nucleic acid by separation of two strands using heat or sodium hydroxide and hybridization with a probe. The specific binding between nucleic acid and complementary probe is known as hybridization. The term *in situ* is applied when the nucleic acid probes are used for whole cells or sections of tissues. The advantage of *in situ* hybridization technique is not only the detection of viral genome but also its location in the cell.

The labelling of nucleic acid probe with radioisotope can be achieved by Nick translation method. Commonly used radioisotopes labelled with nucleic acid probes are 32P, 3H, 125I and 35S. An alternate to radioisotopes is biotin; the biotinylated probes can be made visible using avidin tagged with an enzyme like peroxidase and application of suitable substrate like DAB. (Ref: immunoperoxidase techniques). The hybridization through radio labelled nucleic acid probes is visualized by autoradiography while and biotinylated probes by light microscopy or electron microscopy.

Procedure

For *in situ* hybridization technique, smears of cell culture, tissue impressions or tissue sections are required. The cell smears or tissue impressions are fixed with ethanol acetic acid (3:1, (v/v) for 5-10 min which also eliminates the interference of some basic proteins. Either the smears of cells and tissue impressions are dipped into 0.4% agarose at 60^{0}C or the slides are precoated with gelatin and chrome alum in order to prevent the detachment of cells from the slides. For sections, the tissues are fixed in 10% buffered formaldehyde and processed similar to the methods used in histopathological techniques through paraffin embedding. Briefly, take tissue sections in water after removal of paraffin and hydration, clean the slides and remove artefacts. The steps required for hybridization of nucleic acid are as follows.

1. Place the slide in 0.07 N NaOH for 2 min for denaturation of nucleic acid present in cells.
2. Wash the slide twice in 70% ethanol for 5 min each.
3. Rinse in 95% ethanol followed by absolute alcohol for 5 min each.
4. Apply radiolabeled or biotinylated probe in 0.1 ml of 2 X SSC (0.15 M NaCl + 0.015 M trisodium citrate).

5. Put coverslip gently on section or smear.
6. Keep slide in chamber wet with 6 X SSC for 24 hours at 65^{0}C.
7. Wash it in 2 X SSC three times for 5 min each.
8. Treat it with 20 µg/ml RNAase for 30 min at 37^{0}C.

A. For radiolabeled nucleic acid probes

i. Wash the slide in 70% ethanol (2 changes of 5 min each) followed by 95% ethanol for 10 min and absolute ethanol 3 changes of 5 min each.

ii. Dry the slide and observe the hybridization using autoradiography.

B. For Biotinylated probes

i. Wash the slide in 2 X SSC for 5 min

ii. Apply avidin tagged with peroxidase conjugate in optimum dilutions on smears or sections for 1 hour at 37^{0}C in humid chamber.

iii. Wash the slide in PBS-Tween for 15 min (3 changes or 5 min each).

iv. Apply 0.5% diaminobenzidine tetrahydrochloride containing 0.01%, H_2O_2 in citrate buffer for 5 min.

v. Wash the slide in PBS for 5 min

vi. Dehydrate by placing in 70%, 95% and absolute ethanol for 5 min each; clear in xylene (2 changes of 5 min each) and mount using DPX or Canada balsam.

vii. Examine the slide under light microscope for hybridization which is visualized as brown dots.

The *in situ* hybridization technique is more useful in detection of nucleic acid of those viruses which are not expressed as cytopathogenic effects in the cells, e.g. retrovirus or episomal DNA in parvovirus infection. The probes can be made highly specific by selection from a collection of cloned fragments of viral genome. This technique is particularly advantageous over virus isolation in cases of viruses which are not cultivable, slow growing and dangerous. Though the *in situ* hybridization technique is quite sensitive and specific; but it is not routinely used for diagnosis and is confined to the research laboratories. Thus, the readers are advised to consult relevant literature before carrying *in situ* hybridization particularly for preparation of short length nucleic acid probes and their labelling. The nucleic acid probes are commercially available for some infectious diseases.

17

Toxins and Poisons

- General considerations
- Cyanide poisoning
- Nitrate poisoning
- Nitrite poisoning
- Oxalate poisoning
- Strychnine poisoning
- Arsenic poisoning
- Lead poisoning
- Thalium poisoning
- Ergot poisoning
- Carbon monoxide poisoning
- Phenothiazine poisoning
- Pesticide poisoning
- Organochlorine group of pesticides
- Organophosphate group of pesticides
- Carbamate group of pesticides
- Lantana poisoning
- Bracken fern poisoning
- Aflatoxins

General Considerations

Rapid advancement in human civilization have brought up many synthetic chemicals in our environment. With the increasing and indiscriminate use of chemicals in various agricultural and animal husbandry practices, the possibilities of toxicosis in animals have increased considerably. A large number of chemicals including pesticides, heavy metals, rodenticides and other chemicals are in use, which may be taken up by animals either accidentally or due to negligence of man.

These chemicals may also accumulate in the body tissues and clinically toxicosis appears after sometime. The chemical poisons are taken by animals through weeds, grass, fodder of the field in which these chemicals have been used. Certain cases of malicious poisoning in animals have also been observed during last few years. It is, however, very difficult to investigate and confirm the malicious nature of the toxicity. The veterinarians are fortunate enough as their clients do not commit suicide like in medical sciences; however, they fall sick of toxicity due to human negligence or error. The investigations of toxic conditions in animals are not only important for the accurate diagnosis and proper medication but also from the veterolegal point of view. The veterinarians should collect the proper samples from the suspected cases of toxicosis and forward them to the appropriate labora-tory for confirmation and diagnosis after proper labelling. However, the veterinarian may also carry out certain simple tests at his own level in order to provide a rapid diagnosis and initiate the treatment. For this purpose, some of the simple diagnostic tests are described here, so that these can be performed in a clinical pathology laboratory or disease investigation laboratory with minimal facilities.

Cyanide Poisoning

Cyanide poisoning occurs in animals due to sorghum and/or other chemicals and characterized by ataxia, incoordination, cystitis, paralysis, and death. Cyanide is detected in tissues/ruminal contents through chemical tests (Fig.17.1).

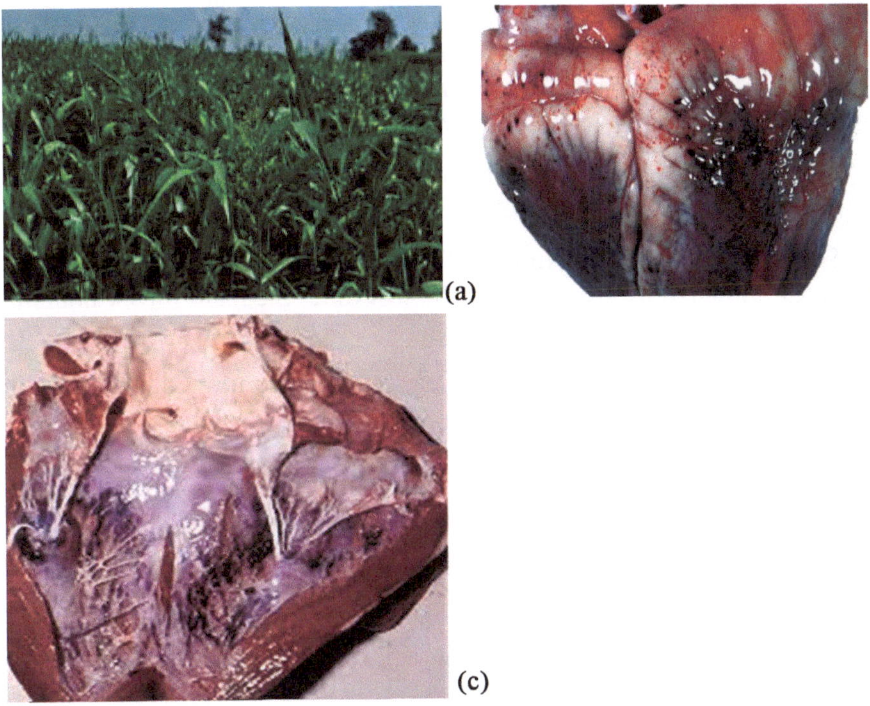

Fig.17.1: Sorghum crop – source of cyanide poisoning **(a)**, epicardial **(b)** and endocardial hemorrhage **(c)**.

Test-1

- Take 1 ml supernatant of centrifuged gastrointestinal contents in a test tube.
- Add 2 ml of 10% sodium hydroxide solution.
- Add 2 ml of 10% ferrous sulfate solution (freshly prepared in distilled water).
- Add 10% hydrochloric acid in sufficient quantity, which can dissolve the precipitate formed in the mixture due to ferrous oxide formation.
- Blue colour will develop due to formation of ferri-ferrocyanide complex (Prussian blue) in the test tube if cyanide is present in the sample of gastrointestinal contents.

Test-2.

- In a flask, take 5.0 gm sodium carbonate and 0.5 gm picric acid; dissolve in 100 ml distilled water. The filter paper strips (1 cm wide x 5 cm long) are wet in the solution and dried in air.
- Take about 5.0 gm of moist plant or rumen content and grind into small pieces and keep in test tube. Add few drops of chloroform.
- The strip is placed at the mouth of test tube, 2/3 part of which should be in test tube. Apply stop cork on the test tube. Incubate for 24 hours at 37°C.
- In cyanide positive cases, the filter paper strip becomes reddish brown in colour.

Nitrate Poisoning

Test-1

a. In a 100 ml volumetric flask, take 20 ml distilled water and dissolve 0.5 gm diphenylamine.

b. Add sufficient quantity of sulfuric acid to make it 100 ml. Store the solution in a dark coloured bottle.

c. For testing of nitrate in plants, put one drop of above solution on the cut surface of plant; in positive cases, the cut surface of plant will become green or blue in colour.

Test-2

a. It is applied on prepared and grinded folder and feed.

b. In this test, take about 5 gm grinded feed and mix it with 5-10 ml distilled water in a beaker, mix well and keep for 15-30 minute.

c. Centrifuge the contents and take out 2.0 ml supernatant in a test tube

d. Add 2 ml of 0.3% sulfanilic acid prepared in 20% glacial acetic acid, mix well.

e. Add 2 ml of 0.15% alphanaphthylamine hydrochloride in 20% glacial acetic acid.

f. Development of a pink to red colour is an indication of the presence of nitrate in the sample.

Test-3

a. This type of test can be applied to stomach or intestinal contents and in urine.

b. In a test tube take 0.1 ml of the clear stomach contents after centrifugation or urine.

c. Add 0.1 ml sulfanilic acid reagent and mix well.

d. Add 0.1 ml imipramine solution and 0.2 ml concentrated sulfuric acid and mix thoroughly.

e. Development of a blue colour confirms the presence of nitrate in the sample.

Nitrite Poisoning

a. Take 1 ml clear stomach contents or urine in a test tube and add 0.1 ml imipramine solution. Mix well.

b. Add 0.2 ml hydrochloric acid.

c. The development of a blue colour in the tube is indicative of nitrite in the sample.

Oxalate Poisoning

a. In a test tube, take 1 ml clear stomach contents or urine and add 0.2 ml concentrated ammonium hydroxide and heat it on flame of a burner or spirit lamp to evaporate the solution.

b. Add 40 mg thiobarbituric acid crystals and gently reheat on burner or spirit lamp.

c. Formation of an orange red colour, which is soluble in ethanol is indicative of oxalates in the samples.

Strychnine Poisoning

Strychnine poisoning occurs is animals as a malicious poisoning caused by baits of strychnine and characterized by nervous signs, convulsions and death within few hours (Fig.17.2). The following test can be performed to detect strychnine in tissues and/ or stomach contents.

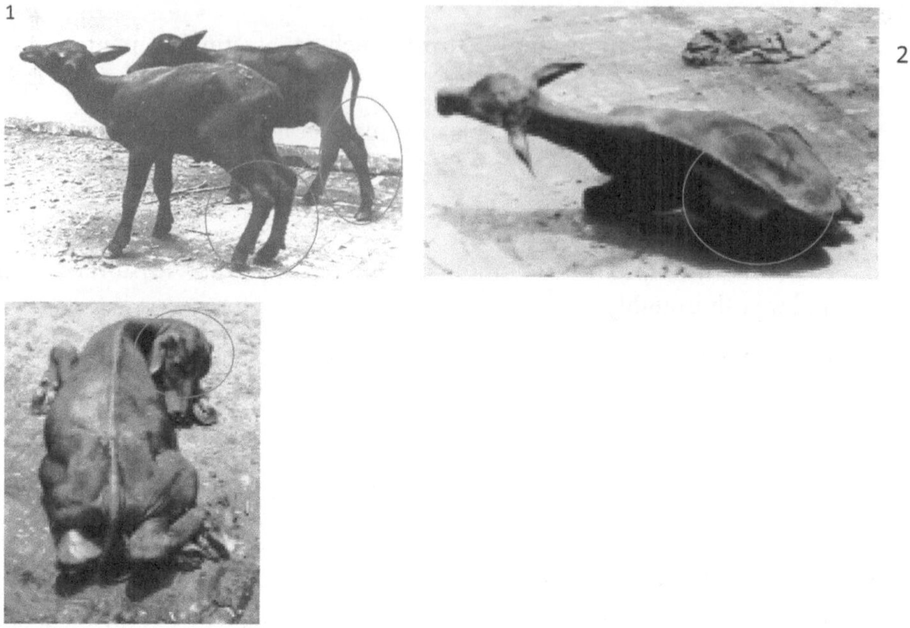

Fig. 17.2: Strychnine poisoning in animals-1.Stiffness in legs and neck, 2.Prostration and staggers and 3. Torticollis in buffalo calves.

a. Strychnine can be detected in stomach con-tents, intestinal contents, serum and urine.

b. In a clean and dry petri dish, take 1-2 ml clear stomach contents or urine and serum.

c. Add equal quantity of concentrated sulfuric acid and mix well with the glass rod.

d. Add few crystals of potassium dichromate in the contents of petri dish. Mix the contents.

e. Examine the plate for change of colour for 5-10 minute. A change in colour from yellow orange to greenish blue is indicative of the presence of strychnine.

Arsenic Poisoning

a. Take 1 ml of the stomach content fluid in a test tube. Add small crystal of zinc and 2-3 ml hydrochloric acid and 0.5 ml iodine (Lugol's iodine).

b. Place an absorbent cotton plug and put a filter paper strip wet in silver nitrate solution.*

c. If arsenic is present in the sample, the filter paper becomes yellow which may turn black if water is applied on it.

*Note: In place of silver nitrate strip at step above, one can also use filter paper strip impregnated in mercuric chloride.

Lead Poisoning

Lead toxicity occurs in animals due to its excess in environment and is characterized by gastroenteritis, muscle tremors, immunosuppression and death. The source of lead is smoke of automobiles and generator (Fig.17.3).

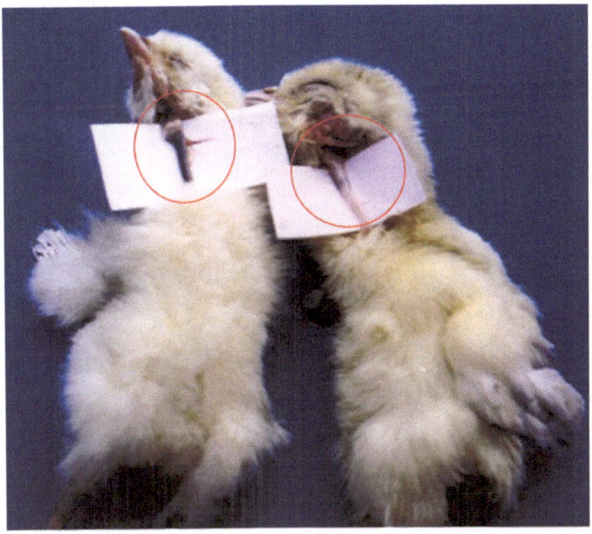

Fig. 17.3: Lead poisoning- diesel generator smoke in trachea

a. Collect about 1.0 ml of scrapings of mucosal surface of the stomach (abomasum in ruminants).

b. Mix 1 ml of concentrated nitric acid and heat gently the contents till it becomes dry.

c. Add about 0.5 ml water and 0.1 ml of 10% potassium iodide in the test tube. In case lead is present in the sample, it may give yellow colour in the test tube.

Thalium Poisoning

a. Take one ml urine in a test tube and add 1 ml of 10% potassium iodide in a petri dish. Mix them properly.

b. A yellow precipitate will appear in the tube.

c. Add 1 ml of 2% sodium thiosulfate in the test tube, if the yellow precipitate do not dissolve in it, it confirms the presence of thalium in the sample.

Ergot Poisoning

a. Take 1 ml clear supernatant of centrifuged stomach contents

b. Add 1 ml of sulfuric acid and 0.1 ml of ferric chloride solution.

c. It becomes orange red to deep red in colour with margin deep blue to greenish blue in colour, if the sample is positive for ergot poisoning.

Carbon Monoxide Poisoning

a. Take 15 ml distilled water in a small beaker and add 2-3 drops of freshly collected blood; the colour of water be-comes faint pink.

b. Add few drops 20% sodium hydroxide and mix well.

c. Observe the colour

   - Pink colour persists for 30 second— More than 20% carboxyhemoglobin
   - Pink colour changes to strain yellow colour — Less than 20% carboxyhemo-globin.

Phenothiazine Poisoning

a. Take 2 ml urine and add 6 drops of sulfuric acid and 2 drops of 10% ferric chloride.

b. Light pink to purple colour is indicative of phenothiazine compound in the sample.

Pesticide Poisoning

Organochlorine Group of Pesticides

The organochlorine group of pesticides can be detected in body tissues, stomach contents, stomach washings, urine and in blood (Fig.17.4). These are first extracted from the samples and then detected by thin layer chromatography or other available procedure. The method of extraction of organochlorine pesticides is as follows.

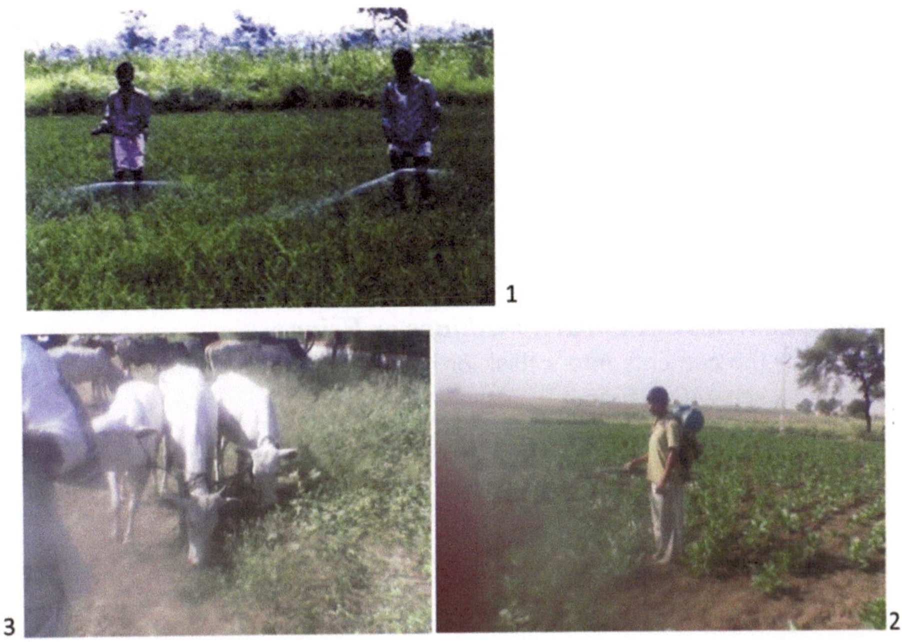

Fig. 17.4: Pesticide toxicity in animals-1. Pesticide spray on fodder crop, 2. Pesticide spray in front of grazing animals and 3. Grazing animals in pesticide spray area directly consuming the pesticide.

Tissues

a. Take 20 gm tissue, macerate into a slurry and transfer into a conical flask having air condenser.

b. Add 30 gm sodium sulfate and 50 ml acetone into slurry and place the flask in boiling water bath for 30 minute; cool and filter the contents.

c. The process of step (b) is repeated with 25 ml acetone and keeping in water bath for 30 minute, cool and filter; mix all filtrates.

d. Transfer all acetone filtrates into a separating funnel, containing 100 ml distilled water and 20 ml saturated sodium sulfate solution.

e. Extract the solution using 20 ml, 10 ml and 10 ml chloroform for 3 times after shaking 5 minute each time and transfer the separated chloroform layer in another funnel.

f. Add 20 ml of 5% potassium hydroxide solution and mix the contents for one minute.

g. Separate the chloroform layer and repeat the process as detailed in step (f) twice. Wash the chloroform layer with 20 ml distilled water for 5 times.

h. Dry the chloroform layer by passing it through 2 gm of anhydrous sodium sulfate and concentrate to 2 ml in a water bath.

i. Dry in air, solvent will evaporate and dissolve the residue in 1 ml acetone from which spot the 10 microliter on TLC plates.

Stomach contents or Stomach washings or Urine

a. Filter the contents into a flask or beaker and place about 20 ml filtrate into a separating funnel.

b. Add 10 ml saturated solution of sodium sulfate and shake with 20 ml n-hexane. Filter the n-hexane layer through 2.0 gm of anhydrous sodium sulfate.

c. Extract the aqueous layer twice with 10 ml of n-hexane and mix all the extracts.

d. Concentrate the extracts to 2 ml by keeping the contents in a flask in boiling water bath; dry in air.

e. Dissolve the residues in 1.0 ml acetone and spot 10 microliter aliquot on TLC plate.

Blood

a. Place 10 ml blood in a conical flask containing 20 ml concentrated sulfuric acid. Add 10 ml of 10% sodium tungstate and keep the flask at room temperature for 10 minute.

b. Filter the contents and transfer the filtrate into a separating funnel. Wash the residues with 10 ml distilled water and mix with the contents in separating funnel.

c. Extract the residues as in stomach contents from step (2) onward.

Thin Layer Chromatography (TLC)

a. In a flask, take 60 gm silica gel and 110 ml distilled water and mix well.

b. With the help of pipette about 10 ml of silica gel is coated on (20 x 20 cm) glass plate. A coating of 0.3 mm is sufficient. Note the direction of coating. With the available solution, one can prepare about 10 plates.

c. Dry the plates at room temperature and the plates can be preserved in desiccator.

d. Just prior to use, activate the coated plates at 90-110° C for 30 min by placing them in hot air oven.

e. Spot the plates with 10 microliter test sample as well as positive control, about one to two inches above the bottom line.

f. Dry the spot and place the plate in a chamber having solvents, close the chamber and saturate it for 2 hours. Care should be taken that the spot should be above the layer of solvent.

g. Remove the plate after the solvent reach the 10 cm point; dry the plate at room temperature.

h. Spray the plate with chromogenic reagent and dry it for 30 minute at room temperature.

i. Expose the plate to UV light (366 nm) for 10 minute.

j. Grey to black spots are observed against a white background, measure the Rf value and compare with standard organochlorine pesticide. If the Rf value is similar, the toxicant is identified as organochlorine pesticide.

Organophosphate Group of Pesticides

a. Take 20 gm tissue and macerate into a slurry by mixing 20 gm anhydrous sodium sulfate. Transfer the slurry into a conical flask fitted with air condenser. One can also use blood or stomach content, etc. in this method.

b. Add 50 ml n-hexane and heat the flask in boiling water bath for 1 hour. Filter the n-hexane layer after cooling. The extraction process is repeated twice with 25 ml n-hexane.

c. Combine all extracts and place them in a separating funnel and shake vigorously for 5 minute with 15, 10 and 10 ml of acetonitrite saturated with n-hexane.

d. Place acetonitrite layer in another separating funnel and dilute it ten times with distilled water. Add 25 ml saturated solution of sodium sulfate.

e. Extract the mixture with 25 ml of n-hexane saturated with water. Combine the extracts and keep in boiling water bath to reduce the volume to 2 ml.

f. Dry in air and dissolve the residues in 1 ml acetone.

g. Prepare the TLC plates as described in "organochlorine group of pesticides" and activate at 120°C for 30 minute in a hot air oven.

h. Spot 10 microliter residue on plate one to two inches above the border line along with a positive control.

i. Place in saturated glass chamber containing solvents; care should be taken that the spots should be above the layer of solvents. Mark the 10 cm point above.

j. Remove the plate after a run of solvent up to 10 cm mark; then dry at room temperature.

k. The plate can be seen with UV light (254 nm) for spots of P-nitrophenyl derivatives (ethyl parathion, methyl parathion and sumithion).

l. Spray the plate with 1% solution of silver nitrate, dry in air and irradiate it with UV light (366 nm) for 10 min.

m. Examine for black spots of phosphamidon and DDVP.

n. Spray with 0.5% solution of pallidium chloride in 0.1 N HC1, dry in air and keep the plate at 80°C for 20 minute. Yellow spots turning brown on heating are observed for malathion, dimethoate, diazinon, metasystox, baytex, disyston and desanit based on their Rf values.

Carbamate Group of Pesticides

a. In a 500 ml flask, take 50 gm of sample, properly grinded or chopped into a slurry and 180 ml ethanol and 120 ml distilled water is mixed into the contents. Mix the contents properly and filter.

b. Place the filtrate in a separating funnel and add 100 ml petroleum ether, 10 ml saturated sodium chloride and 500 ml distilled water and mix gently.

c. Discard the lower water layer and filter the upper ether layer through 2 inches of sodium sulfate and concentrate it to 5 ml.

d. The extraction can be repeated and combine all the extracts.

e. Concentrate all the extracts to 0.5 ml.

f. Prepare the TLC plate and activate as described in organochlorine group of pesticides. Ten microliter of the extract is spotted on TLC plate along with standard. Develop the plate in solvent ether xylene in 1:3 ratio. Calculate the Rf value and compare with extract.

g. The plate is sprayed with anisaldehyde to visualize the spot.

Lantana Poisoning

Lantana poisoning occurs in animals due to feeding of *Lantana camara* plant and characterized by Sore month, photosensitization, hepatopathy, icterus and death (Fig.17.5). Chemical tests are done for detection of lantana toxins in tissues, blood and ingesta. Its diagnosis is mainly based on the fact of grazing/ feeding of lantana and appearance of the signs and lesions of icterus in animals.

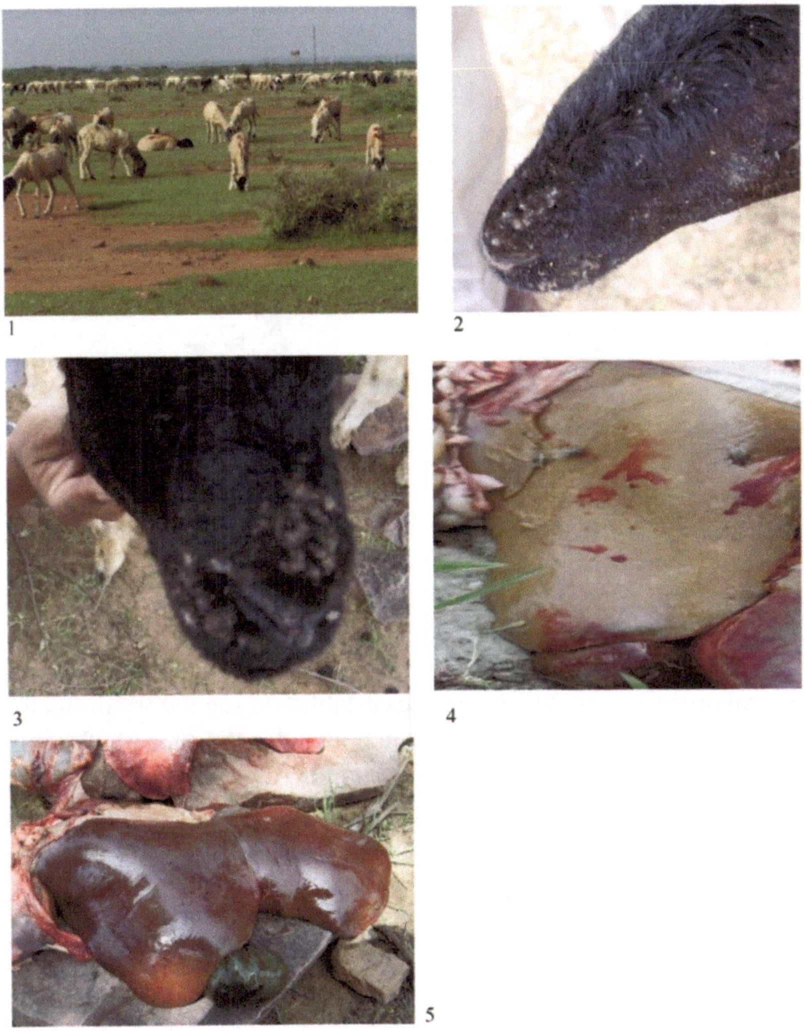

Fig. 17.5: Lantana poisoning in sheep-1. Sheep grazing in field with new growth of lantana plants just after first rain, 2.&3. Presence of scabs on mouth and face, 4.& 5. Icteric liver.

Bracken Fern Poisoning

Bracken fern poisoning occurs is animals due to ingestion of fern along with grazing or fodder and characterized by hematuria, neoplasm in urinary bladder and death (Fig.17.6). Ptaquiloside present in fern causes hematuria in cows which is presence of blood in urine and can be differentiated from that of hemoglobinuria as described earlier in this book.

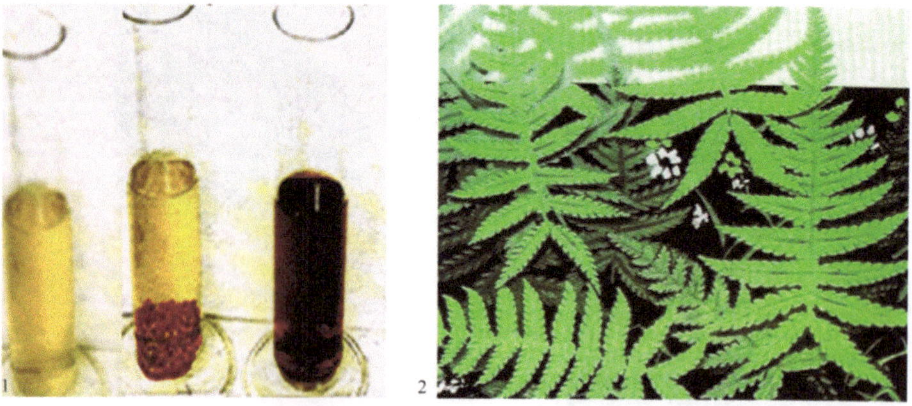

Fig. 17.6: Bracken fern poisoning in animals- 1. Hematuria and 2. Bracken fern

Analysis and Detection of Aflatoxins

In view of the evidence, particularly the carcinogenic effects of aflatoxin in several animal species, and the association between aflatoxin exposure levels and human liver cancer, exposure to aflatoxins should be kept as low as practically achievable. The tolerance levels for food products have been established in several countries, intended to facilitate the implementation of aflatoxin control programmes. Most countries established regulatory limits for either aflatoxin B1 or for total aflatoxins, which includes the sum of aflatoxin B1, B2, G1, and G2, as well as regulatory limits for Aflatoxin M1. Aflatoxin is measured in terms of parts per billion (ppb). Acceptable levels in importing countries are generally in the range 30-100 ppb.

Sampling of the food and feed samples is the first hurdle before proceeding to the detection or analysis of aflatoxins or any other mycotoxins present. The sample preparation is often challenging and remains a considerable source of error in the analytical identification of aflatoxins. It is thus crucial that sampling is carried out in a way that ensures that the analytical sample is truly representative. Therefore a systematic approach is necessary for the determination especially at low toxin levels in agricultural commodities. After the sampling procedure, all methods of detection have in common the extraction with organic solvents followed by a clean-up step before separation by various chromatographic methods. Thin layer chromatography (TLC), is a technique, which is easy to use and to identify and quantitate aflatoxins at very low levels. Another widely used reference method of aflatoxin analysis is High Performance Liquid Chromatography (HPLC) after a variety of clean up procedures. Fully quantitative aflatoxin determination is mainly performed in government laboratories, using TLC and sophisticated techniques such as high-performance liquid chromatography (HPLC) and high-performance thin-layer chromatography (HPTLC). For the purpose of aflatoxin screening, immunochemical methods like enzyme-linked immunosorbent assay (ELISA) and immunoaffinity column assay (ICA) are also commonly used. Apart from these commonly used techniques, recently, detection of toxins and toxigenic fungi were performed using biosensors and polymerase chain reaction (PCR) respectively.

A strong and accurate awareness of the level of contamination of aflatoxin in natural products and commodities can only be obtained by developing good and rapid analytical methodologies which in the future could enable to dwindle the aflatoxin menace. Taking it to account all these factors the procedures starting from sampling of food or feed commodities to the analysis and quantitation of aflatoxins are described in detail.

Sampling of Food and Feed Commodities for Aflatoxin Detection

Mycotoxins are often distributed in food commodities in a very heterogeneous manner, as they are formed by moulds that occur either in isolated pockets in bulk materials or in individual grains or nuts. When procedures are carried out to ensure concordance with statutory or guideline maximum limits, it is vital that the analytical result be a true value for the consignment. If this is not achieved, satisfactory consignments may be rejected or contaminated loads may be accepted. In addition to health and safety concerns, this can have serious financial implications for the trader and may lead to costly legal disputes. Thus the importance of sampling on the analytical result cannot be underestimated. Sample preparation procedures play a key role and are dependent on the physico-chemical properties of the sample and the toxin that should be determined.

Mycotoxins are usually present at the spot at which toxigenic fungi have developed. Samples can be taken at various stages viz. from growing crops, during transport or storage. They should be collected after particulate size has been reduced by grinding. Sampling is most effective if small samples are taken at periodic and predetermined intervals. The first consideration is the size of sample as distribution of mycotoxin between and within batches depends on type of raw material and extends of contamination. Smaller quantities are required for liquid samples than for grain samples. The individual samples should be combined and mixed thoroughly, after which a subsample of 10 lb (4.5 kg) should be taken. A larger sample is required for large size kernels like peanuts and other nuts. Since contamination of fungi in foods and feeds in a batch occurs in pockets, therefore, to get a representative sample, random sampling should be chosen. Since sample size is generally large, sub-sampling is done. It is very important step to reduce sample size while maintaining it as representative of the original sample as possible. It should be done after the sample is crushed into an appropriately reduced size suitable for extraction.

The official first action method specified by the Association of Official Analytical chemists (AOAC) does not designate sample size, but it requires that the entire sample ground should pass a No.14 sieve, and that a 1-2 Kg. sub-sample of this material be ground to pass a No. 20 sieve. U.S. Food and Drug Administration (FDA) have advocated a minimum of a 15 lb. (6.8 kg.) sample size to be taken while sampling.

Factors Required to Achieve "Representative Sampling" are Summarized Below

- Samples should be taken by qualified, suitably trained personnel, who understand the importance of sampling for obtaining an accurate test result.
- Appropriate, clean and well-maintained tools should be used. Adverse conditions such as poor weather, environment and factors such as cross-contamination should be avoided.
- Incremental samples have to be drawn from various spots randomly distributed throughout the entire lot or sub-lot.
- Samples should be taken when all parts of the lot are easily accessible, all parts of a lot must have an equal chance of being selected.
- Transportation and storage facilities for samples must be adequate and storage time must be as short as possible.
- Good sampling practice necessarily requires clear and secure labeling of samples, giving essential information such as name of sampler, place of sampling, lot number, conditions, applied tools, time, date and observations.

Extraction and Clean up Procedures

Extraction usually involves conventional procedures using polar solvent like acetone, chloroform and methanol or their mixtures. Small amounts of water in addition give higher extraction efficiencies. For aflatoxin extraction the common extraction solvents used are Aceto-nitrile/water, methanol/water combinations. Other solvent mixtures like acetone: hexane: water azeotrope; acetone: water (70: 30), hexane: alcohol etc. have been found to be effective in removing aflatoxin from contaminated material especially oilseeds. Clean-up procedures are generally used for the removal of interfering compounds such as lipids, carbohydrates and proteins. The extracted sample is usually cleaned up by liquid-liquid extraction, solid liquid extraction or column chromatography before the final analysis step. A portion of the extract is placed on a column of silica gel and the lipids and pigments are eluted from the column before elution of the aflatoxins. The use of solid-phase extraction (SPE) with C_{18} cartridges, or immunoaffinity columns (IAC) is now well established in aflatoxin determination. Mycosep columns (ROMER LABS), which remove matrix components efficiently and can produce a purified extract within a very short time, are also available. Conventional clean-up with silica columns has also been reported. After the aflatoxins are eluted they can be analyzed by TLC, HPLC, or gas chromatography-mass spectrometry (GC-MS). The column cleanup procedure should use three washes to eliminate impurities before elution of aflatoxins. The final extract obtained can be used for the desired quantitative analytical procedure. In the extraction process it is important to mix the citric acid and diatomaceous earth, if aflatoxin has to be determined from animal tissue samples and filtering should be done to squeeze as much of the extract from the mixture as possible.

Cleanup for Aflatoxins by Immunoaffinity Columns

Immunoaffinity columns (IAC) are widely used for cleanup and isolation of mycotoxins extracted from foods and biological fluids, particularly aflatoxins. The columns are prepared by binding antibodies specific for aflatoxin to a specially activated solid-phase support. The mycotoxin in the extract or fluid binds to the antibody, impurities are removed with water or aqueous solution, and then the mycotoxin is desorbed with a miscible solvent such as methanol. Further separation can be performed with IAC, followed by liquid chromatographic (LC) quantitation, either in an automated system or by fluorometry. Immunoaffinity columns are nowadays used conjunction with HPLC or TLC for detection of aflatoxin B_1, B_2, G_1 and G_2 in a wide range of commodities.

Other Clean-up Techniques Used are

Defatting

It is carried out prior to the toxin extraction step and uses petroleum ether or hexane to extract lipids from the sample using a Soxhlet extractor. This step is only required when the subsequent clean-up step is not capable of removing the lipids.

Column Chromatography

This technique has very wide application, and is used in a number of regulatory or officially approved methods. A glass column is packed with one or more adsorbent materials and the crude extract is added to the top of the column. The column is then eluted with a series of solvents or solvent mixtures which are designed to first wash off interfering compounds and then elute the desired mycotoxins, whilst other interfering compounds remain strongly bound on the column. A miniature column, called a mini-column is used in many rapid aflatoxin assay methods to remove interfering compounds and to qualitatively detect aflatoxin down to a few parts per billion (ppb)

Precipitation

It is an extremely useful technique whereby certain chemicals, sometimes in colloidal form, are added to the crude extract and these absorb certain pigments, proteins and other interfering compounds onto their surface. The complex so formed precipitates out of solution and can be filtered off, leaving a "cleaned-up" solution. Useful precipitating agents include: cupric carbonate, ammonium sulfate, lead acetate, and ferric gel.

Liquid-liquid Partition

It is commonly used, often in conjunction with one of the other clean-up procedures, to provide additional clean-up and also to transfer toxins from one solvent system to another whilst at the same time effecting a considerable increase in concentration of the toxins. The partition is carried out in a separating funnel which contains the two immiscible solvents. The funnel is shaken for a few minutes to allow the dissolved compounds, including the mycotoxins, to partition between the two phases. The solvents are selected so that the mycotoxins are preferentially partitioned into one of the solvents. Care must be taken in the choice of solvents in order to minimize the risk of emulsion formation.

Thin Layer Chromatography (TLC)

Although this technique is used mainly for detection and quantification of toxins it is also useful for separating the mycotoxins from interfering compounds in the extract. Sometimes it is necessary to try a range of developing solvents in order to separate the toxins of interest from the interfering compounds. If this proves impossible, or too time consuming, then two dimensional TLC may be applied.

Detection of Aflatoxins

I. Immunochemical Method

Rapid methods for analysis of aflatoxins have been developed and are commercially available. Most of these techniques employ immunologic (ELISA) procedures that are semiquantitative.

Enzyme-linked Immunosorbent Assay (ELISA)

ELISA is an immunoassay technique involving the reaction of antigen and antibody *in vitro*. It is a sensitive and specific assay for the detection and quantification of antigens or antibodies against various infectious diseases in humans and animals. The utility of this technique is also exploited for detection of aflatoxins and many other mycotoxins. Nowadays, ELISA has been routinely used for detection of Aflatoxin B1 in cereals, and is becoming an increasingly important clean-up technique in combination with chromatographic detection methods. Monoclonal antibody-based ELISA of aflatoxin B1 has been developed which can be utilized for specific detection of the toxin. In most assays, the monoclonal antibodies specific to aflatoxins are conjugated to horseradish peroxidase for a direct competitive ELISA. Assays using competitive ELISA are also becoming popular among many analytical laboratories. Typically, the competitive ELISAs are based on competitive assay that either uses a conjugate of an enzyme-coupled mycotoxin or a primary antibody specific for the toxin analyte. The sequence of reactions is as follows: (i) a pre-optimised toxin-coupled enzyme is added to the sample extract; (ii) the mixture is added to the corresponding surface-immobilised antibody (e.g. microtitre plate sensitised with antibodies); (iii) the amount of toxin-coupled enzyme that binds to the immobilised antibody is dependent on the amount of toxin in the sample; higher the amount of toxin in a sample, lower will be the amount of the enzyme conjugate bound to the surface and *vice versa* and finally (iv), the enzymic activity of the conjugate bound to the surface is determined by adding a corresponding substrate which results in a chromogenic product, the concentration of which is inversely proportional to the concentration of the toxin in the sample.

For cleanup for the ELISA procedure, water is added to the acetonitrile extract and then the mycotoxins re-extracted with chloroform. The chloroform extract was evaporated to dryness and redissolved in Tris HCl buffer for performing ELISA.

Recently, the use of catalyzed reporter deposition method of signal amplification called “tyramide signal amplification”, which can be used in immunoassays to increase the specificity of aflatoxin detection and to reduce the assay time.

II. Chromatographic Techniques

Thin layer chromatography (TLC)

TLC is the oldest of all the chromatographic methods, requires less advanced and expensive equipment than other chromatographic methods, while achieving a considerable speed in detection of samples. After separation, target components can be detected visually or by using UV light, and can more or less be selectively colored for quantification. Aflatoxins can easily be detected by fluorometry, because they are strongly fluorescent themselves without any further treatment. Most solvent systems used for TLC method are based on chloroform and small amounts of methanol or acetone, but recently, more environmentally friendly mixtures like toluene/ethyl acetate or acetone/iso-propanol etc. has been used. One of the advantages of TLC in the detection of aflatoxins is that confirmation of identity can be conducted directly on TLC plates. However, the samples should be spotted and developed on two-dimensional plates and then derivatized using trifluoracetic acid in hexane. Thin-layer chromatographic analysis of milk samples can be accomplished by spotting on plates. The residues from the extraction and cleanup are dissolved in benzene : acetonitrile (9:1), this solution is spotted on the plate along with the aflatoxin M1 standard.

High Performance Liquid Chromatography (HPLC)

For aflatoxins, HPLC is currently the most widely used technique even though it requires costly equipments and standardization of the analytical laboratory. HPLC is a chemistry-based tool for quantifying and analyzing the amount of any toxin or chemical compounds within a mixture of substances. The sample to be analyzed is dissolved in a solvent such that a liquid mobile phase is created. The mixture is forced through a chromatographic column under high pressure where separation occurs. This is conducted utilizing the fact that certain compounds have different migration rates given a particular column and mobile phase. The mobile phase is isopropanol: acetonitrile: water. Stationary phases for aflatoxins (B and G derivatives) are mainly C_{18}

materials. A sensor, called a detector, usually UV, fluorescence, etc. emits a response corresponding to the eluting sample compound to a data system viz. computer, integrator, or recorder and subsequently signals a peak on the chromatogram. These peaks are correlated to specific mycotoxins. New techniques for HPLC have improved separation, identification, purification, and quantification far beyond other techniques for aflatoxin analysis. For the detection of aflatoxins by fluorescence, derivatisation is performed with strong acids like trifluoro-acetic acid, which results in an increase of fluorescence. Fluorescence detection is possible in the μg/kg range at 435 nm (excitation at 365 nm). For fluorescent detection, a fluorescence detector containing a UV light source, the flow cell which is coupled to the HPLC and a detector are essential. HPLC using fluorescence detection has already become the most accepted method for the determination of aflatoxins due to its several advantages over other analytical methods. Both normal- and reversed-phase HPLC can be used. However the reversed-phase HPLC methods are more popular. Recently, a diode array detection system has also been developed to enhance the detection spectrum of HPLC. An array detector is a multichannel system that measures all detection wavelengths simultaneously. The solvent usually interferes with the spectral measurements and only a limited number of wavelengths are accessible for detection. To make the detection more easier, minimum wavelengths have been defined for most solvents used in HPLC (e.g. acetonitrile at 190 nm, methanol at 210 nm).

Gas Chromatography (GC)

Gas chromatography works similarly to other chromatographic methods. One or more high purity gases are supplied to the GC. One of the gases, called the carrier gas, flows into the injector through the column, where the eluting compounds are separated, and then into the detector and finally the data is processed. GC used as the method of analysis for aflatoxin testing will always have to face instability problems during injection and chromatographic separation, because the toxins are generally nonvolatile. To be suitable for GC analysis, a compound must have sufficient volatility and thermal stability.

III. Other Methods

Mass Spectral Confirmation

Absolute identification of the aflatoxins and the other mycotoxins can be accomplished with MS analysis. Currently, identification of aflatoxins with mass spectroscopy (MS) particularly the combination of liquid chromatography and MS (LC/MS) is becoming increasingly popular. MS feature high specificity, good reliability and wide possibilities for automation. They are sensitive enough to operate in concentration ranges, where legal limits are established for agricultural commodities. Nevertheless, the application of these methods is expensive and requires expert knowledge and skilled personnel. MS has been used for identification of aflatoxinB_1, B_2, G_1 and G_2. Derivatisation is not necessary, but may enhance the sensitivity. In Selected Ion Monitoring (SIM) mode, levels as low as picograms can be detected. The addition of sodium bisulfite as a derivatisation agent leads to the formation of adducts in case of B_1 and G_1 metabolites. Recently, the optical waveguide light mode spectroscopy (OWLS) has also been used for the detection of aflatoxins in immunoassays

Plastic Mini Column for Aflatoxin Detection

An inexpensive method for determination of aflatoxin in food and agricultural products has been developed which is suitable for quality testing of the agricultural products. The method is easy to operate by inexperienced persons, and is sensitive enough to detect aflatoxin to a limit of 20 ppb. The technique used plastic mini column, a kind of small chromatographic tube, was devised in Thailand. Plastic mini column was made using clear polyethylene straw with a diameter of 6 mm. and a length of 25 cm. The precipitating solution was a mixture of zinc acetate and saturated ammonium sulfate which will increase the precipitation property in the interaction to reduce interfering substances in the extraction. Saturated NaCI was used as precipitating solvent that will precipitate more in higher acidity while aflatoxin will be extracted more easily. With this method, aflatoxin could be measured within two hours with an accuracy of lower than 10 ppb.

Gold-labeled Antibody Probe

An antibody-colloidal gold probe conjugate has been recently developed for rapid and specific detection of aflatoxin B1. Mono-dispersional nanogold colloid was synthesized and nanogold-labeled polyclonal antibody was prepared to probe aflatoxin B1 under optimal condition. Combination of antibody with nanogold particles was characterized by UV-visible light absorption spectra, transmission electron microscopy (TEM), fluorescence spectroscopy, cross reactivity and stability measurements. Later, the nanogold-labeled probe was used to develop an immunochromatographic method for aflatoxin B1 analysis which could be completed in less than 10 min. Detection time using this procedure was reduced 6-10 times compared with ELISA technique and the lower test limit was found to be around 2.5 ng/ml aflatoxin B1, which was increased to two times to that of ELISA.

Identification of Toxigenic and Non-toxigenic Fungi by Media Growth Characteristics

Media growth characteristics of various Aspergilli have been documented which can help in the specific identification of species. This will enable the differentiation of toxic and non-toxic species and thus will be useful in detecting the specific presence of toxigenic fungi in food and feed stuffs. In determining whether a fungal species isolated from an agricultural commodity is toxigenic, the substrate and experimental conditions used for its culture also appears to be extremely important. Listed below are the diagnostic characteristics of a number of mould species in common fungal media.

- *Aspergillus flavus:* Colonies are bright green often with black sclerotia; conidiophores with usually 2 sets of sterigmata and with spiny stalks. Conidia globose and spiny.
- *Aspergillus parasiticus*: Colonies are bright green but without sclerotia. Conidiophore has only one set of sterigmata and stalk is spiny only at the top. Globose spiny conidia are produced.
- *Aspergillus fumigatus:* Colonies are bluish green and produce columns of conidia. Conidiophores have one set of sterigmata and conidiophore vesicles and sterigmata are pigmented blue. Colony reverse is also blue to black.
- *Aspergillus oryzae:* In the A. flavus group but colony color is yellow green. Just one set of sterigmata with smooth conidiophore stalks. Conidia are usually smooth and elliptical and larger than those of A. flavus.
- *Aspergillus tamarii:* Colonies are bright green, but quickly become deep chocolate brown. Conidiophores are the same as *A. flavus* but conidia are unique, having a double wall and color bars rather than spines.
- *Aspergillus ochraceus:* Colonies are bright yellow and sometimes produce purple sclerotia Conidiophores have 2 sets of sterigmata, the stalk is spiny with definite yellow pigment in the walls. Conidia are usually smooth walled and globose to slightly elliptical.
- *Aspergillus versicolor:* Colonies are dark green and with highly and variously colored mycelial sectors. Conidiophores with 2 sets of sterigmata, smooth and colorless stalk, and small vesicles. Conidia are slightly roughened.

- *Aspergillus sydowi:* Colonies are consistently blue and produce no highly colored mycelial sectors. Conidiophores similar to *A. versicolor*, but conidia are very definitely spiny.
- *Aspergillus nidulans:* Colonies are dark green and produce long columns of conidia. Conidiophores and conidia similar to *A. versicolor* but stalk and vesicle are pigmented brown.
- *Aspergillus terreus:* Colony color is tan to beige. Produces long columns of conidia. However, conidiophores are colorless and smooth, have a small vesicle and 2 sets of sterigmata.
- *Aspergillus glaucus*: colonies are blue-grey and contain numerous bright shiny yellow balls. Conidiophores are smooth with slight blue pigmentation and one set of sterigmata. Conidia are spiny.

Biological Assays of Mycotoxins

Bioassays are the oldest and most primitive types of analysis for toxicity testing as they are conducted using biological organisms. Bioassay means administration of suspected commodity or its solvent extracts to any biological test systems and then determination of the degree and nature of the effect produced. Although the biological species used invariably differs, demonstration of toxicity greatly improves the diagnostic confidence. In addition to confirm the presence of toxin, use of various test systems can also provide valuable insights into its nature, thus enabling an efficient chemical approach to be adopted for its identification and quantification. Different species have been used in some areas to examine the suspected commodity for contamination.

Bile Duct Hyperplasia in Duckling Liver

The characteristic bile duct hyperplasia produced by aflatoxins in liver of ducklings has led to widespread use of this species for bioassay. In this method, feed is first extracted with methanol; the residues are dispersed in water and re-extracted with chloroform. An aqueous suspension of the extract is administered to day-old ducklings by oral route over 4 days and the surviving birds are examined on 7th day. On histopathological examination, bile duct hyperplasia is seen as cord of cells which is related to aflatoxin content in the suspected material. This method produced liver lesion at 20 μg aflatoxin/kg diet when fed to day old ducklings. It was also noticed that concentration of 150 μg aflatoxin/kg diet killed all ducklings in 9-11 days.

In Chick Embryo

The use of chicken embryos has proved extremely useful in mycotoxin research because of its great sensitivity to numerous mycotoxins. This method involves administration of methanol-chloroform extracts of commodities dissolved in ethanol sub germinally into eggs or through a hole in shell into the air sac. After normal incubation, death and abnormalities in hatched chicks are noted. This system yield LD_{50} as 0.064 μg aflatoxin B1. For optimum sensitivity, dose response and reproducibility, an injection volume of 10 μI into air sac on day 1 or 2 of incubation with a minimum of 20 egg/ dose level and incubation of eggs until hatching was recommended.

Brine Shrimp Larvae

Brine shrimp larvae are the most widely tried and used species for toxin bioassays. A number of workers have evaluated this species as a bioassay organism. Two basic methods are being used for this assay. The toxin is placed directly in a medium containing the shrimps or a paper disc inoculated with toxins brought in contact with larvae after the solvent has evaporated. The activity of larvae using a photocell and photoelectric counter to count interruptions of light through a cell containing the larvae; more precise results could be obtained as inhibition of larval movements occurs at a lower dose than death.

The methodology used and interpretation of data are the vital aspects of bioassays. Many of the factors influencing toxicity like species, sex, age, method and route of administration of extract, nutrition, etc. can be controlled in test design. However, since bioassays are generally conducted on crude extracts of commodities, there is possibility of interference by compounds other than fungal toxins. Effective control of bioassays will require a number of precautionary measures, i.e. the vehicle used for administration of toxin must be pretested for lack of toxicity. Also solvent and negative commodity control should be included in test design. However, these bioassays are time consuming requiring days for completion; therefore, their use is very much limited as far as routine analysis of commodities is concerned. These cannot be used for programme of quality control.

Advanced Techniques for Rapid and Specific Detection of Aflatoxins and Toxigenic Fungi

Bright Greenish-yellow Fluorescence (BGYF) Test

A new method has been developed which uses fluorescence detection for the detection of Aflatoxins in grain. Since most samples do not contain a detectable amount of aflatoxin, there is a need for a method which correctly identifies the many negative samples with minimum expenditure of time and money. This newly evolved method is able to solve the problem and it is known as the BGYF test or black light test. In this method, feed samples are inspected under the UV lamp (365 μm) for a characteristic bright greenish yellow fluorescence in damaged kernels for the presence of aflatoxin or kojic acid produced from *Aspergillus flavus* or *A. parasiticus*. It is postulated that the BGYF resulted from the action of heat labile peroxidase in the living plant tissues and from some microorganisms on kojic acid produced by the fungal species. Thus the BGYF test indicates the growth of the fungi that may have resulted in the production of aflatoxin. As the BGYF test very easy to perform, attempts have been made to establish aflatoxin levels by numbers of BGYF particles or by the weight and by area of BGYF particles in whole samples. Although a relationship existed between numbers of BGYF particles and kernels and aflatoxin levels, the correlation was not high enough to encourage use of the numbers as an indication of aflatoxin content (2). So BGYF test could not provide a satisfactory quantitative estimation for aflatoxin but could be very well used for qualitative analysis.

Biosensor Assay

Common methods for mycotoxin determination including TLC, ELISA and HPLC, even though are very sensitive method, is also costly and time consuming due to extraction and cleanup procedures that are unavoidable in any mycotoxin analysis. To counter these drawbacks, recently an assay has been developed in which the principle of detection is based on surface plasmon resonance (SPR) and monoclonal antibody technique. In principle, SPR is a measurement of mass concentration changes that occur at the sensor surface due to binding of toxin molecules. Biosensors monitor interactions by measuring the mass concentration of biomolecules close to a surface. One of the interacting molecules is the monoclonal antibody (MAb), which is attached in order to make the surface specific to the analyte of interest. The sample, which contains the interacting reaction molecule, is pumped to the surface, where the sample binds to the MAb on the surface. The concentration of the analyte can be detected by the surface changes and can be quantified by SPR. Recognizing the utility of this novel system, sensors and sensor systems are being developed for food analysis, environmental applications, and for pharmaceutical purposes. A number of sensors are the subject of ongoing research. Other sensor systems that are currently being investigated include fiber-optic sensors, chemo-luminescence systems and "electronic noses" for the detection of aflatoxins.

Detection of *Aspergillus* Using Polymerase Chain Reaction

Development of molecular methods and advanced techniques for the identification of aflatoxigenic Aspergilli, Primers for PCR and RT-PCR were designed for aflatoxin biosynthetic pathway genes. Genomic DNA isolated from aflatoxigenic, non-aflatoxigenic *Aspergilli* were subjected to PCR using aflatoxin regulatory (*afl R)*, o-methyltransferase (*omt*) and oxidoreductase (*ord*) primers. PCR amplicons were obtained for aflatoxigenic *A. flavus* and *A. parasiticus* with *afl R* and *omt* gene primers. Nowadays, aside from detection of feed samples, PCR is widely used for the detection on aflatoxigenic fungi in the lung tissues and serum samples of suspected human cases. A nested PCR has also been recently reported using primers for 18S rRNA gene of *Aspergillus fumigatus*. Very recently, PCR-ELISA and Real time-PCR has also been developed for the detection of *Aspergilli* in human cases.

Biochip Technology

MicroSERS is a new biochip technology that uses surface-enhanced Raman scattering (SERS) microscopy for label-free transduction and thereby detection. The biochip itself comprises pixels of capture biomolecules immobilized on a SERS-active metal surface. Once the biochip has been exposed to the sample and the capture biomolecules have selectively bound their ligands, a Raman microscope is used to collect SERS fingerprints from the pixels on the chip. Therefore, pathogens can be individually identified by microSERS, even when organisms that cross-react with the capture biomolecules are present in a sample. MicroSERS is capable of sensitive and highly specific detection of toxins. Aflatoxins B1 and G1 could be detected and individually identified when biochips bearing pixels of antibody or enzyme capture biomolecules were incubated in samples containing one or both aflatoxins, and the spectra were then collected from an area of the biomolecule pixel approximately 1 μm in diameter. In the future, hyperspectral imaging Raman microscopy may be used for collecting fingerprints from all the pixels on the biochip, individually yet simultaneously, to enable the rapid detection of diverse fungal pathogens and their toxins in a sample, using a single biochip.

Detection by Gene Expression

Green fluorescent protein (*gfp*) was used for this detection technique, as a reporter to monitor gene expression and food colonization by *Aspergillus flavus*. Transformants of *A. flavus* containin 303g the *Aequorea victoria gfp* gene fused to a viral promoter or the promoter region and 483 bp of the coding region of *A. flavus* aflR, expressed green fluorescence detectable without a microscope or filters. Expression of green fluorescent protein fluorescence was correlated with resistance to aflatoxin accumulation in five crop genotypes inoculated with these transformants.

Aflatoxin Detection Protocols

Estimation of Total Aflatoxins by Velasco Fluorotoxinometer

This quantitative technique is followed for routine purpose for aflatoxin estimation in mixed feeds. Briefly, in this method, 50 g of the properly mixed sample is taken in flask. To this 250 ml of acetone water (85 : 15) is added. The mixture is blended at high speed for 5 minutes or kept overnight and then filtered through Whatman filter paper No. 1. Ninety ml of the filtrate is transferred in flask containing ferric gel (prepared by adding 10 ml of 10% ferric chloride solution to 100 ml of distilled water followed by addition of 4.83% sodium hydroxide with pH of gel adjusted to 5.0±0.2). The flask is closed with a stopper, shaken vigorously and then the contents are filtered. Approximately 180 ml of filtrate is taken in separating funnel. To this 180 ml of distilled water and 50 ml of chloroform is added. The separating funnel is shaken and different layers are allowed to separate. Collect lower chloroform layer and dry it on a water bath. Add 2 ml of chloroform-methanol (96 : 4) solution and swirl gently to dissolve residues. Transfer this in a vial. Repeat this procedure twice, each time adding 2 ml of chloroform methanol solution and transferring to the beaker so as to make total volume 6 ml in vial.

Preparation of Mini Column

Plug one end of mini column with glass wool. Place a small funnel on the other end and add a layer of sea sand (5-7 mm) followed by fluorosil 100-200 mesh (5-7 mm), sea sand (5-7 mm), silica gel (15 mm) and finally neutral alumina (15 mm). Wet the mini column by placing it in chloroform and allowing chloroform to seep up through various layers. Then add, from top, one ml of sample residue solution from vial (having six ml) and allow it to drain. After this add one ml of chloroform-methanol (96: 4) solution and allow it to drain.

Calibrate the instrument with 20 ppb standard column at least half an hour before taking reading of unknown sample. The instrument has calibrations from 1-50 ppb. The mini column which is still wet, is placed in sample holder and digital reading in parts per billion (ppb) are read directly in front panel meter. The column is turned around 1800 so that front now faces back and take second reading. The final reading is the average of two readings. If reading on the front panel meter exceeds 50, dilute the sample 10 or 25 times and take reading and multiply it with 10 or 25 as the case may be to get final result, which indicates total aflatoxins in a sample.

Aflatoxin B1 in Mixed Feeds by Enzyme-linked Immunosorbent Screening Methods

Aflatoxin B1 in mixed feeds can be estimated by ELISA using method of AOAC. This method is based on the principle of conjugation of APB1 to enzyme and the conjugate is used as known antigen. Antibodies specific to aflatoxins are coated onto microtitre wells. Aflatoxins are extracted from unknown samples and extract is mixed with enzyme conjugated AFB1. The mixture is then placed in well of antibody coated microtitre plate. Aflatoxin from unknown sample and enzyme conjugated AFB1 compete for binding sites on antibodies. Excess of unbound aflatoxin and enzyme substrate added to each well is catalyzed by bound enzyme and changes from colourless to coloured solution. Intensity of colour depends on the amount of enzyme conjugated AFB1 bound to antibodies present. Dark colour indicates less aflatoxins in unknown sample. Colour intensity can be used to rate toxin level in product by comparing with colour obtained using AFB1 standard solution. This is used for quantitative as well as qualitative screening of aflatoxins in mixed feeds. Positive samples can be determined visually or by microtitre well reader. Assay is not confirmatory method because antibodies cross react with other aflatoxins (B2, G1 and G2).

Feed Sample (50 gm) + acetone: water (85 : 15) – (250 ml)
Keep overnight and filter

↓

Take 90 ml filtrate and add ferric gel

↓

Shake well and filter
Take 180 ml filtrate in separating funnel

↓

Add equal amount of distilled water and 50 ml chloroform

↓

Shake well and allow to stand

↓

Drain out lower chloroform layer in beaker

↓

Evaporate in water bath or keep it overnight at room temperature

↓

Residues in beaker + Chloroform-Methanol (96:4)
2-2-2 ml for thee times
Total volume 6 ml in a vial

↓

Take 1 ml
Place in minicolumn

↓

Allow to drain
Take reading in fluorotoxinometer

Reagents Required

a. AFB1 enzyme conjugate (HRD).

b. Enzyme conjugate hydration solution.

c. Antibody coated solid support 12 well microtitre strips or 96 well ELISA plate.

d. Enzyme substrate ABTS/ OPD.

e. Hydrogen peroxide.

f. Colour stopping solution.

g. AFB1 standard prepare 15 and 50 ng/g standard of AFB1.

h. Methanol solution- methanol: water (55 + 45).

i. Hexane

Working solutions: These solutions are to be prepared fresh and used within an hour of preparation for better results.

a. Enzyme conjugated AFB1 working solution: Add two ml of enzyme conjugate hydration solution to AFB1 enzyme conjugate. Mix well to dissolve pellet.

b. ABTS substrate working solution: 5 mg in 10 ml citrate phosphate buffer containing a few drops of hydrogen peroxide.

Extraction

Weigh 5 g of unknown sample in the tube. Add 25 ml methanol solution and 10 ml of hexane. Shake well and filter or centrifuge for 5 min at 3000 rpm. Let the layers separate, draw off upper hexane layer and discard.

Enzyme Assay

1. Set up mixing wells. Do not use antibody coated microtitre wells. Pipette 0.01 ml of enzyme conjugated AFB1 working solution into control wells and into 1 well for each unknown sample. Add 0.1 ml AFB1 standard solution and unknown sample filtrate to separate wells and mix thoroughly. At least 1 AFB1 control well should be used with each strip.

2. Set up antibody-coated wells. Transfer 0.1 ml solution from each mixing well to corresponding antibody coated well and let it stand for 10 min.

3. Take solution out of antibody coated wells into waste receptacle decontaminating solution. Do not let decontaminating solution enter the wells. Rinse wells 10 times with water and shaking out wash solutions. After final wash, invert wells on adsorbent paper and remove excess of water drops.

4. Add 0.1 ml ABTS substrate working solution to each antibody coated well and let it stand for 10 min Wells may be agitated slowly several times during assay.

5. Then add 0.1 ml of colour stopping solution to each antibody well. Compare colour development of controls and unknown samples. For better result, hold micro titre well strip against white background. While

using ELISA reader, negative control should be prepared by adding 0.1 ml ABTS substrate working solution and 0.1 ml colour stopping solution to empty well as blank.

Interpretation

Visual: AFB1 control well for 15-50 μg/g level will show light grey green to pink colour.

Unknown samples: Dark green colour indicates aflatoxins less than 15 ng/g and light green pink colour indicates level more than 15 ng/g.

ELISA reader: Insert 405 nm filter and calibrate instrument with blank. Record percent absorption or the optical density for each well.

DOT ELISA for Aflatoxin B1, B2, G1 in Corn, Cottonseed or Peanuts

This procedure is applicable to screening aflatoxin B1, B2 and G1 in whole cottonseed and peanut butter at ≥20 ng/ g and in corn and raw peanuts at ≥30 ng/g.

Principle antibodies specific to B1, B2 and G1 are mobilized on filter and toxin (AFB1) is labelled with enzyme horse radish peroxidase. Presence of free aflatoxin in test/ unknown sample inhibits the binding of toxin enzyme conjugate by immobilized antibodies. As the fixed number of antibody reaction sites is available, the enzyme activity is proportional to the amount of bound toxin enzyme conjugate. Antibody toxin enzyme complex concentration is inversely proportional to the concentration of free toxin added. Bound enzyme catalyses oxidation of substrate to form blue complex. Development of colour indicates that test sample contains aflatoxin ≤20 ng/g and if no colour then ≥20 ng/g.

Specificity of Antibodies

Antibodies have specific ability to bind structurally related compounds like B1, B2 and G1. Specificity of purified rabbit anti aflatoxin B1 polyclonal antibodies is determined by direct competitive ELISA. Coat serially diluted antibodies on micro titer plates. Prepare standard solution of aflatoxin and add to individual micro titre well. Then add solution of aflatoxin B1 conjugated to horse radish peroxidase to each well. Add substrate solution of tetra methyl benzidine and hydrogen peroxide. Development of colour is measured. Development of the least colour indicates highest reactivity of toxin antibody reaction.

Reagents

a. Antibody coated filter material attached to analytical cup made of porous polyethylene.

b. AFB1 horse radish peroxidase conjugate at toxin enzyme molar ratio of 10-15 : 1.

c. Wash solution: Phosphate .buffer saline solution. Dissolve 0.23 g (sodium dihydrogen phosphate), 1.95 g (dipotassium hydrogen phosphate), 8.70 g sodium chloride, 0.125 ml tween 20 and 10 mg thiomersal (ethyl mercurithio salicylic acid sodium salt) in 900 ml water, adjust pH to 7.2 and dilute to 1 litre.

d. Buffer: 0.1% bovine serum albumin in phosphate buffer saline solution containing 0.05% thiomersal.

e. Substrate solution A: Diaminobenzidine (DAB) in citrate phosphate buffer (pH 5.0) 10 mg/10-15 ml and few drops of 30% H_2O_2.

f. Methanol, hexane and chloroform.

g. Standard AFB1 solution: Approx. 28 μg as dry film. Add 3 ml chloroform to vial having 28 μg AFB1. It acts as stock solution. For working solution, dispense 300 μg stock solution in vial. Add 2400 μL methanol (1 ng/μL), mix and store. Prepare daily. Dispense 10 μL diluted standard (1 ng/μL) into test tube. Add 300 μL methanol and 700 μL buffer. Always prepare fresh.

Assay

a. Prepare fresh substrate.

b. It is better to run one negative control cup and one positive control (standard) cup each time. Negative control cup can be run by applying 100 μL of buffer to the centre, of cup. Apply working standard to cup as unknown sample.

c. Add 200 μL test extract to 400 μL buffer to make total 600 μL.

d. Thoroughly mix diluted test extract and apply 150 μL aliquot to centre of cup. After one min, apply 150 μL again.

e. Apply 100 μL enzyme substrate solution to centre of cup.

Dot Immunobinding Assay

Dot immunobinding assay is an enzyme based immunological test by which aflatoxin can be detected in animal feed. This is qualitative method and indicates the presence of aflatoxins in feed.

Requirement

a. Dip sticks
b. Antibody to aflatoxin labelled with peroxidase enzyme
c. Substrate:

   DAB (brown)

   4-chloro 1-naphthol (blue)

3-amino-ethyl-carbazol (red)

d. PBS (pH 7.2)
e. PBS-TWEEN
f. 5% milk in PBS-TWEEN
g. Hydrogen peroxide

Procedure

a. Dipsticks are washed in PBS for 1-2 min and air dried.
b. Place a drop of processed feed in the centre with the help of micropipette or microcapillary and dry in air.
c. Place the dipstick in 5% milk for 15 min and wash in PBS-TWEEN.
d. Place the dipstick in anti-aflatoxin (AFB1) antibody conjugated with HRP for 15 min and wash in PBS-TWEEN.
e. Place the dipstick in substrate solution containing few drops of hydrogen peroxide and look for development of coloured dot in the centre.

Interpretation

Positive results are visualized by the presence of coloured dot at the site of sample deposition.

Estimation of Aflatoxin M1 in Milk and Cheese

Aflatoxin M1 is potential hepatocarcinogen which is the hydroxylated metabolite of aflatoxin B1 and is secreted in milk of mammals receiving aflatoxin B1 in diets.

Apparatus

a. Blender

b. Chromatographic column: Glass column of 30 x 1.0 cm (internal diameter) with porous polyethylene frit and nylon stopcock.

c. Thin layer plate: 10 x 10 cm or 20 x 20 cm coated with 0.25-0.5 mm of silica gel.

d. Filter paper (24 cm)

e. Developing tank

f. Viewing cabinet with long wave UV range

Reagents

a. Solvents: Acetic acid, acetone, methyl cyanide, benzene, chloroform, diethyl ether, hexane, isopropanol and toluene.

b. Saturated salt solution.

c. Silica gel for column chromatography: 70-230 mesh and activate it by drying 1 hat 105°. Add water 1 ml/100 g, shake -and store.

d. Sodium sulfate (Na_2SO_4)

e. Diatomaceous earth.

f. Aflatoxin M standards: 0.25 μg M1/ml of benzene CH_3CN (9 + 1).

g. Densitometer

h. Urea 6 M: 360 g Urea/litre water.

Extraction

For Fluid Milk

a. To 50 ml of milk, add 10 ml saturated salt solution and 120 ml chloroform. Shake and let layers separate for approximately 2 min.

b. Drain lower chloroform layer into 125 ml flask.

c. Add 10 g Na_2SO_4 in it, stir for approx. 3 min and filter it.

For Powdered Milk

a. Reconstitute 5 g of powder with 50 ml water in 250 ml separator.

b. Add NaCI and $CHCl_3$ as in fluid milk.

c. Break emulsions by centrifugation or by substituting 60 ml 6 M urea for 50 ml water and 10 ml salt solution.

Cheese

a. Blend 15 g cheese with 1 ml salt solution, 5 g diatomaceous earth and 100 ml chloroform.

b. Filter mixture in 120 ml flask and treat extract as in fluid milk.

Column Chromatography

a. Fill column half full with $CHCl_3$ and add 2.0 g silica gel.

b. Add 3-4 ml $CHCl_3$ and make silica slurry and drain $CHCl_3$ to settle silica.

c. Add 2.0 g Na_2SO_4 to supernatant solvent above silica gel and drain excess $CHCI_3$.

d. Add product filtrate in portions and drain the entire solution through column and rinse column sides with chloroform and drain.

e. Wash column with 25 ml toluene- CHCOOH (9+ I), 25 ml hexane, 25 ml hexane either- CH_3CN (5+3+2) and discard washes.

f. Elute AFM1 with 40 ml $CaCl_3$- acetone (4+1) and evaporate eluate to dryness.

g. Dissolve in $CHCl_3$ and transfer to vial and dry under pressure.

Thin Layer Chromatography

Add 100 μl benzene CH_3CN (9+1) to sample residue and mix per/min. This amount is sufficient either for visual or densitometric analysis.

Visual: On TLC plate, spot 20 μl of sample extract and 2, 4, 6, 8, 10 μl of M1 standards. Develop plate in $CHCl_3$-acetone -isopropanol (87+10+3) or ether methanol-water (95+4+1) or ether-hexane-methanol-water (85+10+4+1). Quantify visually using formula:

μg/kg = (S x Y x V) / (X x W)

Where,

S = μl aflatoxin M1 standard equal to unknown

Y = Concentration of aflatoxin M1 standard

V = μl of final dilution of sample extract

X = μI of sample spotted giving florescent intensity equal to S.

W = The volume or weight of milk product represented in final extract for TLC (original volume or weight sample x filtrate volume/ 720).

In this method, the fluorescent intensities of spots from sample extract are compared with standard spots and the sample portion matching the standard is determined. To aid in determination, move plate away from lamp to alternate UV light so that any particular pair of spots can be compared. If spot of sample extract is too intense to match standard, dilute the sample and re chromatograph.

Densitometric (milk)

On TLC plates, spot two 20 μl aliquot of sample extract and 5, 5 and 10 μI aliquot of M1 standard. Develop plate as in 'a', according to manufacturer's instruction and calculate concentration as in 'a' or as

μg/kg = (B x Y x S x Y)/ (Z x X x W)

Where,

B = average area aflatoxin M1 in sample aliquots

Y = concentration of aflatoxin M1 standard

S = μI aflatoxin M1 standard spotted

V = final dilution of sample extract (μI)

Z = Average area aflatoxin M1 peaks in standard aliquot

X = μI sample extract spotted

W = gm sample represented by final extract

Visual and Densitometric analysis (Cheese): Spotting and scoring pattern of two dimensional TLC:

Spot 20 μL of sample extract and either 1.5, 0.5, 1.0 and 1.5 ng of M1 standard (visual) or 2.5, 1.25, 1.25 and 2.5 ng of M1 standard (densitometric). Plates in first direction are developed in ethyl ether-methanol-water (95+4+1) and in second direction in $CHCI_3$-acetone-isopropanol (87+10+3). After developing in first direction remove the plate, air dry and heat at 50°C for 2 min cool and then redevelop in second direction. Quantify visually or densitometrically as for milk except that W = original weight of sample x filtrate volume/ 100.

Estimation of Aflatoxin B1 in Eggs

Apparatus

Items (a), (c), (d), (e) and (f) as in milk and in addition Butt tube -32 x 200 rpm.

Reagents

a. Solvents: Acetonitrile, Acetone, Alcohol, benzene, chloroform, hexane, acetic acid, methanol and petroleum ether.

b. Sodium sulfate.

c. Diatomaceous earth.

d. Saturated salt solution.

e. Lead acetate solution: Dissolve 200 g lead acetate in distilled water with warming and add 30 ml acetic acid and dilute to 1 liter.

f. Silica gel.

g. Aflatoxin B1 standard: 0.5 pg AfB1/ ml benzene-methyl cyanide (98 + 2).

Extraction and Lipid Removal

a. Weigh egg and add water into blender jar as indicated below:

	% Water	Sample Weight (g)	Water added before extraction (ml)	Sample equivalent in final extract (g)
Whole egg	74	100	0	45
Egg white	88	100	0	44
Egg yolk	51	100	20	46

b. Add 42 ml of saturated salt solution and blend for 1 min.

c. Add 300 ml acetone, mix and filter in cylinder.

d. To 235 ml of filtrate add 20 ml lead acetate solution; 150 ml water. Mix and let stand for 3 min. To it add 10 g diatomaceous earth and filter.

e. Transfer 525 ml filtrate in separating funnel, add 100 ml petroleum ether and shake for 1 min and let layers separate.

f. Drain aqueous layer into another separator and add 50 ml $CHCl_3$ to it. Shake and let layers separate.

Butt Tube/ Column Chromatography

a. Insert loose plug of glass wool in butt tube followed by 2 cm layers of sodium sulfate, 10 g silica gel slurried 50 ml chloroform.

b. Drain chloroform and add 2 cm layers of Na_2SO_4.

c. Filter lower chloroform layer through tube, and collect filtrate in flask.

d. Add 20 ml acetone to aqueous layer in previous separator and extract with 50 ml chloroform.

e. Filter lower chloroform layer of the column followed with 25 ml $CHCl_3$-acetone (9 + 1).

f. Evaporate combined filtrates to near dryness and transfer contents to vial.

g. Evaporate to dryness and reserve for TLC.

h. Final extract represents weight egg product as :

Weight egg = 100 g x [235/(300 + 42 + 74)]

x [325/ (235+ 20+ 150)] = 45 g

Thin Layer Chromatography

Add 100 μL benzene-CH_3CN (98 + 2) to sample residue and shake. For screening analysis, use 10 x 10 cm thin layer plates using 20 μL extract and 2 μL aflatoxin B1 standard solution. If sample is positive, re-spot extract for quantitation on 20 x 20 cm plate. The sample may be over spotted with 1 ng aflatoxin B1 as internal standard. Develop plates in first direction with anhydrous ethyl ether-methanol-water (96+3+1) in unequilibrated tank. Remove plate and over dry at 50°C for 1 min. Cool and develop in second direction with acetone-chloroform (1+9). Evaporate solvent at room temperature and observe in dark under longwave UV light. For positive samples aflatoxin B1 from sample plus added internal standard are perfectly super imposed. The fluorescence of the combination spot is more intense than that of sample or 1 ng reference standard, quantitate visually or by densitometry as previously described using following formula:

$$\mu g/kg \text{ of AFB1} = (S \times Y \times V) / (X \times W)$$

Estimation of Aflatoxin B1 and M1 in liver or Tissue Samples

Apparatus

a. Shaker

b. Meat grinder

c. Chromatographic column

d. Filter paper 32 cm Whatman No. 2

e. Thin layer plates-10 x 10 cm or 20 x 20 cm coated with 0.25-0.5 mm thick silica gel dried at 105°C for 1 hour.

Reagents

a. Solvents: Glacial acetic acid, acetone, methyl cyanide (CHCN), benzene, chloroform, CH_2CI_2, ether, hexane, isopropanol and toluene.

b. Citric acid solution 20%.

c. Silica gel for column chromatography- 70-230 mesh. Stir 1 hr in methanol, filter and treat with chloroform. Activate at 105°C for 1 h. Add water 1 ml/100g.

d. Sodium sulfate

e. Diatomaceous earth.

f. Aflatoxin standards to contain 0.25 µg AFB1, and M1/ml of benzene-CH_3CN (9+1).

Extraction

a. To 100 g of homogenized meat, add 10 ml citric acid, mix and after 5 min add 20 g diatomaceous earth.

b. Add 200 ml CH_2Cl_2 and shake flask on shaker for 30 min.

c. Filter contents in flask containing 10 g Na_2SO_4 and compress entire filter to obtain maximum filtrate.

d. Shake flask, refilter and record volume. Evaporate to near dryness after transferring in flask.

Column Chromatography

a. Fill column half full with CH_2Cl_2 and add 2.0 g silica gel.

b. Add 3 µI CH_2Cl_2 and slurry silica.

c. Drain CH_2Cl_2 to settle silica.

d. Add 2.0 g Na_2SO_4 above silica to cap column and drain excess CH_2CI_2.

e. Re-dissolve concentrated filtrate with 25 ml CH_2Cl_2 and add to column.

f. Rinse flask with additional CH_2Cl_2 and drain this through column.

g. When filtrate reaches Na_2SO_4 rinse column sides with CH_2Cl_2 and drain it.

h. Wash column with 25 ml toluene-acetic acid (9+1), 25 ml hexane and 25 ml hexane-ether-CH_3CN (6+3+1) and discard washes.

i. Elute aflatoxin with 40 ml CH_2Cl_2-acetone (4+1) and evaporate eluate to near dryness and transfer contents to vial and evaporate to dryness.

Visual and Densitometric Analysis

a. Add 100 µl of benzene-CH_3CN (9+1) to residue contents in vial and mix.

b. Perform TLC as for eggs.

c. 20 µl of sample extract is spotted on sample spot and either 1.5, 0.5, 1.0 and 1.5 ng of reference standard (visual) or 2.5, 1.25, 1.25 and 2.5 ng of standard (densitometric).

d. Develop plate in ether-methanol-water (95+4+1) in first direction and when solvent reaches score line, air dry and heat at 50°C for 2 min, cool and redevelop in second direction in $CHCl_3$-acetone-isopropanol (87+10+3) to score line. Quantitate visually or densito metrically as for eggs and calculate concentration of B1 or M1 as µg/ kg = (S x Y x V) / (X x W).

Protocol for Biosensor Assay of Aflatoxins

The assay method presented here is designed as an inhibition assay in which a fixed concentration of mycotoxin specific antibodies is mixed with a sample containing an unknown concentration of mycotoxin. The mixture is then passed over a sensor surface on which a mycotoxin is immobilised. Non-complexes antibodies are then measured as they bind to the mycotoxin on the sensor surface. The sensor surface contains four serial connected flow cells, making it possible to detect four mycotoxins in a single measurement and will contribute to an efficient monitoring and control of mycotoxins in the food and feed chain.

Materials

- Aflatoxin B1, zearalenone, ochratoxin A, DON and fumunosin B1 toxins
- Monoclonal antibodies against the toxins.
- Carboxymethoxylamine, N-hydroxysuccinimide(NHS), hexanediamine,
- 2-[N-morpholino]ethanesulfonic acid, guanidine chloride
- Dimethyl sulphoxide (DMSO), pyridine, ethanolamine and acetonitrile.
- 1-ethyl-3-(3-dimethylaminopropyl) carbodiimide (EDC)
- Boric acid and glycine
- HEPES buffered saline
- MycoSep 224 cleanup columns
- The CM5 sensor surfaces
- BIACORE-2000 instrument used for sensor analysis

Procedure

1. For immobilizing aflatoxin on the sensor chip surface, aflatoxin B1 was carboxylated using carboxymethoxylamine (10/5 mg of mycotoxin) in pyridine (7.5 ml).
2. This mixture was shaken overnight at 200 rpm protected from light.
3. The pyridine was evaporated to dryness and the aflatoxin was redissolved in DMSO.
4. Immobilization on the CM5 sensor surface took place using a modification of the standard EDC–NHS reaction
5. Before use, each flow cell is regenerated 20 times with a 6 M guanidine chloride solution in 50 mM glycine pH 2.0.
6. Every flow cell of a docked sensor chip was immobilized separately.
7. A diamine spacer was coupled to a EDC–NHS activated CM5-sensorchip after which EDC–NHS activated aflatoxin was injected.
8. For blocking of non-reacted group, an ethanolamine injection was used.
9. Calibration and sample concentration determinations on the BIACORE 2000 equipment were done according to a standard method, using a buffer flow of 20 μl/min and an injection of 70 μl the appropriately

diluted sample, mixed 1:1 with an antibody solution-mix consisting of antibodies against the aflatoxin B1 that was determined.

10. This injection was followed by a regeneration, which consisted of an injection of 6.0 M guanidine chloride solution in 50 mM glycine pH 2.0 during 1 min.
11. Extraction and clean-up of the sample require approximately 15 min and the measurement takes 10 min, including regeneration of the sensor chip surface, making a total of approximately 25 min for the complete detection of Aflatoxin in a sample.

Protocol for Fungal Genomic DNA Isolation

CTAB method for fungal DNA isolation of *Aspergillus flavus*

- Add 500μl of freshly prepared CTAB (cetyltrimethyl ammonium bromide) buffer to 1.5ml eppendorf tubes and add one scoop of glass beads (425-600μ; Sigma G9772) to the tubes.
- Collect spores from fungal colony by pipetting 50 μl of Triton-X100 up and down several times over the same spot on the plate
- Add spore/Triton-X100 mix to 1.5ml tubes and vortex using disruptor for 2 minutes
- Incubate at 65°C for 15 minutes
- Add 233 μl of isopropanol and 32 μl of 7.5M ammonium acetate into a new 1.5ml tube and keep aside
- Again vortex the primary tube using disruptor for 1 minute
- Incubate at 65°C for 15 minutes
- Add 500 μl of 24:1 Chloroform : isoamyl alcohol
- Mix well by shaking and centrifuge for 5 minutes at maximum speed
- Transfer 400 μl of aqueous phase into tube containing isopropanol and Ammonium acetate (second tube)
- Mix well by shaking and centrifuge for 5 minutes at maximum speed
- Pour off the supernatant and add 500 μl of chilled 70% Ethanol
- Centrifuge again for 5 minutes at maximum speed
- Pour off supernatant, being careful not to lose pellet.

- Dry pellet in speed vac and resuspend samples with 20 μl of DNase free water
- From this total amount, 5 μl can be used for performing polymerase chain reaction.

CTAB Buffer (for use within 1 week)

CTAB stock-20ml

Polyvinyl pyrrolidone- 0.8g

Mercapto ethanol- 100μl

CTAB stock (1L)

100ml 1M Tris pH 8

280ml 5M NaCl

40ml 0.5M EDTA

20g CTAB

Commercial Diagnostic Kits For Aflatoxin Detection

Card tests

A qualitative screening card Total Aflacard (R-BIOPHARM RHONE LTD) for detection of total aflatoxins at various levels in food and feed commodities using a specific monoclonal antibody to detect aflatoxins has been developed. Aflatoxins are extracted from the sample, filtered and passed through a cleanup column before being diluted and applied to the card. Aflatoxin conjugate is applied to the membrane and unbound conjugate is removed by washing. A colourless substrate is added and the card is incubated for five minutes. Finally a stop solution is applied to the membrane. If a coloured reaction develops with the sample, this indicates a negative aflatoxin result, a colourless reaction with the sample indicates that the total aflatoxin content is above the screening level of the card. A coloured reaction should always develop with the control spot to confirm that the test has been performed correctly. The whole assay will be completed in ten minutes and the detection limit is 4ppb.

Another card test to identify the specific presence of Aflatoxin B1 is the Aflacard B1 (R-BIOPHARM RHONE LTD), which involves qualitative screening of food and feed commodities for aflatoxin B1 using a specific monoclonal antibody. The assay time is about ten minutes and the detection limit is 2ppb. The advantage of card test is that the cards can be stored in the dark for long time, to provide a permanent record of results.

ELISA Kits

A quantitative ELISA for detection of Aflatoxin B1 in a wide range of commodities, has been developed (Afla Elisa, R-BIOPHARM RHONE LTD). The sample to be analyzed should be first extracted with 60% methanol, filtered and applied directly to the plate. Aflatoxin B1 specific conjugate is added to wells, followed by the addition of standards and samples. The solutions are mixed and transferred to the clear antibody coated wells. The plate is incubated, washed and a colourless substrate is added. The substrate produces a coloured product in the presence of the aflatoxin-enzyme conjugate but no colour in the presence of free aflatoxin. The colour produced is inversely proportional to the concentration of aflatoxin B1 in the sample. Stop solution is added and the plate is read at 450nm with a microplate reader. The results are obtained within 45 minutes and the test is having a detection limit of 2ppb.

Another diagnostic kit called MycoMonitor Total Aflatoxin Assay (HELICA BIOSYSTEMS) uses a solid phase direct competitive enzyme immunoassay for detection of total aflatoxins in the samples. An aflatoxin specific antibody optimized to cross react with all four subtypes of aflatoxin is coated to microwell plates. In this test the samples should be extracted with 70% methanol. The extracted sample and HRP-conjugated aflatoxin B_1 are mixed and added to the antibody-coated microwell. Aflatoxin from the extracted sample and HRP-conjugated aflatoxin B_1 compete to bind with the antibody coated to the microwell. Microwell contents are decanted and non-specific reactants are removed by washing. An enzyme substrate (TMB) is added and color develops. The intensity of the color is directly proportional to the amount of bound conjugate and inversely proportional to the concentration of aflatoxin in the sample or standard. Therefore, as the concentration of aflatoxin in the sample or standard increases, the intensity of the blue color will decrease. The results are measured optically by a microplate reader with an absorbance filter of 450nm. The optical densities of the samples are compared to the OD's of the kit standards and an interpretative result is determined. Another ELISA kit using the same procedure has also been developed to assess the levels of Aflatoxin M1 (Quantitative Aflatoxin M1 Detection Elisa Kit- HELICA BIOSYSTEMS) in milk samples.

Immunoaffinity Columns

Aflatoxins in the sample are extracted, filtered, diluted and passed slowly through the AFLAPREP column (R-BIOPHARM RHONE LTD) where binding takes place between the specific antibody and the toxin. The AFLAPREP column is then washed to remove any extraneous unbound pigments. The aflatoxin is released from the column using neat methanol prior to injection onto an HPLC. Another immunoaffinity column with florisil tips was also developed to use in conjunction with UV light for the detection of total aflatoxins in a wide range of commodities. Aflatoxins in the sample after extraction and filtration is diluted and passed slowly through the AFLASCAN® column (R-BIOPHARM RHONE LTD) where antibody-toxin binding occurs. The AFLASCAN column is then washed to remove any unbound material and the aflatoxin is released from the column using 100% methanol. The sample is passed through a florisil tip, which is then viewed under UV light at 366 nm where the natural fluorescence of the aflatoxins is observed as a blue or purple band on the tip. The intensity of the fluorescence on the tip is compared to a non-hazardous fluorescent card to obtain a semi-quantitative result. This test is able to detect as little as 1ppb of total aflatoxin in feeds. Among commercial IACs, Aflatest P (VICAM Pvt. Ltd) is most commonly used as the cleanup step in an LC method and in a solution fluorometry method for corn, peanuts, and peanut which was adopted as an AOAC International Official Method. As part of a fluorometer-based test kit, Aflatest P was further certified by the AOAC Research Institute to measure total aflatoxins in 10 different grains and grain products. Agra Strip total aflatoxin test kit (ROMER LABS), a one-step lateral flow immuno-chromatographic assay based on an inhibition immunoassay format, is also very efficient in giving accurate results in rapid time.

18

Molecular Biological Techniques

- General considerations
- Polyacrylamide gel electrophoresis (PAGE)
- SDS-polyacrylamide gel electrophoresis (SDS PAGE)
- Nucleic acid hybridization
    - Radio labelled probes
    - Biotin labelled probes
- DNA finger printing
- Polymerase chain reaction (PCR)
- Reverse transcriptase polymerase chain reaction (RT PCR)

General Considerations

Progress in the field of life science has been so rapid that molecular biology has become one of the basic pillars on which all biological, medical and veterinary sciences are based. The molecular biological techniques have given new dimensions to understanding the disease process and its etiology. On the basis of molecular biology, the classification of the etiological agents particularly of viruses have been reorganized. These techniques are nowadays very much in use in the sophisticated laboratories world over. Though, these techniques are performed with sophisticated instruments or equipment(s) and require specialized trained personnel; some of them can be undertaken in routine diagnostic laboratories. The aim of this chapter is to give a basic knowledge about some of the molecular techniques in diagnosis of infectious diseases of animals.

The procedures described in this text are standard and typical ones. There are several variations and procedural modifications in molecular biology, all of which cannot be discussed here. Therefore, attempts have been made to give the typical or standard procedure for protein resolution; nucleic acid resolution, blotting and other related techniques to give a preliminary idea, which will help in diagnosis of many bacterial and viral diseases.

Polyacrylamide Gel Electrophoresis

The polyacrylamide gels are prepared by mixing acrylamide and bis-acrylamide. The high molecular weight complex compounds are allowed to pass through gel matrix of the polymer of acrylamide by applying electric current. Various components of the compounds are resolved in the gel system on the basis of their size and electric charge. This method has high resolution capacity which can be further enhanced by addition of sodium dodecyl sulfate (SDS) which allows the resolution on the basis of molecular weight of the compound.

In the polyacrylamide gel electrophoresis, one requires 0.2 M sodium phosphate buffer (pH 7.2), acrylamide-bisacrylamide ratio (22.2:0.6), ammonium persulfate (15 mg/ml distilled water), TEMED (N, N, N', N'-Tetra methylethylene diamine), bromophenol blue (50 mg/100 ml distilled water) and staining solution.

The phosphate buffer is boiled on burner in order to remove the air dissolved in it and cooled at room temperature. In a beaker, take 15 ml phosphate buffer, 13.5 ml acrylamide bisacrylamide solution and 1.5 ml ammonium persulfate solution (freshly prepared). Add 50 µl TEMED solution and mix the contents. Perform these procedures in dark or with minimal light source. Take clean and dry gel tubes (10 x 6 mm) and fill them with 2 ml of the above solution after closing one end with rubber stopper or the tubes are closely fitted on the rubber of the chamber of electrophoresis apparatus. After filling the tubes with acrylamide solution, a few drops of distilled water are placed on the top of the gel solution. Place these tubes under the fluorescent light at one feet distance. After about 30 min, an interface can be seen between water and acrylamide which indicates the solidification of gels. The water layer is then removed and the tubes are placed in gel apparatus.

In 40 µl solution of protein (sample, which may be bacteria/ virus/ rickettsia/ chlamydia/ mycoplasma in purified form), add 10 ml of tracking dye (bromophenol blue 0.05%) to each gel. Also use positive control to compare the results. The gel buffer is prepared with dilution of stock solution with distilled water in the ratio of 1:1. Layer the gel buffer over each tube to fill the tubes; both the chambers of apparatus are filled with buffer. Apply current at the rate of 5 mA per gel tube with positive in lower chamber and negative in upper chamber. Under normal circumstances, tracking dye takes about 5 hours to resolve. After the electrophoresis, the gels are removed from the tubes by pushing water from fine needle and syringe between gels and glass. The length of gel and the distance by the dye is measured.

The gels are kept in test tubes or culture tubes with screw cap and the tubes filled with coomassie blue solution (0.2% coomassie blue in 50% ethanol) for 2 hours. Thereafter, de-stain the dye by keeping the gels in de-staining solution of methanol-acetic acid solution (454 ml of 50% methanol + 46 ml glacial acetic acid). Gels can be stored in 7.5% acetic acid. The bands of protein can be observed with naked eyes. The standard can also be run along with sample for comparison.

Sds-Polyacrylamide Gel Electrophoresis

Sodium dodecyl sulfate is added in polyacrylamide gel solution in order to have better resolution on the basis of molecular weight of the molecule. The SDS-PAGE methodology given here is used for the diagnosis of rotavirus infection of calves. The rotavirus genome segments in polyacrylamide gels are detected by ultrasensitive silver staining instead of coomassie blue. This procedure involves the direct nucleic acid extraction from feces by diluting the feces of diarrhoeic calves 1:4 with 0.1 M sodium acetate buffer (pH 5.0) containing 1% sodium dodecyl sulfate, the normal sample size used being 0.25 gm feces, which provides enough extracts for analysis. An equal volume of 3:2 phenol chloroform mixture is added to the fecal suspension and the sample is mixed for 1 min. The emulsified mixture was then centrifuged for 10 min at 200 x g and the resulting clear upper aqueous layer is taken in a sterile vial. The sample is then prepared for electrophoresis by addition of 10 μl of 25% sucrose containing 0.2% bromophenol blue to 40 μl of the aqueous layer.

The 50 μl samples are loaded on to 5% polyacrylamide gel tubes (acrylamide: bisacrylamide ratio 37:5:1), which are polymerized with 0.01% TEMED and 0.05% ammonium persulfate. The gel and electrode buffer is 0.036 M Tris-0.03 M sodium hydrogen phosphate and 0.001 M EDTA (pH 7.8). The gel tubes are 11 cm long and have 0.4 cm diameter. The electrophoresis is performed at room temperature for 12 hours at 20 mA.

The gels are stained by using a washing with 10% ethanol – 0.5% acetic acid for 30 min and then soaked in 0.01 M silver nitrate for 15 min. The gels are then rinsed briefly in distilled water and the reduction step is performed with a solution of 0.75M sodium hydroxide containing 0.1 M formaldehyde and 0.0023 M sodium borohydride. Although the bands appear at this stage, the reduction is continued for a maximum period of 10 min until the bands are clearly visible. The gets are then placed in 0.07 M sodium carbonate and the intensity of staining of both the bands and the background increases slightly in 20-30 min. After that the gels are placed in fresh carbonate solution which can be stored in screw cap culture tubes for a longer period.

On SDS-PAGE, 11 bands of ds RNA genome appear in gel which can be grouped into four classes based on their electrophoretic mobility. Class I consists of segments 1-4, class II of segments 5 and 6; the tightly migrating triplet of segments, 7, 8 and 9 fall into class III and class IV includes segments 10 and 11. This unique grouping of ds RNA segments in polyacrylamide gels is considered as characteristic of rotavirus genome (Fig.18.1).

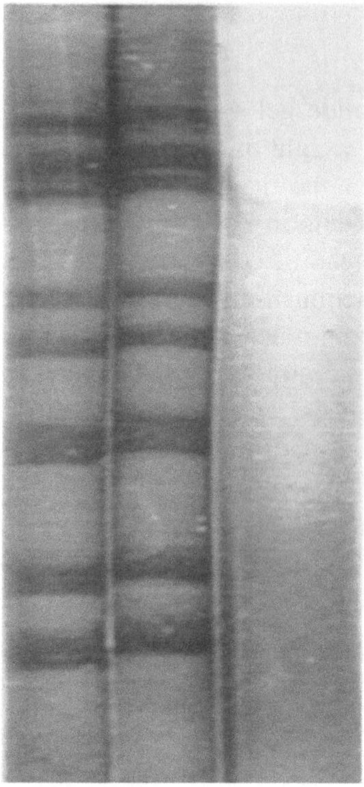

Fig. 18.1: SDS-PAGE in tube- rotavirus segments of ds RNA

In place of tube gels, one can also use the vertical slab gels for the resolution of protein or nucleic acid (Fig.18.2). The dimensions of the gels can be standardized according to the materials used for resolution.

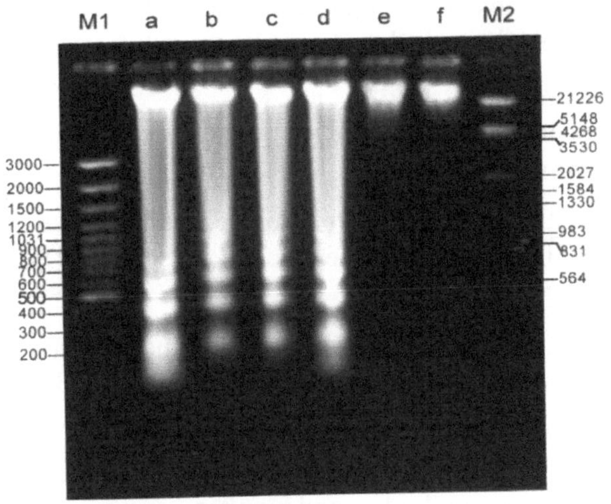

Fig. 18.2: Slab gel electrophoresis

Nucleic Acid Hybridization

After electrophoresis, the gels are blotted on the nitrocellulose paper. For this the nitrocellulose paper is applied on both sides of the gels to get duplicate blots of the gel. After overnight blotting, the nitrocellulose membranes are slightly rinsed in distilled water and heated at 80^{0}C for 2 hours. The membranes are then kept at room temperature till hybridization. For hybridization, specific probes are used in order to make a confirmatory diagnosis. The probes are purified, characterized, nucleic acid sequence, which can be specific for a given species of organisms. The probes are of two types.

Radio Labelled Probes

The probes are labelled with radioactive material like ^{32}P, ^{125}I or ^{3}H, which facilitate the identification and detection of the probe after hybridization. The blotted membranes are hybridized with the radio labelled probes for 16-18 hours at 50^{0}C. It varies from organism to organism like bacteria/virus/ mycoplasma which have separate procedures. It requires a specific procedure unique for each disease causative agent. The hybridized nitrocellulose membranes are exposed to X-ray film for autoradiography and characterization of the blots.

Biotin Labelled Probes

Instead of radioactive material, the probe is labelled with biotin which is detected by avidin-peroxidase conjugate by using an enzyme substrate like diaminobenzidine tetrahydrochloride. The details of avidin biotin complex assays are given elsewhere in this book. The colour developed by the substrate at the reaction site is visible by naked eye; and the blotted nitrocellulose sheets can be stored for long period.

The electrophoresis of nucleic acid and protein blotting and its detection by using probes is classified into three types.

1. *Southern blotting* When the DNA is electrophoresed and blotted on nitrocellulose paper and is detected by the nucleic acid probe. It is known as southern blotting.
2. *Northern blotting:* When the RNA is electrophoresed and blotted on nitrocellulose paper and is detected by nucleic acid probe, it is known as northern blotting.
3. *Western blotting:* When protein is electrophoresed and is detected by using monoclonal or polyclonal antibodies and enzyme conjugates and substrate and by producing a coloured visible reaction; it is known as western blotting or immunoblotting.

DNA Finger Printing

The nucleic acid of the causative organisms is isolated and cut into fragments by using restriction endonucleases. These fragments are resolved in agarose or polyacrylamide gels by electrophoresis and are stained by ethium bromide or silver stain, which gives an endonuclease fragment pattern specific to particular organism, it is known as DNA finger printing.

Polymerase Chain Reaction

This is for the amplification of nucleic acid so that the small amount of nucleic acid present in the clinical sample may also be detected. In this the DNA is denatured at 90-98^{0}C into two segments through de-annealing process. By using two primers complementary to each strand and bordering sequence to be amplified, the DNA template are mixed, cooled to 40-60^{0}C for annealing of primers to the complementary sequence. Addition of DNA polymerase and nucleotide triphosphate allows the synthesis of complementary strands to each primer. The process is continued and new copies are synthesized, thereby increasing the number of DNA fragments. The amplified DNA fragments are electrophoresed into gel system and can be detected by probes. This technique can detect the very small amount of nucleic acid present in the clinical sample. Since, this technique is quiet cumbersome and requires sophisticated equipment(s), its use is limited only to the well-equipped laboratories having trained manpower.

PCR is used to amplify the specific DNA fragment that lies between two regions of known sequences. It consists of repetitive cycles of DNA denaturation, primer annealing and extension by DNA polymerase. The amplification is achieved by extension of short single stranded oligonucleotide primers on single stranded DNA template by a DNA polymerase. Each new strand of DNA synthesized becomes a template for any further cycle of amplification. However, the first two cycles of amplification do not produce any target sequences of defined length. Such target sequences are synthesized in the third cycle only and it increases exponentially from the fourth cycle onwards. So the final number of copies of target sequence is expressed by the formula $(2^n - 2_n)$ x, where n is number of cycles, 2n is products of undefined length obtained in cycle 1 and 2 and x is the number of copies of the original template. At the end of 20 cycles it is expected that there is two fold increase in the product under standard conditions.

Requirements

1. *Thermostable DNA polymerase*

The use of thermostable DNA polymerases in PCR has made it simple because single addition at the beginning is sufficient for the entire amplification process without any further requirement. These enzymes are obtained from thermophilic bacteria that have capacity to replicate at higher temperatures. Such enzymes are also produced in *E. coli* through recombinant DNA technology and at present both natural and recombinant enzymes are commercially available. These include Taq polymerase, AmpliTaq, Vent, pfu DNA polymerase, Tth DNA polymerase, UITma etc.

2. *Deoxynucleoside Triphosphates (d NTPs)*

It is used in 200 μM concentration which is enough to synthesize 12.5 μg DNA. Each batch of dNTP should be checked for pH and pH 7.0 should be adjusted using 1N NaOH.

3. *Primer*

Primer is oligonucleotide sequence with 17-30 nucleotides having 50% GC content 5' end primer is used for PCR product modification like addition of restriction site but 3' end should be intact without any inter or intra-primer complementarity which may lead to primer dimmer formation in PCR. Various kinds of primers are as under:

Random primers- These are random hexamers of four nucleotides A, T, G and C and are used for c DNA synthesis.

Universal primers- Primer sequences flanking the cloning sites of plasmids are termed as universal primers.

Degenerate primers- Every possible combination of nucleotides that code for a given aminoacid sequence are called degenerate primers.

Specific primers- Primers designed to amplify a specific target DNA of defined length.

Nested Primers- Primers used to amplify a segment interval to the previously amplified PCR product.

4. *Buffers and Magnesium Chloride*

The most commonly used buffers (10x) include 100 mM Tris hydrochloride, 500 mM potassium chloride and 15 mM magnesium chloride. It also contains 0.1% (w/v) gelatin and has pH 8.5 at room temperature. It is used with taq or AmpliTaq DNA polymerase. However, buffer should be used as per the recommendations of supplies and it may vary with DNA polymerase. Magnesium chloride is very critical in PCR and is responsible for formations of soluble complex with d NTPs which is essential for incorporation. It also stimulates polymerase activity, increases Tm of ds DNA and promotes primer annealing. Low concentration of magnesium chloride results in low yield while excess concentration may lead to accumulation of non-specific products. The EDTA used for dissolving DNA should not have more than 0.1 mM concentration otherwise it will affect magnesium ion concentration.

5. *Template DNA*

Sample is prepared by lysing the cells through boiling in hypotonic solution. Care should be taken to avoid contamination of template DNA with PCR inhibitors which include heparin, proteinase-K porphyrin, ionic and nonionic detergents and phenol.

Procedure

1. In a 0.5 ml PCR tube, prepare a reaction mixture as follows:

   a. Nuclease-free water – 59.0 μl

   b. 10 x PCR buffer – 5.0 μl

   c. dNTPs (2mM each) –1.0 μl

   d. Primer I (100 p moles) – 1.0 μl

   e. Primer II (100 p moles) – 1.0 μl

   f. Template DNA – 2.0 μl

2. Mix well and centrifuge at 5000 rpm for 15 sec and add 1 μl enzyme Taq polymerase (2.54/Ml).
3. Mix well and again centrifuge at 5000 rpm for 15 sec.
4. Heat the PCR mixture at 94^{0}C for 4 min for denaturation.
5. Again heat the PCR mixture at 94^{0}C for 1 min.
6. Incubate the mixture at 55^{0}C for 1 min.
7. Incubate the PCR mixture at 72^{0}C for 3 min.
8. Repeate the process from step 5 to 7 for 54 cycles, However, the number of cycles depends on denaturation temperature, duration and amount of template DNA. At higher denaturation temperature, enzyme activity is lost and more number of cycles would not help. If the template concentration is low, the number of cycles can be increased.
9. After 54 cycles, incubate the mixture at 72^{0}C for 5 min. This is the final extension step to ensure all PCR products are blunt ended.
10. Cool the product in ice. It should be immediately chilled and should not be left at room temperature as the residual enzyme activity may lead to formation of non-specific product.
11. For amplification of RNA by PCR, complementary DNA (cDNA) is synthesized first using reverse transcriptase and then cDNA is amplified in PCR as given above.
12. Confirmation of PCR product is the ultimate result of PCR standardization. The PCR amplified product is confirmed through either of the following methods.
    a. *Agarose gel electrophoresis.* It can confirm the size of product when run in 1% agarose with molecular weight markers and dye.
    b. *Restriction enzyme analysis*: The product can be fragmented using restriction enzyme and then run on agarose gel for expected fragments.
    c. *Nested PCR*: In this, amplify a region of PCR product using nested primers that flank the region internal to the product and confirm the specific PCR product.
    d. *Nucleotide sequencing* : Sequence the PCR product for confirmation.
    e. *Southern blotting*: Transfer the PCR product on nitrocellulose after electrophoresis and carryout hybridization using DNA probe.

For standard PCR, a DNA polymerase, magnesium, nucleotides, primers, DNA template to be amplified and a thermocycler are required. The PCR mechanism is as simple as its purpose: 1) double-stranded DNA (dsDNA) is heat denatured, 2) primers align to the single DNA strands and 3) the primers are extended by DNA polymerase, resulting in two copies of the original DNA strand. The denaturation, annealing, and elongation process over a series of temperatures and times is known as one cycle of amplification. Each step of the cycle should be optimized for the template and primer set used. This cycle is repeated approximately 20-40 times and the amplified product can then be analyzed. PCR is widely used to amplify DNA for subsequent experimental use. PCR also has applications in genetic testing or for the detection of pathogenic DNA.

Guanine/Cytosine-rich (GC-rich) regions represent a challenge in standard PCR techniques. GC-rich sequences are more stable than sequences with lower GC content. Furthermore, GC-rich sequences tend to form secondary structures, such as hairpin loops. As a result, GC-rich double strands are difficult to completely separate during the denaturation phase. Consequently, DNA polymerase cannot synthesize the new strand without hindrance. A higher denaturation temperature can improve this and adjustments towards a higher annealing temperature and shorter annealing time can prevent unspecific binding of GC-rich primers. Additional reagents can improve the amplification of GC-rich sequences. DMSO, glycerol and betaine help to disrupt the secondary structures that are caused by GC interactions and thereby facilitate separation of the double strands.

Hot Start PCR

Unspecific amplification is a problem that can occur during PCR. Most DNA polymerases that are used for PCR, work best at 68 - 72°C. Therefore, the chosen extension temperature should be in this range. The enzyme can, however, also be active to a lesser degree, at lower temperatures. At temperatures that are far below the annealing temperature, primers tend to bind non-specifically, which can lead to non-specific amplification, even if the reaction is set up on ice. This can be prevented by using polymerase inhibitors that dissociate from the DNA polymerase only once a certain temperature is reached. The inhibitor can be an antibody that binds the polymerase and denatures at the initial denaturation temperature.

Reverse Transcriptase Polymerase Chain Reaction (RT-PCR)

Reverse transcriptase polymerase chain reaction (RT-PCR) is a molecular biology technique by which RNA molecules are converted into their complementary DNA (cDNA) sequences by reverse transcriptase followed by the amplification of the newly synthesized cDNA by standard PCR procedures. This approach to study gene expression is universally known as RT-PCR, because of the role of reverse transcriptase (RT) in the synthesis of first-strand cDNA. RT-PCR is a two-step process. It involves reverse transcription of purified RNA by RT via an appropriate method for priming and amplification of first-strand cDNA using some variant of PCR. Normalization of samples is very important in RT-PCR, and the efficiency of first-strand cDNA synthesis is one of the most important determinants in the success or failure of this method. For this reason, it is strategically better to make a large cDNA pool from which aliquots may be drawn for individual applications rather than repeating the same cDNA synthesis reaction over and over.

RT – PCR uses RNA as starting material for *in vitro* nucleic acid amplification. The discovery of retroviral reverse transcriptase in the early 1970s ultimately made RT-PCR possible. Reverse transcriptase is an RNA-dependent DNA polymerase, catalyzing DNA synthesis using RNA as the template. The end product is known as complementary DNA (cDNA). cDNA is not degraded by RNase , making it more stable than RNA. In RT-PCR, the starting RNA is subsequently degraded, dsDNA is produced, and PCR amplification proceeds in the usual manner. RT-PCR is commonly used in the diagnosis and quantification of RNA virus infections and the analysis of mRNA transcripts such as those produced by translocations commonly associated with leukemias, and sarcomas. Gene expression profiling is likely to have a major impact on molecular diagnostics in the coming years and will depend on RNA analysis using RT-PCR. RT-PCR is sensitive enough to enable detection and quantitation of RNA from even a single cell. In contrast, two other commonly used techniques for quantifying mRNA levels Northern blot analysis. A potential problem with RT-PCR is contamination of the RNA with genomic DNA, which can result in false positive results. Consequently, primers should be designed to span introns or bridge an exon–exon junction. When they span one or more introns, the amplified product from genomic DNA will be bigger than expected, or there will be no product at all if the distance between the primers exceeds the DNA polymerase processing. When they bridge an exon–exon junction, they will not amplify genomic DNA template because the intron will hinder the annealing.

RT-PCR is used to amplify RNA targets. The RNA template is converted into complementary (c)DNA by the enzyme reverse transcriptase. The cDNA serves later as a template for exponential amplification using PCR. RT-PCR can be undertaken in one or two steps. One-step RT-PCR combines the RT reaction and PCR reaction in the same tube. Only sequence-specific primers may be used. During two-step RT-PCR, the synthesized cDNA is transferred into a second tube for PCR. Oligo deoxythymine (dT), gene-specific primers can be used. Oligo (dT) primers are generally preferred as they hybridize to the 3′ poly adenylation (polyA) tails in mRNAs transcribed gene sequences, whereas random primers prime anything including ribosomal RNA. There are advantages and disadvantages to both methods. One-step reactions are easier to set up and ideal for screening, while two-step reactions are ideal for detection of several messages from a single RNA sample. RT-PCR is a sensitive in vitro method and has a crucial role in medical and veterinary applications. RT-PCR is used for detecting and comparing the levels of mRNA and the surface proteins. PCR can be performed in real-time PCR and end-point PCR. Relative and absolute quantification (aqPCR) are two models of real-time RT-PCR. The main role of end-point PCR in biomaterial fields is the measurement of gene expression. The absolute quantification is preferred to end-point PCR for detecting levels of gene expression but end-point PCR is usually used because it has low cost and needs simple equipment.

RT-PCR is becoming an increasingly important tool for the diagnosis of Classical Swine Fever Virus. Evaluation of RT-PCR can be performed either by agarose gel electrophoresis, or by real-time techniques (RT-qPCR). As laboratory equipment is becoming reliable and also more affordable, coupling of liquid handling robotics for nucleic acid isolation and RT-qPCR is becoming practicable. Another advantage of both the standard gel-based RT-PCR and the RT-qPCR is that, due to their high sensitivities, pooled samples can be tested. In particular, the use of RT-qPCR allows rapid and reliable testing of herds at the perimeter of an outbreak in order to avoid preemptive slaughter. Despite the advantages that RT-PCR methodology may have over conventional diagnostic tests, it is extremely vulnerable to false negative or false positive results. False negative results can arise when the nucleic acid is degraded, or when the reaction mixture contains inhibitors. Due to its high sensitivity, false positive results may arise from contaminations, either from sample to sample or from other sources. This implies that before diagnostic laboratories can replace any test, their RT-PCR protocols have to be validated, and regular participation in proficiency testing must prove that performance of the methods used is accurate. In addition, specification concerning sensitivity of the detection must be defined. This is important when samples are pooled. In summary, analytical performance must be equal to or better than that of the standard method.

RT-PCR, allows the use of RNA as a template. An additional step allows the detection and amplification of RNA. The RNA is reverse transcribed into complementary DNA (cDNA), using reverse transcriptase. The quality and purity of the RNA template is essential for the success of RT-PCR. The first step of RT-PCR is the synthesis of a DNA/RNA hybrid. Reverse transcriptase also has an RNase H function, which degrades the RNA portion of the hybrid. The single stranded DNA molecule is then completed by the DNA-dependent DNA polymerase activity of the reverse transcriptase into cDNA. The efficiency of the first-strand reaction can affect the amplification process. From here on, the standard PCR procedure is used to amplify the cDNA. The possibility to revert RNA into cDNA by RT-PCR has many advantages. RNA is single-stranded and very unstable; most commonly, it serves as a first step in qPCR, which quantifies RNA transcripts in a biological sample.

qPCR and RT-qPCR

Quantitative PCR (qPCR) is used to detect, characterize and quantify nucleic acids for numerous applications. Commonly, in RT-qPCR, RNA transcripts are quantified by reverse transcribing them into cDNA first, as described above and then qPCR is subsequently carried out. As in standard PCR, DNA is amplified by 3 repeating steps: denaturation, annealing and elongation. However, in qPCR, fluorescent labeling enables the collection of data as PCR progresses. This technique has many benefits due to a range of methods and chemistries available. In dye-based qPCR (typically green), fluorescent labeling allows the quantification of the amplified DNA molecules by employing the use of a dsDNA binding dye. During each cycle, the fluorescence is measured. The fluorescence signal increases proportionally to the amount of replicated DNA and hence the DNA is quantified in "real time". The disadvantages to dye-based qPCR are that only one target can be examined at a time and that the dye will bind to any ds-DNA present in the sample. In probe-based qPCR, many targets can be detected simultaneously in each sample but this requires optimization and design of a target specific probe(s), used in addition to primers. There are several types of probe designs available, but the most common type is a hydrolysis probe, which incorporates the use of a fluorophore and quencher. Fluorescence resonance energy transfer (FRET) prevents the emission of the fluorophore via the quencher while the probe is intact. However, during the PCR reaction, the probe is hydrolyzed during primer extension and amplification of the specific sequence it is bound to. The cleavage of the probe separates the fluorophore from the quencher and results in an amplification-dependent increase in fluorescence. Thus, the fluorescence signal from a probe-based qPCR reaction is proportional to the amount of the probe target sequence present in the sample. Probe-based qPCR is more specific than dye-based qPCR.

Real-time PCR has revolutionized the way clinical and laboratory diagnosis laboratories diagnose animal and human microbial infections. This testing method combines PCR chemistry with fluorescent probe detection of amplified product in the same reaction vessel. In general, both PCR and amplified product detection are completed in an hour or less, which is considerably faster than conventional PCR detection methods. Real-time PCR assays provide sensitivity and specificity equivalent to that of conventional PCR combined with Southern blot analysis, and since amplification and detection steps are performed in the same closed vessel, the risk of releasing amplified nucleic acids into the environment is negligible. The combination of excellent sensitivity and specificity, low contamination risk, and speed has made real-time PCR technology an appealing alternative to culture- or immunoassay-based testing methods for diagnosing many infectious diseases.

RT-PCR assays that have been developed for the detection of RNA viruses that cause diseases in animals and poultry that are notifiable to the World Organization for Animal Health (OIE). The detection and diagnosis of veterinary infectious diseases is an area in which the potential of Real-time PCR has been best demonstrated. In particular Real-time PCR has been successfully applied as a front line tool in the diagnostic laboratories for notifiable veterinary viral pathogens such as Avian Influenza, classical swine fever, foot-and-mouth disease, bluetongue virus, rabies and Newcastle disease virus. The rapidly transmissible nature of these agents necessitates near real-time detection and diagnosis in suspected infected animals to allow implementation of control procedures. The importance of Real-time PCR in facilitating the rapid diagnosis has had on containing and controlling veterinary infectious disease outbreaks.

For the sake of accuracy and precision, it is necessary to collect quantitative data at a point in which every sample is in the exponential phase of amplification (since it is only in this phase that amplification is extremely reproducible). Analysis of reactions during exponential phase at a given cycle number should theoretically provide several orders of magnitude of dynamic range. Rare targets will probably be below the limit of detection, while abundant targets will be past the exponential phase. In practice, a dynamic range of 2-3 logs can be quantitated during end-point relative RT-PCR. In order to extend this range, replicate reactions may be performed for a greater or lesser number of cycles, so that all of the samples can be analyzed in the exponential phase. Real-time PCR automates this otherwise laborious process by quantitating reaction products for each sample in every cycle. The result is an amazingly broad 107-fold dynamic range, with no user intervention or replicates required. Data analysis, including standard curve generation and copy number calculation, is performed automatically. With increasing numbers of labs and core facilities acquiring the instrumentation required for real-time analysis, this technique is becoming the dominant RT-PCR-based quantitation technique.

Real-Time PCR Chemistries

Currently four different chemistries, TaqMan® (Applied Biosystems, Foster City, CA, USA), Molecular Beacons, Scorpions® and SYBR® Green (Molecular Probes), are available for real-time PCR. All of these chemistries allow detection of PCR products via the generation of a fluorescent signal. TaqMan probes, Molecular Beacons and Scorpions depend on Förster Resonance Energy Transfer (FRET) to generate the fluorescence signal via the coupling of a fluorogenic dye molecule and a quencher moiety to the same or different oligonucleotide substrates. SYBR Green is a fluorogenic dye that exhibits little fluorescence when in solution, but emits a strong fluorescent signal upon binding to double-stranded DNA.

TaqMan Probes

TaqMan probes depend on the 5'- nuclease activity of the DNA polymerase used for PCR to hydrolyze an oligonucleotide that is hybridized to the target amplicon. TaqMan probes are oligonucleotides that have a fluorescent reporter dye attached to the 5' end and a quencher moiety coupled to the 3' end. These probes are designed to hybridize to an internal region of a PCR product. In the unhybridized state, the proximity of the fluor and the quench molecules prevents the detection of fluorescent signal from the probe. During PCR, when the polymerase replicates a template on which a TaqMan probe is bound, the 5'- nuclease activity of the polymerase cleaves the probe. This decouples the fluorescent and quenching dyes and FRET no longer occurs. Thus, fluorescence increases in each cycle, proportional to the amount of probe cleavage. Well-designed TaqMan probes require very little optimization. In addition, they can be used for multiplex assays by designing each probe with a spectrally unique fluor/quench pair. However, TaqMan probes can be expensive to synthesize, with a separate probe needed for each mRNA target being analyzed.

Molecular Beacons

Like TaqMan probes, Molecular Beacons also use FRET to detect and quantitate the synthesized PCR product via a fluor coupled to the 5' end and a quench attached to the 3' end of an oligonucleotide substrate. Unlike TaqMan probes, Molecular Beacons are designed to remain intact during the amplification reaction, and must rebind to target in every cycle for signal measurement. Molecular Beacons form a stem-loop structure when free in solution. Thus, the close proximity of the fluor and quench molecules prevents the probe from fluorescing. When a Molecular Beacon hybridizes to a target, the fluorescent dye and quencher are separated, FRET does not occur, and the fluorescent dye emits light upon irradiation. Molecular Beacons, like TaqMan probes, can be used for multiplex assays by using spectrally separated fluor/quench moieties on each probe. As with TaqMan probes, Molecular Beacons can be expensive to synthesize, with a separate probe required for each target.

Scorpions

With Scorpion probes, sequence-specific priming and PCR product detection is achieved using a single oligonucleotide. The Scorpion probe maintains a stem-loop configuration in the unhybridized state. The fluorophore is attached to the 5' end and is quenched by a moiety coupled to the 3' end. The 3' portion of the stem also contains sequence that is complementary to the extension product of the primer. This sequence is linked to the 5' end of a specific primer via a non-amplifiable monomer. After extension of the Scorpion primer, the specific probe sequence is able to bind to its complement within the extended amplicon thus opening up the hairpin loop. This prevents the fluorescence from being quenched and a signal is observed.

SYBR Green

SYBR Green provides the simplest and most economical format for detecting and quantitating PCR products in real-time reactions. SYBR Green binds double-stranded DNA, and upon excitation emits light. Thus, as a PCR product accumulates, fluorescence increases. The advantages of SYBR Green are that it is inexpensive, easy to use, and sensitive. The disadvantage is that SYBR Green will bind to any double-stranded DNA in the reaction, including primer-dimers and other non-specific reaction products, which results in an overestimation of the target concentration. For single PCR product reactions with well-designed primers, SYBR Green can work extremely well, with spurious non-specific background only showing up in very late cycles. SYBR Green is the most economical choice for real-time PCR product detection. Since the dye binds to double-stranded DNA, there is no need to design a probe for any particular target being analyzed. However, detection by SYBR Green requires extensive optimization. Since the dye cannot distinguish between specific and non-specific product accumulated during PCR, follow up assays are needed to validate results.

Real-time Reporters for Multiplex PCR

TaqMan probes, Molecular Beacons and Scorpions allow multiple DNA species to be measured in the same sample (multiplex PCR), since fluorescent dyes with different emission spectra may be attached to the different probes. Multiplex PCR allows internal controls to be co-amplified and permits allele discrimination in single-tube, homogeneous assays. These hybridization probes afford a level of discrimination impossible to obtain with SYBR Green, since they will only hybridize to true targets in a PCR and not to primer-dimers or other spurious products.

Quantitation of Results

Two strategies are commonly employed to quantify the results obtained by real-time RT-PCR; the standard curve method and the comparative threshold method.

1. Standard Curve Method

In this method, a standard curve is first constructed from an RNA of known concentration. This curve is then used as a reference standard for extrapolating quantitative information for mRNA targets of unknown concentrations. Though RNA standards can be used, their stability can be a source of variability in the final analyses. In addition, using RNA standards would involve the construction of cDNA plasmids that have to be in vitro transcribed into the RNA standards and accurately quantitated, a time-consuming process. However, the use of absolutely quantitated RNA standards will help generate absolute copy number data. In addition to RNA, other nucleic acid samples can be used to construct the standard curve, including purified plasmid dsDNA, in vitro generated ssDNA or any cDNA sample expressing the target gene. Spectrophotometric measurements at 260 nm can be used to assess the concentration of these DNAs, which can then be converted to a copy number value based on the molecular weight of the sample used. cDNA plasmids are the preferred standards for standard curve quantitation. However, since cDNA plasmids will not control for variations in the efficiency of the reverse transcription step, this method will only yield information on relative changes in mRNA expression. This, and variation introduced due to variable RNA inputs, can be corrected by normalization to a housekeeping gene.

2. Comparative Ct Method

Another quantitation approach is termed the comparative Ct method. This involves comparing the Ct values of the samples of interest with a control or calibrator such as a non-treated sample or RNA from normal tissue. The Ct values of both the calibrator and the samples of interest are normalized to an appropriate endogenous housekeeping gene. The comparative Ct method is also known as the 2–delta Ct method, where 2 delta Ct is equal to deduction of delta Ct of reference from delta Ct of sample. Here, delta Ct of sample is the Ct value for any sample normalized to the endogenous housekeeping gene and delta Ct of reference is the Ct value for the calibrator also normalized to the endogenous housekeeping gene. For the 2delta Ct calculation to be valid, the amplification efficiencies of the target and the endogenous reference must be approximately equal. This can be established by looking at how delta Ct varies with template dilution. If the plot of cDNA dilution versus delta Ct is close to zero, it implies that the efficiencies of the target and housekeeping genes are very similar. If a housekeeping gene cannot be found whose amplification efficiency is similar to the target, then the standard curve method is preferred.

Real-Time RT-PCR Methodology

1. **Sample Collection:** To start the diagnostic test, a trained Veterinarian / laboratory technician should collect proper specimens from the animal into a sterile tube containing viral transport media to keep the virus viable.

2. **Sample Preparation:** Once the specimens arrive at the laboratory, researchers will use available commercial purification kits to extract RNA from the sample. Next, the RNA sample is added into one reaction mixture containing all the ingredients required to complete the diagnostic test, also known as "one-step RT-PCR". The ingredients inside this mixture includes DNA polymerase, reverse transcriptase, DNA building blocks, and specific fluorophore probes and primers that recognize the desired virus.

3. **Reverse Transcription:** As mentioned earlier, PCR only works on DNA templates. Thus, the role of reverse transcriptase inside the reaction mixture is to convert all the RNA present within a given sample into cDNA.

    a. **Step 1 – Denaturation/Separation:** To begin, it is important to remember that DNA is a double-stranded structure. Thus, the next step is to unwind the DNA molecule into separate DNA strands. This is accomplished by heating the DNA to high temperatures (> 90°C) for about 10 min.

b. **Step 2 – Primer Annealing:** Next, is the addition of short fragments of DNA, called primers. Primers are designed with high specificity and will attach to specific targets within cDNA of the RNA virus. The specific lower temperature is needed for primer annealing too.

c. **Step 3 – Primer Extension/Elongation:** Since DNA is a double stranded structure, there are two primers in this reaction mix, each one is designed to target one of the two DNA strands. Once the primers attach to their target DNAs, they will direct the DNA polymerase on where to begin and finish amplification on the DNA segment. This step results in an identical DNA copy of the target DNA.

d. **Repeat:** Real-Time PCR will repeat the cycle multiple times (usually for 40 cycles). Every time RT-PCR completes a cycle, it will double the target DNA. Additionally, there are also fluorescent probes that bind specifically to the DNA targets, downstream of each primer. Every time DNA polymerase amplifies the DNA target, it will activate the probe to release a fluorescence signal. Thus, as the amount of target DNA increases, the fluorescence intensity will also increase.

What is the Readout of Real-time RT-PCR?

The emitted fluorescence is then captured as a signal to generate a 'cycle threshold' (Ct) value. The Ct values refers to the amount of cycles required for the fluorescent signal to exceed background levels. Generally, the more target DNA that is in the sample, the faster its amplification will be and thus, the fewer cycles required before the fluorescence signal crosses the background threshold (lower Ct value). Conversely, if there are low amounts of target DNA, it will require more cycles before the fluorescence can cross the background threshold (higher Ct value).

Why are Ct values Important?

Ct values are useful because they provide information about the pathogen's genetic material load. A low Ct value indicates high viral genomic load, whereas a high Ct value indicates low viral genomic load. Veterinary health professionals can use Ct values in conjunction with clinical symptoms and history to find the stage of disease. Furthermore, serial Ct values generated from repeated testing can also help clinicians monitor the disease progression and predict stages of recovery and infection resolution. Animals with the highest viral genomic load indicates a high risk for transmissibility.

19

Investigation of an Outbreak

- General considerations
- First hand information and constitution of a team
- Gathering the disease information from records and the owner
- Animal data
- Previous illness
- Present disease
- Proforma for animal examination report
- Observation of team
- Logical clinical examination of animals
- Disease investigation kit

General Considerations

Disease investigation is an art which comes with time and experience. For identification of diseases, it involves number of steps. Right from getting the call for investigation, going to the spot, collecting the history of affected animals and their environment (out door and indoor), conducting the clinical examination, collecting the blood/ serum, body fluids and tissues from sick and necropsied animals in different transport media, transporting them to laboratory, the whole process involves lot of time, money and trained manpower. The cost of one sample from field cases to laboratory comes in thousands of rupees. If the same sample is originating from wildlife under forest, one can imagine its cost!! Over and above if these steps are not followed in scientific manner, the diagnostic efforts in the laboratory would badly jeopardize, and of course huge money and man power would again go waste. This in turn would cause bad impact on the implementation of control and containment measures in the field, and again huge economic losses! So it is a vicious cycle, if the steps are not followed strictly and scientifically. We can fight out the diseases by scientific investigation, precise and timely diagnosis. Let us follow the steps given below:

First Hand Information and Constituting the Team

Whenever disease outbreak or any sub acute disease problems occur, information for attending the same is generally received in Diagnostic laboratory through letter, telephone, telegram or fax from animal husbandry department of state governments. Soon after, the Officer In-charge of laboratory constitutes a team of scientists (2-4 scientists) involving persons from Pathology, Parasitology, Toxicology, Bacteriology and Virology, depending upon the suspected cause (s). A veterinary pathologist is invariably included in the team to guide other team members and conduct the investigation. Sometimes contents of message regarding the disease are not clear and written ambiguously or in some cases general health check up are required to find out the cause of production losses; in such situation experts from Medicine or any other related discipline are also included in the team. The team gets approval of tour programme and sets out for investigation by vehicle/ train, etc, carrying with investigation kits/bags which are kept ready in the laboratories (Table 19.1). Information regarding arrival of team is sent in advance to the client, so that someone should be available on the disease investigation site to assist the team during disease investigation.

Gathering the Disease Information from Records and the Owner

After reaching on the spot, the team or Disease Investigation Officer (DIO) discusses disease problem with concerned persons *e.g.* veterinary officer, livestock owner, farm manager etc. This type of discussion is helpful to understand and to make guess about the disease/ condition. In later part of investigation one should go by to know when, where and which animals are affected that would make way for correct diagnosis. The team should gather information about the animals (age, sex, breed, species, etc) affected, their environment (outdoor and indoor) and possible abiotic (physical and chemical) and biotic (microorganisms) factors, contributing to the cause of illness or mortality from the animal records and from the owners

Tricky conversation: During the investigation several kinds of versions about disease occurrence are anticipated from the owners, villagers, veterinarians and media persons. So it is the wisdom of DIO that he/she should not be misled by them, instead keep on recording every bit of information without getting biased and keep on making cross questions. DIO should satisfy himself/ herself regarding the history of animal illness revealed by the owner. It will lead to some possibilities/ probabilities about the disease (s). It has been observed that some owners/ farmers do not yield exact information and hide some aspects due to some vested interest or unwillingly, which ultimately give a misleading picture of the disease. Therefore, DIO should handle the animal owners/

attendants diplomatically and tactfully in their local language. He should avoid using technical terminology as most of the owners/ farmers are not able to understand the technical words. DIO should ask the questions in a friendly and cordial manner and avoid arguments. It has been observed during investigation that some animal owners hesitate in revealing accurate history, so it is very important to ask them in such a way that they should not feel shy. From the right kind of history one can reasonably make out what system (s) is involved, which requires special attention for examination.

Be friendly and cordial while collecting the history: In country side, mostly female members of the family look after the livestock. As they are not much educated, they even cannot understand Hindi. Therefore, DIO should use local language for communication, if not, he can take help of his stock assistant/ pharmacist/ attendant or any other person from village who knows both local language and Hindi/ English and may act as interpreter between owner and DIO. Although these things may be appearing minor or of low importance, but may have sometimes profound effect on confirmatory diagnosis.

Don't mix up the versions with your observations: It is also important for DIO that he should try to keep separate the owner's observations from his own interpretations. Whenever DIO is misled by the animal history (anamnesis), the careful clinical and laboratory examination is essential in such cases. If the anamnesis does not conform to the results of examination, it should be accepted with utmost care/ attention to avoid any misinterpretation.

Have a set of questionnaire in mind for better information: DIO must know the right order and type of questions (have a list in mind) to be asked from animal owners which comes with time and experience, practicing the art of disease investigation. The owners usually describe the symptoms/signs in a disorderly manner and remained focused only to anorexia, fever and loss in production. It is the task of DIO to ask a set of questions including patient data, previous illness history, about present illness, herd position, previous treatments, vaccination, control and preventive measures adopted, mortality and morbidity rates, management, nutrition and environment. He can also use pre-designed proforma (Box 2) for recording history and observations, which maintains homogeneity in the data recorded and useful for retrospective as well as perspective studies. While filling up the proforma, DIO should consider following points:

Animal Data

Animal Data Sheet should record the owner's name and address along with species, breed, sex, age, name and number of animals, identification and colour marks in the proforma. The identification number of the animal is very essential, particularly in vetrolegal cases.

Previous Illness

In this column, record the previous suffering of animal, if any, along with treatment (name of the drug, its duration and frequency) given and preventive and control measures taken. It will indicate whether the animal is suffering from the same disease or a new one. The previous vaccinations, if any, should be included in this part of proforma. It is pertinent to have the clinical signs, clinical pathology, post-mortem lesions and diagnosis of previous illness of the animals recorded. This information will be helpful in determining the disease diagnosis.

Present Disease

DIO should select a typical case showing overt sings during the clinical period and ask the questions to farmer about its onset and progress. During the outbreak, usually animals are found in different phases of illness (incubation period, prodromal period, clinical period, and convalescent period), so in such cases it is more important to select a typical case showing frank sings, which would give indication of the disease. The owner's observation about the onset of the disease mostly starts when animal(s) becomes anorexic or its milk production or draught capacity is reduced. In many diseases, the early signs are missed by owners; therefore, one should be very careful regarding onset of disease. It is also advisable to examine few typical cases along with other incontact animals, which look apparently normal. In some diseases, fever lasts for 1-2 days then other signs appear. If fever is missed, it will become a confused state of mind for DIO who may end up with wrong diagnosis. The behaviour of animals, feeding, watering, production, growth, respiration, defecation, urination, sweating, activity, gait, posture, voice and odour should be noted. After recording the history on general aspects, one should ask the owner about total number of animals kept the premises, number of animals affected from present disease and number of animals dead due to disease to calculate morbidity, mortality and case fatality rates. **Morbidity rate** is calculated by dividing the number of affected animals by total number of animals kept at the farm and is expressed in per cent. The total number of dead animals divided by total number of animals is the **mortality rate** which is also expressed in per cent. The **case fatality rate** is calculated by dividing the number of dead animals due to the disease by number of animals affected with same disease and is expressed in per cent. The morbidity, mortality and case fatality rates indicate about the type of disease involved as in contagious diseases, the morbidity rate is very high because of rapid transmission while in non-infectious diseases the morbidity rate is low. The DIO should ask the owner about treatments given to animals and its response; the vaccination and/ or other control measures taken by the owners to contain the disease.

After recording the animal data on present disease, one should see the management aspect, which includes nutrition, feed and fodder, status of toxins in feeds, *e.g.* aflatoxins, pasture grazing or stall feeding, climate, housing, drainage of water, sources of water supply and ventilation in animal houses that should be recorded properly.

Besides, one should also examine the host environmental, which includes vegetation, soil type, soil composition, population density, environmental temperature, moisture, prevalence of insects, fauna and flora and status of pollution. At certain places soil is deficient in certain minerals and trace elements which may give rise to clinical illness. Similarly, the environmental pollution may lead to immuno-pathological/ immuno-toxicological diseases, *e.g.* immuno-suppression, glomerulo-nephritis in animals while improper disposal of waste and unhygienic conditions at farm may be responsible for occurrence of an epidemic of infectious disease; prevalence of flies and insects may cause outbreaks of hemoprotozoan diseases and arboviral infections. The presence of ticks in poultry houses is indicative of the presence of spirochetosis in flock.

Box 1. Proforma for Recording History/ Animal Examination Report

Animal Examination Report*

Case No. ______________________________ Date ______________

Owner's Name and Address ________________________________

Animal species ________________ Breed __________ Sex ________

Animal No. __________________ Identification marks ___________

Age of Animal _____________ Date of start of illness ______________

Previous history (previous illness, treatment, control measures, etc.)

Present history (clinical signs, lesions, behaviour of animal, nutrition, management, environment, morbidity, mortality).

Observations of the veterinarians (clinical signs, lesions and tentative diagnosis).

Signature of owner

Signature of veterinarian

**One copy of this must be accompanied with the forwarding of clinical specimens to laboratory investigations.*

Observations of the Team/ DIO

Apart from the history revealed by the owners, expert team/ DIO should make his own assessment about the disease under investigation, sequence of disease process, clinical signs and managemental conditions. It should not wholly depend on the revelations of the owners. DIO must make his/her own judgement based on observations. This is particularly important in case of toxic conditions of malicious nature, e.g., if animal suffers from fever, then veterinarian should take the temperature of affected as well as normal animals by thermometer. The lesions and other clinical signs, which owner is not able to describe, should also be taken into account by him or DIO. By doing so, DIO establishes faith in owners/ farmers. He/ she should talk with them preferably in local language or use local versions of the technical terms which not only shows the affection but also very useful for accurate anamnesis. It is well said that ***"anamnesis is a base line for accurate diagnosis of disease"***.

Logical Clinical Examination of Animals

Once microbes overcome the host, development of the disease follows a set pattern whether the disease is acute or chronic. These patterns are: incubation period (entry to first sign), prodromal period (relatively of short period; early anorexia and malaise), clinical period (most acute with overt signs) and convalescent period (body start regaining pre diseased state followed by complete recovery. During period of incubation, period of illness and convalescence, infection can be spread. In some diseases like FMD the convalescent period is very long up to 2 months. At the time of outbreak investigation, animals are found in different stages of disease development. However, in point source of infection (like parasitic, food borne and water borne infections) many animals exhibit similar stage of clinical signs/ symptoms. DIO should observe and record various stages of clinical development in animals and select the animals exhibiting overt clinical sings for disease identification. The owners/ farmers often record only dullness, inappetence and decreased production in animals usually in prodromal and convalescent phase of illness that are not sufficient to identify the disease. So animals exhibiting the most severe clinical illness should be examined clinically for their behaviour and general appearance, voice, eating, defecation, urination, mucus discharges, posture, gait, conformation and then for pulse, rectal temperature and respiration. Usually people omit to see the oral mucosa and tongue surfaces and do not go for auscultation and percussion the body parts right from head to thorax and abdominal areas, thereby loose the diagnosis even the animal is in clinical period.

It is also advisable to examine few typical cases along with other incontact animals, which are apparently normal. In some diseases, fever lasts 1-2 days, and then other signs appear. If fever is missed, it will be a confused state for DIO who may end up with wrong diagnosis. The clinical signs/ symptoms in various infectious and non infectious conditions/ diseases have been shown in Table-1. After recording the history on general aspects, one should ask the owner about total number of animals on the premises, number of animals affected and number of animals dead due to disease to calculate morbidity, mortality and case fatality rates. The DIO should ask the owner about treatments given to animals and its response; vaccination and/or other control measures taken to contain the disease. During the clinical examination, collect blood in EDT and also for serum in sterile tubes, prepare blood smears. Also make smears from aspirates, collect body fluids (pleural, peritoneum, synovial, CSF) depending upon the situation and scrapings from skin or solid lesions, etc. After clinical examination of sick animals, DIO should look for the dead or moribund animal and should conduct the post-mortem examination.

20

Diagnosis of TB, JD and Sexually Transmissible Diseases (STDs)

- General considerations
- Tuberculosis
- Johne's disease
- Brucellosis
- Infectious bovine rhinotracheitis
- Campylobacteriosis
- Tichomonosis

General Considerations

The Indian livestock industry is in the state of great transformation with the objective of increased production by proper health care, management and breeding programme. There are number of diseases transmitted sexually through natural mating, AI, transfer of embryo, etc. One good bull can be utilized for breeding many cows, either by natural service or AI; if one bull or cow is infected with any of the sexually transmissible disease it can infect a large number of animals. The important sexually transmissible diseases that are of great concern in our country are Brucellosis, Leptrospirosis, IBR, Trichomonosis, Campylobacteriosis, etc. As per the policy of Govt. of India, the breedable animals should be tested for TB, JD, IBR, Brucellosis, Campylobacteriosis and Trichomonosis; before their use in breeding through either natural service or artificial insemination. The diagnosis and minimum standards for management of these diseases are described.

Tuberculosis

Tuberculosis is a chronic bacterial disease of cattle, buffaloes, sheep, goat and pigs caused by *Mycobacterium* sp. and characterized by presence of tubercle nodules in lungs, spleen and lymph nodes.

Etiology

- *Mycobacterium tuberculosis*
- *M. bovis*

Epidemiology

- 3.28% positive reactors out of 8091 cattle and buffaloes tested.

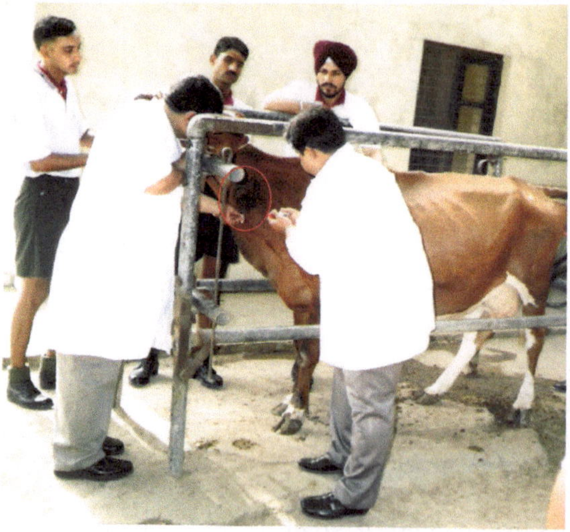

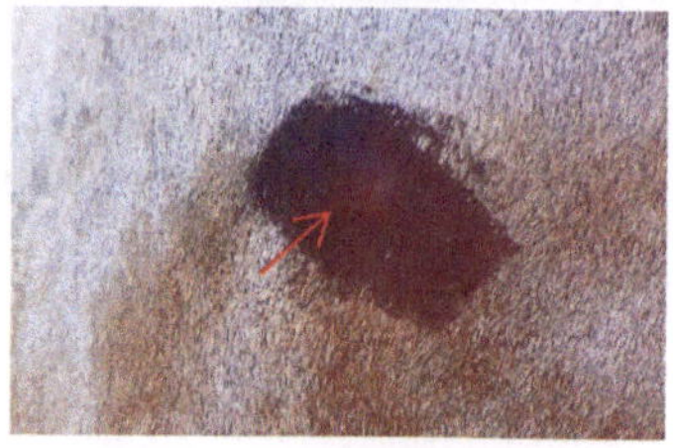

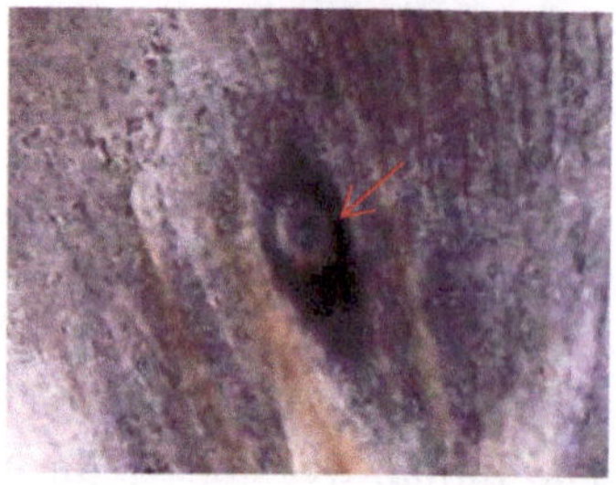

Pathogenesis

Disease spreads through contact with infected animals or their discharges or morbid tissues. The infected animals release the organisms through sputum at coughing and contact animals get infection through droplet inhalation. Besides sputum, faeces, urine, vaginal discharges, semen, milk, lymph and wound discharges may act source of infection. It is also transmitted through contaminated instruments, utensils and beddings. After entry through inhalation or ingestion, bacilli localizes at the point of entry and produce typical tubercle in associated lymph nodes. Mostly pharyngeal and mesenteric lymph nodes are affected. From lymph nodes, infection may extend across body cavities, blood vessels and lymph vessels. The inhaled organism enter in the bronchial tree after lodging in bronchi a tissue reaction takes place. Neutrophilic infiltration is there and when neutrophils are necrosed, macrophages come to destroy the organism but they fail then many macrophages becomes elongated to form epithelioid cells, the hall mark of granulomatous inflammation. Some macrophages are joint together to form giant cells to destroy the acid fast bacilli. As a consequence of this some bacilli are phagocytosed and are destroyed. A zone of lymphocytes, macrophages, epithelioid cells, giant cells and fibrous connective tissues are formed around the central necrosed area.

Characteristic Symptoms

- Low grade fever
- Progressive wasting/weakness, loss of production
- Coughing

Macroscopic Features

- Consolidation of lungs
- Nodules of tubercle present in lungs containing cheesy mass
- Granulomatous lesions in spleen, lymph nodes, liver and intestines.
- Tubercle on pleura and mesentery (***pearly disease***).

Microscopic Features

- Granulomatous lesions characterized by the presence of tubercles in different organs
- Tubercle consists of central caseative necrosed area surrounded by macrophages, lymphocytes, epithelioid cells and giant cells
- In older cases central necrosed area is calcified and surrounded by fibrous tissue capsule.

Diagnosis

- Symptoms and lesions
- Tuberculin testing of animals
- Immunodiagnostic tests for demonstration of antigen /antibody
- ELISA
- Demonstration of acid fast bacilli in impression smears of tubercle or in tissue sections of lungs and lymph nodes.

Note: *The detailed procedures are described in Chapter 14 Immunopathological Techniques.*

Tuberculosis Management

Screening Test Details	
Name of the test	
Primary screening	Single Intradermal test (at middle of neck),
Confirmatory test	Intradermal comparative test in positive reactors, gamma-IFN/LST
Reagents	Bovine tuberculin PPD, Avian tuberculin PPD, Kit for Gamma-IFN
Source of reagents	IVRI, Izatnagar/Private firms
Testing laboratory	Animal farm, RDDLs, CDDL
Positive result criteria	Increase in skin thickness more than double the normal skin thickness with presence of oedema and induration at the site, 72 hours post-inoculation.
Final positive result criteria	Increase in skin thickness at the bovine tuberculin site more than 4 mm greater than the reaction at site of avian tuberculin injection, positive gamma-IFN assay/LST.
Eligible Animals For Test	All animals above 6 months of age.
Frequency of Testing	
Positive herd	Minimum 60 days after isolation and segregation of last positive animal
Negative herd	Annual testing.
Action on Finding A Positive Animal	
Animal	Immediate isolation and segregation of cattle at separate farm. Culling of buffalo, sheep and goat.
Semen	Test semen by PCR/Isolation; if negative, semen can be used in AI (hygienic semen/certified semen). If positive, destroy the semen by autoclaving.
Tuberculosis Free Herd	Herd found negative on two consecutive tuberculin tests at an interval of 6 months, the first being performed 6 months after the segregation of last affected animal.
Quarantine	
Duration of quarantine	Minimum 90 days
Test schedule	Two tuberculin tests (SID and comparative), minimum interval of 60 days between intradermal tests.
Training	Train the person concerned on SID for uniformity in results.

Johne's Disease

Johne's Disease is a chronic bacterial disease of bovines, ovines and caprines caused by *Mycobacterium paratuberculosis* and characterized by dehydration, emaciation, chronic diarrhoea and thickening of the intestine (***corrugations***).

Etiology

- *Mycobacterium paratuberculosis*

Epidemiology

- 3.5% positive reactors out of 7222 cattle and buffaloes tested.

Pathogenesis

Faeces containing the organism is primary source of infection which is acquired by ingestion of contaminated feed and water. It has very long incubation period (15-18 months). The organism has also been isolated from genitalia and semen of infected bulls. Following infection, organism localizes in intestinal mucosa and its associated lymph nodes. The organism penetrate the intestinal mucosa and set up residence within macrophages. The organism multiplies intracellularly without killing host cells and are resistant to intracellular digestion. They grow inside macrophages and distributed through out body. The primary site for bacterial multiplication is terminal ileum and the large intestine leading to decreased absorptive surface, chronic diarrhoea and malabsorption.

Characteristic Symptoms

- Chronic diarrhoea
- Progressive wasting/weakness, loss of production
- Hide bound condition

Macroscopic Features

- Emaciation, cachexia
- Thickening of the intestinal wall
- Presence of '***rugae***' or transverse folds thickened due to chronic inflammatory changes
- Corrugations cannot be removed even after stretching of intestinal wall
- Lymph nodes (Mesenteric) are also enlarged.

Microscopic Features

- Infiltration of macrophages, epithelioid cells and lymphocytes in mucosa and sub mucosa
- Presence of acid fast bacilli in epithelioid cells

- Absence of caseative necrosis and calcification in cattle. However, it is present in sheep and goat.
- Nests of epithelioid cells in mesenteric lymph nodes.

Diagnosis

- Symptoms and lesions
- Demonstration of acid fast bacteria in rectal pinch
- Johnin testing of animals
- Immunodiagnostic tests for demonstration of antigen /antibody
- ELISA, AGID
- Demonstration of organisms in tissue sections using special stains and immunoperoxidase technique.

Note: *The detailed procedures are described in Chapter 14 mmunopathological Techniques.*

Johne's Disease Management

Screening Test Details	
Name of the test	Bovine: Single intradermal test, fecal examination, ELISA Sheep & Goat: Single intradermal test (Skin test), AGID, ELISA
Reagent	Johnin PPD, ELISA kits, antigen for AGID
Source of reagents	IVRI, Izatnagar; ELISA kit from CIRG/private firms.
Testing laboratory	Animal farm, RDDLs, CDDL, CIRG.
Positive result criteria	1. Increase in skin thickness twice the normal with odema and induration at the site of injection, 72 hours post-inoculation. 2. ELISA (depends on the cut off value).
Eligible Animals	
Bovine	All animals above one year.
Sheep & Goat	All animals above six months.
Frequency of Testing	
Positive herd	Minimum 60 days after segregation of last positive animal
Negative herd	Annual test is minimum. Six months (±1 week) after last whole herd negative testing.
Action on Finding A Positive Animal	
Animal	Immediate isolation and segregation of cattle at separate farm. Culling of buffalo, sheep and goat.
Semen	Bulls: Test by culture/ PCR, if negative, semen can be used for AI. If positive, destroy the semen by autoclaving. Sheep & goat: Don't use semen, destroy the semen by autoclaving.

Quarantine	
Duration of quarantine	Minimum 90 days
Test schedule	Bovine: Two Johnin tests and fecal examination/ ELISA, minimum interval of 60 days between tests. Sheep & goat: Two Johnin tests and fecal examination/ AGID, minimum interval of 60 days between tests.
Training	Train the person concerned on SID and fecal examination for uniformity in results.

Brucellosis

Brucellosis is an infectious bacterial disease of animals caused by *Brucella* sp. and characterized by abortion in late gestation and formation of granulomatous lesions in genital organs, joints and fetal liver.

Etiology

- *Brucella abortus*
- *Br. ovis*
- *Br. meletensis*
- *Br. canis*

Pathogenesis

The brucella organism spreads through ingestion of contaminated feed and water with aborted foetal contents or foetal membrane. It is also transmitted through inhalation and may pierce the intact or abraded skin or conjunctivae. Congenital infection may also occur. After entry bacteria multiply in reticuloendothelial cells in regional lymph nodes. The organism enter and travel through intestinal epithelial cells overlaying peyer's patches by endocytosis and then enters into lymphatics. The brucella organism has specific affinity with female and male reproductive organs, placenta, foetus and mammary glands. The organism can also localize in other organs like lymph nodes, spleen, liver, joints and bones. The bacteria proliferates intracellularly and it has high affinity with erythritol sugar which is present in abundance in placenta and foetus. This organism causes abortions in animals in late gestation.

Characteristic Symptoms

- Orchitis
- Accumulation of fluid in scrotum
- Abortion in late gestation (7-9 month)
- Retention of placenta

Macroscopic Features

- Oedema of chorion, thickened and leathery chorion/placenta
- Oedema of foetus, serosanguinous fluid in body cavity
- Pneumonia, necrotic foci in liver
- Enlargement of scrotum in males
- Induration of mammary gland in cows.

Microscopic Features

- Infiltration of phagocytic cells, epithelioid cells and lymphocytes surrounded by fibrous tissue proliferation
- Fetal broncho pneumonia
- Organism in chorionic epithelial cells
- In males, proliferation of fibrous tissue which compresses or replaces the epididymis.

Diagnosis

- Symptoms and lesions
- Immunodiagnostic tests for demonstration of antigen /antibody- CFT, SAT, ELISA, DIA
- Isolation of bacteria
- Demonstration of organisms in tissue sections using special stains.

Note: *The detailed procedures are described in Chapter 13 Immunological and Serological Techniques.*

Brucellosis Management

Screening Test Details	
Name of the test	MRT, RBPT, ELISA, STAT*
Sample	Serum, Milk
Source of reagents	IVRI, Izatnagar / PD ADMAS / Private firms
Testing laboratory	RDDLs, CDDL, PD ADMAS
Positive result criteria for STAT	In vaccinated animals: 200 IU or more is positive In non-vaccinated animals: 100 IU or more is positive
Eligible Animals	• All animals above one year of age • In females paired serum samples 0 and 21 days after calving or abortion

Frequency of Testing	
Positive herd	30 to 60 days after finding last positive animal
Negative herd	**Cattle:** One year (± 1 week) after last whole herd negative testing **Sheep & Goat:** Six months after last whole herd negative testing
Action on Finding A Positive Animal	
Animal	**Cattle:** Immediate isolation and segregation, castration of bulls (retesting not recommended) **Buffalo, Sheep & goat:** Destroy animals and dispose properly.
Semen	Destroy semen since last negative test after autoclaving.
Brucellosis Free Herd	Herd found negative on two consecutive six monthly tests.
Quarantine	
Duration of quarantine	Minimum 30 days
Test schedule	Two tests, serum ELISA, interval of 21 days between tests. Only negative animals to be allowed to mix with the rest of the herd.
Additional Testing at Sexual Maturity	RBPT, Serum ELISA, STAT before bulls are used for semen collection and distribution for AI.
Prevention	**Cattle & Buffalo:** Vaccination of females at 4-6 month with *B. abortus* S-19. Males should not be vaccinated. If incidence of disease is very high at a farm than adult vaccination with a low dose of *B. abortus* S-19 is advised.

Infectious Bovine Rhinotracheitis (IBR)

Infectious bovine rhinotracheitis is an infectious viral disease of cattle caused by herpes virus and characterized by respiratory disease, conjunctivitis, encephalitis in calves and abortions and mastitis in cows.

Etiology

- DNA virus of Herpesviridae family
- Bovine herpes virus –1 (BHV-1)

Pathogenesis

The main source of infection is nasal exudate and coughed up droplets, genital secretions, semen and foetal fluid/ tissues. Aerosol or droplet infection causes respiratory disease. In genital from, venereal transmission occurs. In respiratory disease, after entry virus multiplies in nasal cavity and upper respiratory tract resulting in rhinitis, laryngitis and tracheitis. There is extensive loss of cilia in trachea. This leaves the tracheal epithelium covered with microvilli, which has an adverse effect on the defense mechanism of respiratory tract. The virus spreads from nasal mucosa through trigeminal ganglion, resulting in a non-suppurative encephalitis. Through peripheral leucocytes, virus may reach to placenta and foetus in pregnant animals causing abortion. The foetus is highly susceptible to the herpes virus infection.

Characteristic Symptoms

- Fever (106°F)
- Nasal discharge
- Abortions in late gestation
- Conjunctivitis
- Infectious pustular balanoposthitis in bulls
- Infectious pustular vulvovaginitis in cows

Macroscopic Features

- Rhinotracheitis, pneumonia, mucopurulent exudate in trachea.
- Pustules in vulva/vagina, glans penis and prepuce
- Ulcers in vulva/vagina
- Necrotic lesions in liver of aborted foetus

Microscopic Features

- Hyaline membrane pneumonia
- Erosions/ulcers in mucosa of upper respiratory tract
- Ulcers on vulval mucous membrane
- Infiltration of lymphocytes
- Presence of intranuclear inclusions in mucosal epithelium
- Necrotic lesions in liver, spleen and kidneys of aborted foetus

Diagnosis

Collection and Processing of Sample

Nasal swabs are collected from animals showing respiratory symptoms (serous and mucopurulent discharges) in early phase of infection. In case of vulvovaginitis, vaginal swabs are taken and in case of balanoposthitis prepuce is washed with NSS and collected. The specimens are suspended in transport medium (cell culture medium containing antibiotics and 2-5% FCS) and sent to laboratory after keeping on ice.

During necropsy, mucous membrane or respiratory tract, portion of tonsil, lung and bronchial lymph nodes are collected from animals having respiratory symptoms and fetal liver, lung, spleen, kidney and placenta cotyledons are collected from abortion cases and sent to the laboratory as early as possible on ice.

In the laboratory, swabs are agitated in the transport medium to elute the virus and left at room temperature for 30 min. The transport medium is clarified by centrifugation at 1500 g for 10 min. The tissue samples are homogenized to a 10% suspension in cell culture medium followed by centrifugation at 1500g for 10 min. The supernatant of these specimens are filtered through 0.45µ filters and used for virus isolation.

Virus Isolation

For virus isolation, Madin-Darby bovine kidney (MDBK) cell line is used. MDBK cells are grown in 24 well plates to a confluent monolayer and 100-200 µl of supernatant described above is inoculated into these cell cultures. After 1hr adsorption period, these cells are rinsed with maintenance medium (MM) and finally 1 ml maintenance medium is added. The cells are observed daily for CPE for 3-7 days. When CPE is not observed within 7 days, a blind passage is again given. The cell culture is frozen and thawed 3 times and clarified by centrifugation and supernatant is used for inoculating fresh monolayers. In case of CPE, BHV-1 is further confirmed by neutralization with specific antiserum in micro serum neutralization test (m-SNT) or polymerase chain reaction (PCR).

Virus Isolation from Semen (a prescribed test for international trade)

0.05 ml of freshly collected raw semen is tested by passaging two times in MDBK cells.

Test Protocol

- Dilute 50 µl of fresh semen in 2 ml of FCS (free of antibody against BHV-1) with added antibiotics.
- Mix vigorously and leave for 30 minutes at room temperature.
- Inoculate 250 µl of the semen/serum mixture into a monolayer of susceptible MDBK cells in a 24 wells tissue culture plate. Incubate at 37°C for 1 hour.

- Remove the mixture, wash the monolayer with 1 ml of MM twice and add 1 ml of MM to each well. For each sample at least two wells are taken.
- BHV-1 positive and negative controls are also included in the test.
- The plates are observed daily for the development of CPE. If CPE appears, it is further confirmed by m-SNT.
- If there is no CPE after 7 days, the cultures are frozen, then thawed, centrifuged and supernatant is used to inoculate fresh monolayers.
- The sample is considered negative, if there is no CPE after 7 days of incubation of the passaged cultures.

Serological Tests

Virus Neutralization T est

Test Procedure

- Inactivate the serum samples for 30 min at 56°C.
- Make 1:2 and 1:4 dilution of serum samples in maintenance medium (MM) containing 2% FCS. For this 200 µl of MM in each well of 24 well plates. 200 µl of serum sample is added to the A1 well mix properly and transfer 200 µl of to B1 well. After proper mixing, 200 µl is discarded from B1 well. Similarly, two dilutions (1:2 and 1:4) of the second serum is made in A2 and B2 wells.
- So, 200 µl of diluted serum is remained in each well of 24 well plate. To each well of 24 well plate, 200 µl of BHV1 containing $100TCID_{50}$ is added.
- Incubate the plates at 37°C for 2 hours.
- 100 µl of each dilution of a serum sample is added to two wells of 96 well plate. [100 µl 1:2 dilution of serum sample no 1 is added to A1 and A2 and 100 µl of 1:4 dilution is added to A3 and A4. Similarly, sample no 2 is added to B1, B2 (1:2 dilution) and B3 and B4 (1:4 dilution) and so on.
- Add 100 µl of cell suspension at $3X10^4$ cells/well.
- Incubate the plates for 48-72 h at 37°C.
- In the positive serum control well 1:2 dilution of serum 50 µl, 50 µl BHV1 virus and 100 µl cells. In the negative serum control well 1:2 dilution of serum 50 µl, 50 µl BHV1 virus and 100 µl cells well are

added. In the virus control well, 50 µl virus, 50 µl MM and 100 µl cells well are added. In the cell control well, 100 µl cells and 100 µl MM are added.

- In the cell control wells, there should not be any CPE.
- In the negative control wells, there should be appearance of CPE.
- If the 1:2 dilution serum (final dilution 1:4) does not show CPE, but the 1:4 dilution serum shows CPE, the serum is considered positive and the titre is 2.
- If all the wells [1:2 and 1:4 dilution (³4)] show CPE, the serum is considered negative.

Enzyme Linked Immunosorbent Assay (ELISA) (a prescribed test for international trade)

Indirect ELISA: The principle of an indirect ELISA is that antigen is coated to the solid phase of a microtitre plate and the test sample is subsequently added to the plate. If antibodies are present, these will bind to the antigen and considered as positive and vice versa.

Test Procedure

- MDBK cells are grown in plastic cell culture bottles. When the confluent monolayer is formed, cells are infected with BHV1 and incubated at 37°C for 2 days. When extensive CPE is observed, cells and medium are frozen at -20°C. After thawing, the resulting cellular lysate is centrifuged for 4 h at 8500 g. The virus containing pellet is suspended in a small volume of PBS, cooled on ice disrupted in an ultrasonicator. The sonicated material is centrifuged at 800 g for 10 min and used at an appropriate dilution to coat the plates.
- Coat the plate with 100 µl of diluted antigen in coating buffer and incubate at 4°C overnight.
- Next day, wash the plates with washing buffer at least 3 times. Add 1/10 to 1/100 dilution of each serum samples along with positive and negative serum samples in PBS-T. Shake the plates and incubate at 37°C for 1 h.
- Wash the plates 3 times with washing buffer and add 1:10,000 dilution of anti-bovine Ig-HRPO conjugate to 100 µl and incubate at 37°C for 1 hour.
- Add freshly prepared substrate/chromogen solution @ 100 µl /well.

- Stop the reaction after 10-15 min by adding 50 µl of 3N H_2SO_4 (4 mg OPD/ 10 ml of substrate buffer).
- Take the reading at 492 nm and the OD values of 0.2 higher than negative control serum is considered positive. The test is valid if the positive and weak positive sera are positive and if the negative serum has an absorbance value less than 0.2. Invalid tests should be repeated.

Polymerase Chain Reaction (PCR)

Methodology

The chemicals and buffers required for extraction of DNA and running PCR and electrophoresis are as given below:

i) Proteinase K

ii) SDS

iii) Phenol

iv) Chloroform

v) Isoamyl alcohol

vi) DNA extracted from semen or other material suspected to be infected with BHV 1

vii) Taq polymerase

viii) Deoxyribonucleotide triphosphates (dNTPs)

ix) Primers used are based on the sequences of the gI glycoprotein of BHV 1 and produce PCR product of 468 base pairs (bp). Primer sequences are:

Forward 5'- CAC GGA CCT GGT GGA CAA GAA G – 3'

Reverse 5' – CTA CCG TCA CGT GAG TGG TAC G – 3'

x) Reaction buffers with Mg++ ions

xi) TAE buffer (1X)

xii) Ethidium bromide

A. Extraction of DNA from Suspected Material

1. Aliquot 500 µl semen fluid in 1.5 ml eppendorf tube and add Proteinase K and SDS to a final concentration of 250 µg/ml and 1%, respectively. Incubate for 2 h at 37°C.

2. 500 ul of Tris saturated Phenol is added to the 500 ul of semen. Mixed the content on the Vortex mixer and centrifuged at 12,000 for 5 min.

3. Aqueous supernatant is collected and 250 ul of phenol and 250 ul of ChC13: Isoamyl alcohol was added to it. Mixed the content on the Vortex mixer and centrifuged at 12,000 for 5 min.

4. Aqueous supernatant is collected and 500 ul of ChC13:Isoamyl alcohol was added to it. Mixed the content on the Vortex mixer and centrifuged at 12,000 for 5 min.

5. Aqueous supernatant is collected add sodium acetate, pH 5.2 to a final concentration of 0.3M and two volumes of absolute ethanol to precipitate the DNA. Keep at -20°C for overnight and centrifuge at 12000 rpm for 20 min.

6. Wash the DNA pellet with 70% ethanol and dissolve the pellet in 50 µl of nuclease free water.

B. Polymerase Chain Reaction

1. Preparation of reaction mixture in PCR tube

Primer I	1 µl (10 pmol)
Primer II	1 µl (10 pmol)
dNTP mix(10mM)	1 µl
PCR buffer 10X containing MgCL2 (15 mM)	5 µl
DNA sample	5 µl
Taq polymerase (3 U/ul)	0.5 µl
Distilled water	36.5 µl

2. Tubes are put in thermocycler programmed with following cycling conditions.

Initial heating at 95°C for 5 min followed by 30 cycles of following steps		
Denaturation	95 °C	1 min
Annealing	55 °C	1 min
Extension	72 °C	45 sec
Total 30 cycles followed by		
Final extension	72 °C	7 min
Store at	4 °C	Indefinite

Take out the samples and check for the presence for specific amplified product.

3. Confirmation of the amplified product by Agarose gel electrophoresis:

Agarose gel (1.0%) is prepared containing ethidium bromide to a final concentration of 0.5 ug /ml in mini gel tray of submarine gel electrophoresis system in 1X TAE buffer, pH 8.3.

Load the wells with amplified product along with 100 bp ladder marker in adjacent well and run the gel at 80V for 2 h. The gel is taken out from the apparatus and seen under the UV transilluminator. The presence of band of 468 bp in length in the test sample indicate that the sample is positive for BHV-1 genomic DNA. In the negative sample, there will be no amplification of the DNA and no visualization of specific amplicon.

Infectious Bovine Rhinotracheitis (IBR) Management

Screening Test Details	
Name of the test	ELISA for screening and Serum Neutralization Test (SNT) for confirmation*
Sample	Serum (history of vaccination to be given)
Source of regents	PD ADMAS/Private firms
Testing laboratory	RDDLs, CDDL
Eligible Animals	All animals above 6 month of age.
Frequency of Testing	
Positive herd	Whole herd test, 30 to 60 days after finding of positive animal. Six monthly, after the herd become negative.
Negative herd	Exactly one year. Where the disease has been maintaining a low profile (less than 5% positive), quarterly or six monthly samples could be collected to minimize losses.
Action on Finding A Positive Animal	
Animal	For confirmation seropositive animals should be subjected to PCR/ virus isolation from semen in 3 ejaculates collected at one week interval. If positive for virus, bull should be castrated and segregated.
Semen	Destroy all semen doses since last negative by autoclaving.
IBR Free Herd	Whole herd tested negative on two consecutive occasions at an interval of 2 to 12 months between tests.
Quarantine	
Duration of quarantine	Minimum 30 days
Test schedule	Two tests, serum ELISA or SNT, interval of 21 days between tests. PCR for semen.
Additional Testing at Sexual Maturity	Serum ELISA or SNT, before bulls are used for semen distribution in field AI programmes. PCR for semen.
Prevention	No vaccination in bulls.

Campylobacteriosis

Campylobacteriosis is an infectious disease of cattle and sheep caused by *Campylobacter foetus* and *C. jejuni* and characterized by early abortion, suppurative metritis, cervicitis and vaginitis.

Epidemiology

- A total of 826 preputial washings were analyzed
- 74 (8.9%) *Campylobacter foetus* and 68 (8.2%) *Campylobacter jejuni* were isolated

Characteristic Symptoms and Lesions

- Mucopurulent vaginal discharge
- Retention of placenta
- Abortions at 5-6 month of gestation (*C. foetus*), 6-7 months (*C. jejuni*)
- Purulent exudate in uterine discharges- yellowish
- Congestion of vagina
- Oedema in foetus
- Necrotic foci in liver
- Oedematous placenta

Diagnosis

Sample collection for isolation of *Campylobacter* sp.

1. **Preputial washings, smegma and semen from bulls:** The preputial washings are collected by introducing 20-30 ml of sterile PBS (pH 7.2) into the preputial sac vigorous massage is done for 15-20 seconds, then the infused saline is collected back into the sterile tubes containing transport and enrichment medium (TEM) and sent to the laboratory for further processing. Preputial mucus or smegma can be obtained by suction method using Bartlett's pipette. Smegma can also be collected using artificial vagina and washing it with 20-30 ml of PBS. Semen is collected under aseptic conditions, kept in sterile tubes containing transport and enrichment medium, sealed and sent to the laboratory in insulated container at temperature 4-18°C.

2. **Vaginal mucus in female:** Mucus samples for isolation may be obtained by using swab, suction by Bartlett's pipette or also by washing the vaginal

cavity, then fluid is taken back and collected in sterile container. Sterile speculum can be used to obtain good quality of mucus samples. The vulval region is cleaned and infusion of 50 ml of sterile PBS in vaginal cavity is made to wash the vaginal cavity using a syringe attached to a sterile catheter. The fluid is collected back by suction and reinfused 4-6 times. Finally the fluid containing mucus is collected into the container or tubes containing TEM. Washing fluid of the vaginal cavity can also be collected by using tampon of sterile gauze kept in vagina for 5-10 min which soaks the fluid. Vaginal mucus samples collected by suction are diluted with PBS or can be sown directly onto the culture or enrichment medium.

3. **Aborted fetus and placenta:** In aborted cases the placenta, stomach contents, lungs and liver of the fetus are collected under aseptic conditions and kept at 4-8°C in sealed containers. The amniotic fluid may also be collected.

Treatment of the Samples

The samples received in the laboratory are treated and also sown directly onto the culture medium. Samples can be passed through 65 μm pore sized membrane filters to reduce the contamination.

The vaginal mucus is viscous in nature so an equal volume of filter sterilized cysteine hydrochloride (0.25 G/100 ml conc., pH 7.2) solution is added. It is kept for 5-20 min and then diluted mucus can be directly sown to the isolation medium. If it is not viscous it can be diluted with equal volume of PBS (pH 7.2) also. It is also inoculated into the selective broth and plated on selective agar medium. The preputial washings are centrifuged at 3500 g for concentration. The final reduced samples about 250 μl is sown to the culture medium.

The internal organs like liver, lung of fetus or the pieces are sterilized by flaming only the outer surface and then homogenized. The homogenate is cultured onto culture medium. Stomach contents of the aborted fetus are inoculated or streaked directly on solid agar media plates. The placental membranes are washed to reduce the surface contamination, the chorionic villi are scrapped and these scrapings are transferred to the culture media.

Preparation of Transport and Culture Media

Various types of transport and enrichment media are available for example Clark's Australian Medium. Lander's medium (UK) and SBL medium France, Foley's and Clark's media used in USA. As antifungal agent amphotericin

B can be used instead of cycloheximide which may have toxic effect on *Campylobacter* growth however, most of the TEM use cycloheximide.

Clark's Australian Transport and Enrichment Medium

Australian transport and enrichment medium is a good medium for isolation of *Campylobacter* spp. particularly *C. fetus* but preparation of this medium is laborious and difficult practically, so its routine use in the laboratories is not feasible. Moreover when a number of samples has to be tested it is difficult use it. To prepare this medium following ingredients are needed.

- 5-Fluorouracil in sterile bovine serum (conc. 300 μg/ml)
  - Polymyxin-B sulphate 1 IU/ml
- Brillant green 50 μg/ml
- Nalidixic acid 3 μg/ml
- Cycloheximide 100 μg/ml

The above mixture is distributed into 10 ml with rubber stopper and lid of screwed metal having hole in the top through which a needle can be inserted into the rubber stopper. The filled containers are kept in a water bath at 100°C. When the medium becomes solidified, now a hypodermic syringe is introduced into the rubber stopper. The air present inside is replaced by mixture of 5% O_2, 8% CO_2 and 87% N_2, but this step is performed inside an anaerobic jar. The containers having the medium are stored in a refrigerator for 1 week before use, and it can be stored up to 3 months at 4°C.

One ml of the sample is injected into the medium by using a syringe and the needle is passed through the rubber stopper. Now the bottles are stored at 18°C and sent to the laboratory. The transport time should not be more than 48 hr. After receiving the bottle (container) having sample inside the medium, it is incubated at 37°C for 4 days and then about 3 ml of normal saline is introduced and the medium is shaken vigorously. One ml of fluid from inside is sucked back for isolation purpose and plated to selective media to obtain the colonies after incubation under microaerophilic conditions at 37°C for 3 days.

Processing of Samples after Enrichment into Transport Media or other Selective Media

The samples present in the transport enrichment or other selective broths are incubated at 37°C under microaerophilic conditions for 3 days. Samples after passing through 0.65 μM pore sized filter may also be sown directly on solid selective agar media. The upper layer debris present on filter are discarded, the filtrate can be directly streaked on to the media and incubated as described above for 5-7 days.

Colony Characteristics

The colonies of *Campylobacter* appear within 2-5 days of incubation on a selective medium under favourable conditions. Growth may be at slower rate if other contaminating competing flora is present on the plates. The colonies of *C. fetus* are 1-3 mm in diameter after 3-5 days of incubation. The colonies appear slightly pink, round, convex, smooth and shiny, translucent with a regular edge. *C. jejuni* produce watery dew drop like colonies which swarming along the streaking lines. Circular convex mucoid type colonies may also be seen. *C. coli* mature colonies may show metallic sheen after one week.

Identification of Etiological Agent

Confirmatory diagnosis for campylobacteriosis is possible through identification of the etiological agent as the national trade regulations do not permit import or export of animals having *C. fetus* infection. Veterinary health certification requires certification of bulls and the semen collection centres must test the materials for campylobacteriosis. The prescribed international test is the isolation and identification of the bacterium by cultural and biochemical methods. Although these methods are laborious, time consuming, cumbersome and require selective media and sufficient technical experience for isolation and characterization of the organism, they are considered as a gold standard test for identification of campylobacter species.

Campylobacter infection is diagnosed through isolation by growing the organism in selective broth and plating on to the selective media. Transport and enrichment medium (TEM) is an important requisite to grow this fastidious organism, particularly when samples cannot be processed in the laboratory within 6 hr after collection of the samples. The samples can be collected in a closed container at temperature range within 4-30°C.

Identification of the Isolates

Presumptive colonies are tested for oxidase, catalase, morphology by Gram staining, motility, urease, nitrate tests etc. and then further tested for species differentiation and confirmation. Suspected colonies may be reinoculated in broth and subcultured to get pure culture which are further tested.

Microscopic Examination after Gram Staining

The colonies which show oxidase positive reaction are selected for Gram staining. Carbol or basic fuchsin is used as counter stain inplace of safranin. Under microscope the smear after Gram staining show Gram negative reaction and show typical morphology as curved, comma, S shaped, long helical shape with spirals may be observed. Phase contrast microscope is better to examine the bacteria in living state to see the morphology. Colonies showing oxidase positive, catalase positive, urease negative, nitrate positive, typical morphology resembling to *Campylobacter* as well as motility are selected for further confirmation and species differentiation.

Management of Campylobacteriosis

Screening Test Details	
Name of the test	Bacterial isolation and identification
Sample	Preputial washing, semen, vaginal mucous
Testing laboratory	RDDLs, refer CDDL for confirmation.
Eligible Animals	All male breed able animals. All repeat breeder female animals with early embryonic death (prolonged estrous cycle).
Prevention	Male animal sheath lavage with antibiotics/antiseptics.
Frequency of Testing	
Positive herd	30 days after finding of positive animal.
Negative herd	One year (± 1 week) after last whole herd negative testing.
Action on Finding A Positive Animal	
Animal	Isolate, segregate the positive females and isolate, segregate and castrate the positive bulls.
Semen	Destroy all the semen doses since last negative after autoclaving.
Quarantine	
Duration of quarantine	Minimum 30 days
Test schedule	One test, if age is less than 6 months, else 3 consecutive tests at weekly intervals.

Trichomonosis

Trichomonosis is a protozoan parasitic disease of animals caused by *Trichomonas foetus* characterized by early abortion, vaginitis, metritis and balanitis in cattle.

Epidemiology

- No positive animal

Characteristic Symptoms and Lesions

- Retention of placenta
- Sterility, Pyometra- Metritis, Vaginitis
- Abortion during 3-5 month of gestation
- Balanitis in bulls

Diagnosis

Preputial washing: It is a delicate protozoan parasite and may get destroyed to changes in osmotic pressure like RBCs. It is, therefore, essential to use sterile normal saline solution prepared in glass distilled water. Because metal distilled water may have copper or other metal which can immobilize the organisms. The bottle of two hundred ml capacity containing 100 ml saline is placed for few minutes into warm water before taking the preputial washings, in order to raise the temperature of normal saline to 30-35°C. Saline is allowed to flow in preputial cavity of bull. Washing of mucous content is collected into container. Use of detergent is avoided to prevent immobilization of parasite. Centrifuge the preputial washings at 1000-1500 rpm/min. Discard supernatant and examine the sediment for presence of mobile protozoa with anterior flagella and undulating membrane which is almost diagnostic. This should be differentiated from motile sperm and bacteria. On examination, preputial washings showing ***brownian movement*** of ***free living flagellate*** or ***ciliate*** may be inoculated into (0.1 to 0.2 ml of sediment) glucose broth serum culture/ other *Trichomonas* culture media within 24 hrs of collection. Medium is incubated at 37°C for 7 days and examined 24 hr interval for presence of *Trichomonas foetus*.

Vaginal discharge: Vaginal discharge is collected from female animals by inserting sterilized glass pipette into vagina. It is important to avoid faecal contamination as this may introduce intestinal protozoa which may be confused with *T. foetus*. Use of detergent may be avoided to clean faecal material from vulva. At the upper commissure of vulva by pushing forward at the level of cervix, pipette is moved around vagina to pick up scattered mucous. If possible suction is applied to get 5 ml mucous. Small amount of mucous is examined microscopically for presence of parasites. Cows in oestrus should not be examined as the mucous at this time is unsuitable for *Trichomonas foetus* testing.

For direct examination sample should be taken before 2-3 days of oestrus. For agglutination test samples can be taken even after few days of oestrus.

Identification of organism by direct microscopy and culture (prescribed test for international trade)

A tentative diagnosis is based on the clinical history, sign of early abortion, repeat breeding or irregular oestrous cycles. Confirmation is done by the demonstration of parasites in placental fluid, stomach contents of the aborted foetus, uterine discharges, pyometral discharges and vaginal discharges. The suitable material for diagnosis is vaginal discharge in female and preputial washings and scrapings in bulls.

The number of organisms varies in different situations. They are numerous in aborted foetus, in the uterus after several days of abortion, in recently infected cows and at 2-3 days before oestrous. In the infected bulls the organisms are present in highest number on the mucosa of prepuce and penis. In case of bulls, before samples are collected, it is desirable to allow bull atleast one week sexual rest in order to increase the number of organisms. Preputial smagma either by swabbing the penis with gauze covered rod, douching the preputial cavity with saline or aspiration using a pipette are the methods for collection of material for identification of *Trichomonas fetus.* Artificial insemination pipette is usually used for collection of smagma. For each bull separate and sterile pipette should be used. It is also important to know that during sample collection the surface of the penis and prepuce should be scraped vigorously to dislodge organisms from the epithelial crypts. Scraping the prepuce is better than aspiration and douching.

Samples from cows are collected by washing the vagina or irrigating the uterus with physiological saline/ phosphate buffer saline using a plastic or glass pipette and a long rubber tube. It is important to avoid faecal contamination as this may introduce intestinal protozoa that may be confused with *T. fetus*. Samples should be kept and examined in warm conditions otherwise organisms will become sluggish. Motility of organisms is an important feature in identification of the organisms. When samples cannot be delivered to laboratory within 24 hours, a transport medium should be used.

Transport medium: PBS (pH 7.2) + 5.0% fetal calf serum or 5.0% skimmed milk + penicillin 1000 unit/ml and streptomycin 100 μg/ml.

Collected material is centrifuged and sediment is inoculated in transport medium in the ratio of one part sediment and nine to ten parts transport medium. It is transported in sterile plastic tube at temperature between 5 to 37°C avoiding extreme temperatures.

Culture of the organism is usually required when the number of organism is not enough to make a positive diagnosis by direct examination. Several media can be used. The ***CPLM*** (cysteine peptone liver infusion media) medium, ***BGPS*** (beef-extract/ glucose/ peptone serum) medium. ***Clausen's medium*** (Neopeptone-Lemco-liver extract glucose), ***Diamond's trichomonad medium,*** and ***Oxoid's trichomonad medium***, are the media of choice. It is important that aseptically collected samples be obtained for inoculation into the media and this should be done as soon as possible after collection. It is also important to make sure that the culture media are used before their established expiry date.

The organisms may be identified on the basis of characteristic morphological features. Samples may be examined with a microscope directly. Culture media may be examined microscopically upto one week at 24 hr interval. The organism may be seen under a standard light microscope using a magnification of 100X or more. Phase contrast/dark field microscopy is very valuable in revealing detail features. The pear shaped organisms have three anterior and one posterior flagella and an undulating membrane that extends nearly to the posterior end of the cell. They also have an exostyle that extend beyond the posterior end of the cell.

Preparation of Media

a) Modified Diamond's Medium

Glassware used for culture should be washed in distilled water (avoiding the use of detergent). The Modified Diamond's Medium comprises: 2 gm trypticase peptone, 1 gm yeast extract, 0.5 gm maltose, 0.1 gm L-cycsteine hydrochloride and 0.02 gm L-ascorbic acid and is made up with 90 ml distilled water containing 0.08 gm each of K_2HPO_4 and KH_2PO_4, and adjusted to the pH 7.2-7.4 with sodium hydroxide or hydrochloric acid. Following the addition of 0.05 gm agar, the medium is autoclaved for 10 min at 121°C, allowed to cool to 49°C and then 10 ml inactivated bovine serum (inactivated by heating at 56°C for 30 min), 1,00,000 units crystalline penicillin G and 0.1 gm streptomycin sulphate are added aseptically. The medium is aseptically dispensed in 10 ml aliquots into sterile screw cap vials and refrigerated at 4°C until use. The incorporation of agar into medium confines contaminating organism largely to the upper portion of the test tube, while helping to maintained microaerophillic conditions at the bottom of the test tube where the trichomonads can grow in large numbers.

b) Trichomonas Medium

Suspend 37.5 gm medium in 1 litter of distilled water, boil to dissolve completely, sterilize by autoclaving at 121°C for 15 min, and cool to 50°C. Add 80 ml of inactivated horse serum to this medium and adjust pH at 6.0. Add 1000 unit of penicillin and 500 µg of streptomycin per ml of medium.

The collected samples in media should be properly labeled.

a) Owner's name and address

b) Description of animals: animal number, age, sex, breed, etc.

Management of Trichomonosis

Screening Test Details	
Name of the test	Agent isolation and identification
Sample	Preputial washing, vaginal discharge
Testing laboratory	RDDLs, CDDL.
Eligible Animals	All breed able males, teaser and females with reproductive disorders.
Frequency of Testing	Annual
Action On Finding A Positive Animal	
Animal	Isolation, segregation and castration of the bull
Semen	Destroy the collections since last negative test by autoclaving.
Quarantine	
Duration of quarantine	Minimum 30 days
Test schedule	One test, if age is less than 6 months, otherwise 3 consecutive tests at weekly intervals.
Additional Testing at Sexual Maturity	Protozoa isolation before bulls are used for semen distribution for AI.
Prevention	Breeding rest for positive females for a period of six months and retest before breeding.

21

Validation of A Diagnostic Test

- General considerations
- Steps in validation
    - Step1- Feasibility studies
    - Step 2- Assay development and standardization
    - Step 3- Determining assay performance characteristics
    - Step 4- Monitoring validity of assay performance
    - Step 5- Maintenance and enhancement of validation criteria
- Measurement of uncertainity of a diagnostic test

General Considerations

Validation of a diagnostic test is evaluation of the test to determine its fitness for diagnosis. A validated assay consistently provides test results that identify animals as positive or negative for disease *e.g.*, antibody or antigen and by inference, accurately predicts the infection status of animals with a predetermined degree of statistical certainty. An assay can be recognized as validated if reliable estimates of Diagnostic Sensitivity (DSe) and Diagnostic Specificity (DSp) for a given target population are available. In practical applications, low values of DSe and DSp or diagnostic problems due to low disease prevalence are compensated by the sampling design or by combining multiple diagnostic assays into parallel or serial testing regimens. The selection of assays, the sampling process, the combination of multiple assays into a testing regimen and the interpretation rule for the results define the diagnostic process.

It must be emphasized that an assay, when applied to target populations, will minimize misclassifications of animals as false positive or false negative. A well designed and documented test method and proper standardized reagents, in combination with well trained technicians, will give a stable assay within the laboratory. It assumes a thorough use of the most rigorous experimental design and epidemiological and statistical tools. These are required to reduce bias, random error, and false assumptions about the reference population of animals upon which the assay performance estimates are made. The assay is fitted to the purpose for which it is intended (*e.g.* a confirmatory assay will likely yield many false-positive results if used as a screening assay). The assay is conducted within the context of a rigorous quality assurance programme.

Steps of Validation

Validation of a diagnostic test requires 5 steps to be followed:

Step 1. Feasibility studies

Feasibility studies are the first stage in validating a new assay. They are carried out in order to determine if the selected reagents and protocol have the capacity to distinguish between a range of antibody concentrations to an infectious agent while providing minimal background activity. Feasibility studies also give initial estimates of repeatability, and of analytical sensitivity and specificity.

I. Control Samples

1. Select four or five positive serum samples that range from high to low levels of antibodies against the infectious agent in question.
2. Select a known negative serum sample.
3. The samples ideally should represent known infected and uninfected animals from the population that eventually will become the target of the validated assay.
4. The samples should have given expected results in one or more serological assay(s) other than the one being validated *e.g.*, if brucellosis is being used as infectious disease, they must be positive/ negative with CFT/ STAT.
5. The samples are preferably derived from individual animals, but they may represent pools of samples from several animals.
6. A good practice is to prepare a large volume (*e.g.* 10 ml) of each sample and divide it into 0.1 ml aliquots for storage at or below –20°C. One aliquot of each sample is thawed, used for experiments, and ideally then discarded. If it is impractical to discard the aliquot, it may be held at –4°C between experiments for up to about 2 weeks; however, there is a possibility of sample deterioration under these circumstances. Then, another aliquot is thawed for further experimentation.

This method provides the same source of serum with the same number of freeze–thaw cycles for all experiments (repeated freezing and thawing of serum can denature antibodies). Also, variation is reduced when the diagnostician uses the same source of serum for all experiments rather than switching among various sera between experiments. This approach has the added advantage of generating a data trail for the repeatedly run samples. After the initial stages of assay validation are completed, one or more of the samples can become the serum control(s) that are the basis for data expression and repeatability assessments both within and between runs of the assay. They may also serve as standards if their activity has been predetermined; such standards provide assurance that runs of the assay are producing accurate data. It is highly desirable to include OIE International Standard Sera or other international standard sera if they are available.

II. Selection of Method to Achieve Normalized Results

Normalization adjusts raw test results of all samples relative to values of controls included in each run of the assay. The method of normalization and expression of data should be determined, preferably no later than at the end of the feasibility studies. Comparisons of results from day to day and between laboratories are most accurate when normalized data are used. For example, in ELISA systems, raw optical density (absorbance) values are absolute measurements that are influenced by ambient temperatures, test parameters, and photometric instrumentation. To account for this variability, results are expressed as a function of the reactivity of one or more serum control samples that are included in each run of the assay. ***A simple and useful method is to express all absorbance values as a percentage of a single high-positive serum control that is included on each plate***. A more appropriate method of data normalization could be use of standard curve using several control sera.

Step 2. Assay development and standardization

When the feasibility of the method has been established, the next step is to proceed with development of the assay and standardization of the selected reagents and protocols.

I. Selection of Optimal Reagent Concentrations and Protocol Parameters

Optimal concentrations/dilutions of the antigen adsorbed to the plate, serum, enzyme- antibody conjugate, and substrate solution are determined through 'checkerboard' titrations of each reagent against all other reagents, following confirmation of the best choice of reaction vessels (usually evaluation of two or three types of microtitre plates, each with its different binding characteristics, to minimize background activity while achieving the maximum spread in activity between negative and high-positive samples). Additional experiments determine the optimal temporal, chemical, and physical variables in the protocol, including incubation temperatures and durations; the type, pH, and molarity of diluent, washing and blocking buffers; and equipment used in each step of the assay (for instance pipettes and washers that give the best reproducibility). Optimization of the reagents and protocol includes an assessment of accuracy by inclusion, in each run of the assay, of one or more serum standards of a known level of activity for the analyte in question. ***An optimized assay that repeatedly achieves the same results for a serum standard and the serum controls may be designated as a standardized assay.***

II. Repeatability– preliminary Estimates

Preliminary evidence of repeatability (agreement between replicates within and between runs of the assay) is necessary to warrant further development of the assay. This is accomplished by evaluating results from replicates of all samples in each plate (intraplate variation), and interplate variation using the same samples run in different plates within a run and between runs of the assay. Three-to-four replicates of each sample run in at least five plates on five separate occasions are sufficient to provide preliminary estimates of repeatability. Coefficients of variation, generally less than 20% for raw absorbance values for most samples, indicates adequate repeatability at this stage of assay development. However, if evidence of excessive variation (>30%) is apparent for most samples within and/or between runs of the assay, more preliminary studies should be done to determine whether stabilization of the assay is possible, or whether the test format should be abandoned. This is important because an assay that is inherently variable has a high probability of not withstanding the rigours of day-to-day testing on samples from the targeted population of animals.

III. Determination of Analytical Sensitivity and Specificity

The analytical sensitivity of the assay is the smallest detectable amount of the analyte in question (ab), and analytical specificity is the degree to which the assay does not cross-react with other analytes (cross reacting Ab titre). These assay characteristics are distinguished from diagnostic sensitivity and specificity as defined below. Analytical sensitivity can be assessed by end-point dilution analysis, which indicates the dilution of serum in which antibody is no longer detectable. Analytical specificity is assessed by use of a panel of sera derived from animals that have experienced related infections that may stimulate cross-reactive antibodies.

Step 3. Determining Assay Performance Characteristics

If the feasibility and initial development and standardization studies indicate that the assay has potential for field application, the next step is to establish the assay's performance characteristics.

I. Diagnostic Sensitivity and Specificity (DSe and DSp)

The data on DSe and DSp are the primary parameters established during validation of an assay. They are the basis for calculation of other parameters from which inferences are made about test results. Therefore, it is imperative that estimates of DSe and DSp are as accurate as possible. Ideally, they are derived from testing a series of samples from ***reference animals of known history*** and ***infection status relative to the disease/ infection in question*** and ***relevant to the country or region*** in which the test is to be used. Diagnostic sensitivity is the proportion of known infected reference animals that test positive in the assay; infected animals that test negative are considered to have false-negative results. Diagnostic specificity is the proportion of uninfected reference animals that test negative in the assay; uninfected reference animals that test positive are considered to have false-positive results.

It is desirable to include at least 300 reference samples from known-infected animals, and about 1000 samples from known-uninfected animals to determine initial estimates of DSe and DSp, respectively. Calculations of DSe and DSp are most reliable when the gold standard of comparison is available. Gold standard methods include unequivocal isolation of the agent or pathognomonic histopathological criteria. Because a true gold standard is impossible to achieve, relative standards of comparison are often necessary; these include results from other serological assays and from experimentally infected or vaccinated animals.

Precision is a measure of dispersion of results for a repeatedly tested sample; a precise assay has only a small amount of dispersion. ***Repeatability*** in a diagnostic assay has two elements: the amount of agreement between replicates (usually two or three) of each sample within a run of the assay, and the amount of between-run agreement for the normalized values of each control sample. ***Reproducibility*** is the amount of agreement between results of the same samples tested in different laboratories. ***Accuracy*** is the amount of agreement between a test value and the expected value for an analyte in a standard sample of known activity (*e.g.* titre or concentration). An assay system may be precise, but not accurate, if the test results do not agree with the expected value for the standard.

II. Selection of the Cut-off (positive/ negative threshold)

The test results first must be reduced to positive or negative categories. This is accomplished by insertion of a cut-off point (threshold or decision limit) on the continuous scale of test results.

a) Frequency distributions of test results from uninfected and infected reference animals.

b) Based only on uninfected reference animals

c) An 'intrinsic cut-off' based on test results from sera drawn randomly from within the target population with no prior knowledge of the animals' infection status.

III. Calculation of Diagnostic Sensitivity and Specificity

Calculations of DSe and DSp are aided by associating the positive/ negative data with the known infection status for each animal using a two-way (2 x 2) table (Table 1). After the cut-off is established, results of tests on standard sera can be classified as true positive (TP) or true negative (TN) if they are in agreement with those of the gold standard/ other standard of comparison. Alternatively, they are classified as false positive (FP) or false negative (FN) if they disagree with the standard. Diagnostic sensitivity is calculated as TP/ (TP + FN) whereas diagnostic specificity is TN/(TN + FP); the results of both calculations are usually expressed as percentages.

Test result	**Reference animals**	
	Infected (1000)	**Uninfected (5000)**
Positive	950 (True positive)	500 (False positive)
Negative	50 (False negative)	4500 (True negative)

$$\text{Diagnostic sensitity} = \frac{TP}{TP+FN} \times 100 = \frac{950}{1000} \times 100 = 95\%$$

$$\text{Diagnostic sensitity} = \frac{TN}{TN+FP} \times 100 = \frac{4500}{5000} \times 100 = 90\%$$

IV. Harmonization of assays

When an international standard method is available for detection of an analyte, it is possible to compare the performance of that method with the one under development. This process requires use of the same serum controls and/or standards in both assays.

Step 4. Monitoring Validity of Assay Performance

An assay's test results are useful only if the inferences made from them are accurate. A common error is to assume that an assay with 99% DSe and 99% DSp will generate one false-positive and one false-negative result for approximately every 100 tests on animals from the target population. Such an assay may be precise and accurate, but produce test results that do not accurately predict infection status. For example, if the prevalence of disease in a population targeted by the assay is only 1 per 1000 animals, and the false-positive test rate is 1 per 100 animals (99% DSp), for every 1000 tests on that population, ten will be false positive and one will be true positive. Hence, only approximately 9% of positive test results will accurately predict the infection status of the animal; the positive test results will misclassify the animal 91% of the time. This illustrates that the capacity of a positive or negative test result to predict infection status is dependent on the prevalence of the infection in the target population.

Step 5. Maintenance and Enhancement of Validation Criteria

A validated assay needs constant monitoring and maintenance to retain that designation. Once the assay is put into routine use, internal quality control is accomplished by consistently monitoring the assay for assessment of repeatability and accuracy. ***Reproducibility between laboratories should be assessed at least twice each year***. Proficiency testing is a form of external quality control for an assay. It is usually administered by a reference laboratory that distributes panels of samples, receives the results from the laboratories, analyses the data, and reports the results back to the laboratories. If results from an assay at a given laboratory remain within acceptable limits and show evidence of accuracy and reproducibility, the laboratory may be certified by government agencies or reference laboratories as an official laboratory for that assay.

When a serum control sample is nearing depletion, it is essential to prepare and repeatedly test a replacement before the serum control is depleted. The prospective control sample is included in 10–20 runs of the assay before depletion of the original control to establish its proportional relationship to the nearly depleted control. If the depleted sample was a positive control in ELISAs where the normalized value is expressed as a per cent of that positive control, the proportional difference in ELISA activity between the original and replacement sera must be factored into the normalization algorithm to retain the same cut-off, and thus the same DSe and DSp in the assay. When other reagents, such as antigen for capture of antibody, is to be replaced, they should be produced using the same criteria as for the original reagents, and tested in at least five runs of the assay using a panel of sera that has been designed for this purpose. Reagent lots (serials) need to be evaluated for consistency so variability is not introduced into the assay as new lots are required. Whenever possible, it is important to change only one reagent at a time to avoid the compound problem of evaluating more than one variable at a time.

Measurement of Uncertainty of A Diagnostic Test

Uncertainty is a parameter associated with the result of a measurement that characterized the dispersion of the values that could reasonably be attributed to measurement. Veterinary diagnostic laboratories should be able to estimate the uncertainty of the test methods as performed in the laboratory. This includes methods used by the laboratory to calibrate equipment uncertainty is vital in interpretating the results or deciding if they are fit for purpose.

Uncertainty does not imply doubt about the validity of a test result or other measurement, nor is it equivalent to error. It may be viewed as a quantitative expression of reliability, and is commonly expressed as a number after a +/– sign (*i.e.* the true value lies within the stated range, as measurement uncertainty is expressed as a range). Standard deviation and confidence interval are examples of the expression of uncertainty. An example of the use of standard deviation to express uncertainty is the allowed limits on the test run controls for an enzyme-linked immunosorbent assay, commonly expressed as +/– SD.

Although the determination and expression of measurement uncertainty has not been standardized for veterinary diagnostic laboratories but it should be considered while the test results are interpreted.

Measurement uncertainty must be estimated in the laboratory for each method included in the scope of accreditation. This can be estimated by a series of tests on control samples. Measurement uncertainty can also be estimated using published characteristics, but the laboratory must first demonstrate acceptable performance with the method. Government agencies may also set goals for measurement uncertainty values for official methods.

The requirement for “use of appropriate internal quality control procedures” implies that the veterinary diagnostic laboratory must use quality control procedures that cover all major sources of uncertainty. There is no requirement to cover each component separately. Components can be estimated with experiments in the laboratory (Type A estimates), or from other sources (reference materials, calibration certificates, etc.) (Type B estimates). A traditional control sample procedure, run many times by all analysts and over all shifts, usually covers all the major sources of uncertainty except perhaps sample preparation. The variation of the control samples can be used as an estimate of those combined sources of uncertainty.

ISO 17025 requires the veterinary diagnostic laboratory to identify all major sources of uncertainty, and to obtain reliable estimates of measurement uncertainty. Veterinary diagnostic laboratories may wish to establish acceptable specifications, criteria, and/or ranges at critical control points for each component. Where appropriate, laboratories can implement appropriate quality control at the critical points associated with each source, or seek to reduce the size of a component. Sources of uncertainty include ***sampling, storage conditions, sample effects, extraction and recovery, reagent quality, reference material purity, volumetric manipulations, environmental conditions, contamination, equipment effects, analyst or operator bias***, and other unknown effects. The laboratory would also be expected to account for any known systematic error. Systematic errors (bias) must either be corrected by changes in the method, adjusted mathematically, or have the bias noted in the report statement. If an adjustment is made to the procedure, there may or may not be a need to reassess uncertainty. If there is an adjustment made to correct for bias, then a new source of uncertainty is introduced (the uncertainty of the correction). This must be added to the measurement uncertainty estimate.

There are three principal ways to estimate measurement uncertainty:

1. The components approach (or 'bottom-up' approach), where all the sources of uncertainty are identified, reasonable estimates are made for each component, a mathematical model is developed that links the components, and the variations are combined using rules for the propagation of error (1).

2. The control sample approach (or 'top-down' approach), where measurements on a stable control material are used to estimate the combined variation of many components. Variation from additional sources needs to be added.

3. The method characteristics approach, where performance data from a valid collaborative study are used as combined uncertainties. Laboratories must meet defined criteria for bias and repeatability for the measurement uncertainty estimates to be valid. These should be larger than would be obtained by competent laboratories using their own control samples or components model.

Example: Measurement Uncertainty

1. Measurement of aflatoxin level in feed

1. Sampling
2. Sample storage, packing, forwarding to laboratory
3. Sample preparation
4. Reference material *i.e.* standard aflatoxin
5. Equipment measurement
6. Environmental factors: Temperature, Humidity
7. Diagnostic expert's bias/ effects
8. Computational effects

2. Measurement of antibody titre in serum against brucellosis

1. Sampling of serum
2. Hemolysis
3. Sample storage, preservation, dispatch to laboratory
4. Standard Antigen- Batch, Source
5. Known positive sample- reference material
6. Dilution(s) and procedure
7. Interpretation- Experts' bias *e.g.*: 50% agglutination
8. Computational effects

Use of biostatistics in calculation of uncertainty

- Mean
- Standard deviation- It can be used as the test values ±SD. That is considered as measurement uncertainty of the test.

Ten samples of sera: Test for Brucellosis using ELISA

	Antibody titre				**Mean ± SD**
	Experiment–1	**Experiment–2**	**Experiment–3**	**Experiment–4**	
1.	2.1	2.2	2.0	1.9	2.05±0.12
2.	1.3	1.4	1.5	1.2	1.35±0.12
3.	0.9	0.8	0.7	0.8	0.80±0.08
4.	2.0	2.1	1.9	1.8	1.95±0.12
5.	1.4	1.3	1.6	1.7	1.50±0.18

The standard deviation shows the dispersal of test results from mean values representing uncertainty.

22

Management of Veterinary Clinical Pathology Laboratory: Safety, Accident And First AID

- General considerations
- Ethics for veterinary diagnostic laboratory personnel
- Safety measures in the laboratory
- Accidents
- First aid
  - Acid burns
  - Alkali burns
  - Poisoning
  - Burns caused by heat
  - Injuries caused by broken glass
  - Contamination by infectious materials
  - Bodily damage by electric shock
- Precautionary measures

General Considerations

The veterinary diagnostic laboratory should be designed in such a way that there is enough space for free movement of the people working in it. A cramped laboratory is likely to lead accidents, damaging the equipment and endangering the life of working individuals. The rooms should be adequately ventilated but without strong currents of air. However, clean rooms, fume hoods, etc. should be a part of big laboratory in which infectious or toxic materials can be handled, respectively. The laboratory should have ample of lighting arrangement that is necessary for accurate measurement in any form.

Veterinary diagnostic laboratory should have a good supply of running water.

Working benches that are to be used for sitting should preferably be 2½ feet high and those to be used while standing should be at least 3 feet high. These benches should preferably be acid proofed.

As a rule the place for receiving or withdrawing the specimens should be separate from the working compartment. To avoid specimen mixing, each sample should be carefully labelled. The label should clearly mention the allotted specimen number, the date and time of receipt of specimen, the investigations to be done and most important the name of the owner with species of animal.

Both, the veterinarians and the technical workers are equally at risk of acquiring transmissible diseases through the animal test samples. The risk of these can be lessened by taking appropriate measures. In addition, one should attend to one's general hygiene and prevent fomite transmission of any infectious disease. Disinfect the working benches and as far as possible autoclave various glassware used in the laboratory. Use a rubber teat for sucking/ filling the pipettes. To avoid strain on the eyes, keep both eyes open while doing microscopic work. Before leaving the laboratory one should thoroughly wash one's hands with soap and water, then rinse them well in a disinfectant lotion.

Ethics for Veterinary Diagnostic Laboratory Personnel(s)

1. Place the well-being and service of the sick animal above your own interests.
2. Be loyal to the veterinary profession by maintaining high standards of work and strive to improve your professional knowledge.
3. Work scientifically and with complete honesty.
4. Do not misuse your professional skills or knowledge for personal gain.
5. Never take anything from your place of work that does not belong to you.
6. Do not disclose to any unauthorized person the result of your investigations except the owner of animal.
7. Maintain confidentiality about personal information that you may learn about a farm/ animal(s).
8. Respect and work in harmony with other staff of your laboratory as a team.

9. Be at all times courteous and considerate to the owners of the animals/ farm.
10. Promote personal health care including hygiene for prevention and control of zoonotic diseases.
11. Follow safety procedures and know how to apply first aid.
12. Do not drink alcohol during laboratory working hours.
13. Use equipment and laboratory correctly and with care.
14. Do not waste reagents or other laboratory supplies.
15. Fulfill reliably and completely the terms and conditions of your employment.

Safety Measures in the Laboratory

One must remain alert and cautious while working in the laboratory. Careless handling of reagents, glassware or specimens to be tested in the laboratory can cause serious injury and is dangerous to life.

Safety with Chemicals/ Reagents

Except few reagents, almost all chemicals/ reagents used veterinary diagnostic in the laboratory are lethal poisons if consumed by anyone. Even if they are splashed on the skin/ eye they can cause irreversible damage. There is an appropriate way of handling and storage of hazardous chemicals to avoid injury and damage to self and others. In our country excessive heating can decompose many chemicals, cause explosions, or lead to the formation of toxic fumes.

Proper labeling of all chemicals, reagents, stains, etc. should be done in legible writing or by using printed adhesive lebels. At appropriate places display the prohibition signs and on all dangerous reagents or chemicals stick Hazard warning symbols.

1. Flammable Chemicals

These include ether, xylene, toluene, methanol, ethanol, glacial acetic acid, acetone, acetic acid, acetone, acetic anhydride, alcoholic Romanowsky stains and acid alcohol etc. These chemicals should be stored in a fireproof metal box at ground level, preferably in a cool store. A container well lined with tin foil can also be used. Store only small quantities of such chemicals on the shelves. Ensure that there is no open flame nearby while opening a bottle containing flammable solvent. Nearest flame should be at least 10 feet away. Never heat a flammable liquid over any flame. Use a water bath or electric hot plate.

Use sand, thick blanket or the now available multipurpose fire extinguishers to prevent undesired blaze. Pouring water on such fires will spread them. Every laboratory should be equipped with the commercially available fire extinguishers. If these are not available, there should be sand buckets in accessible places.

2. Corrosive Chemicals

These include strong acids *e.g.*, concentrated sulphuric acid, hydrochloric acid, nitric acid, glacial acetic acid, trichloroacetic acid, orthophosphoric acid, and strong alkalies like sodium hydroxide and potassium hydroxide. Store these at low levels. Never attempt mouth pipetting. Accidental swallowing can be lethal as these chemicals cause destruction of living tissue. Always pour a corrosive chemical at below eye level, slowly, and with great care to avoid splashing. Wear protective eye glasses/ eye shields while opening such containers. Always add the corrosive substance to water not vice-versa and that too slowly. The addition of small amount of water to sulphuric acid is enough to produce sufficient heat to break a glass container, which should be avoided.

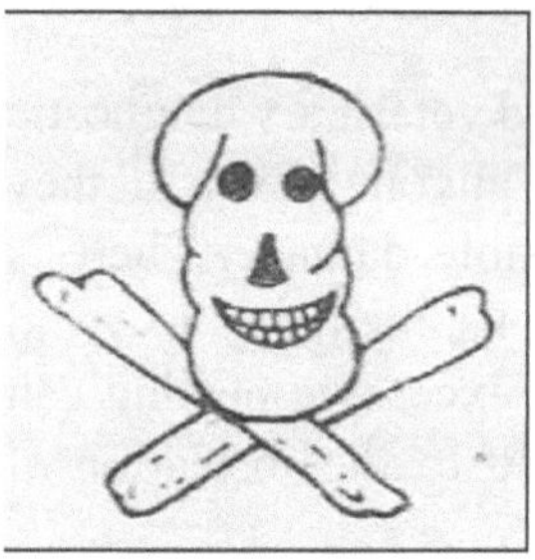

Toxic

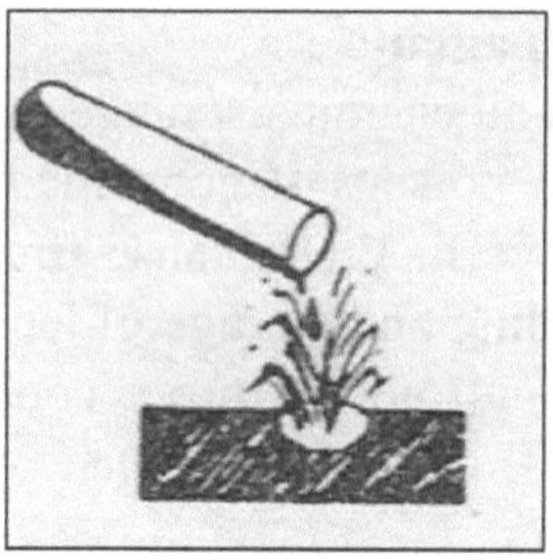

Corrosive

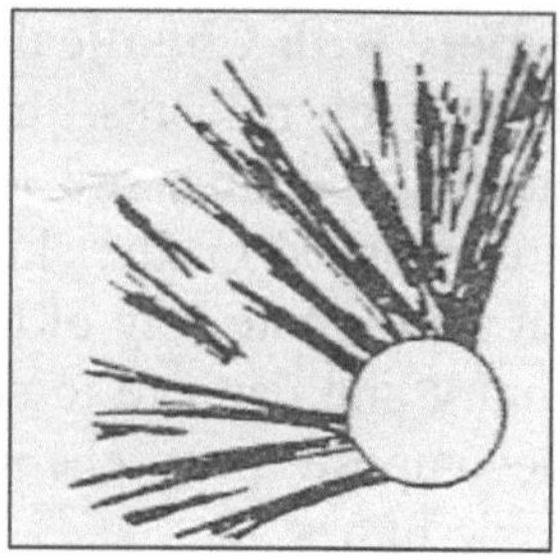

Explosive

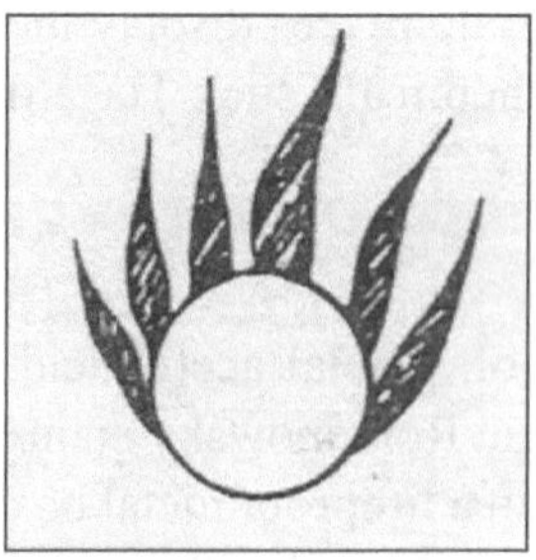

Oxidising

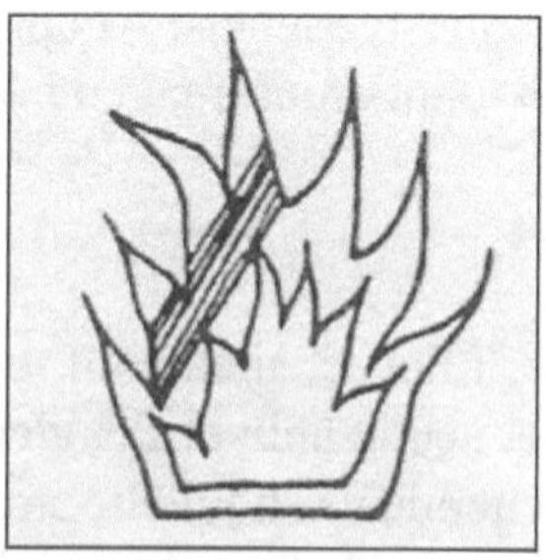

Highly inflammable

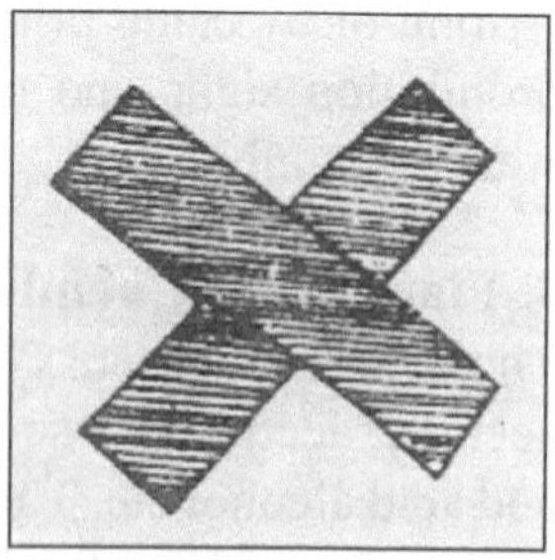

Harmful / Irritant

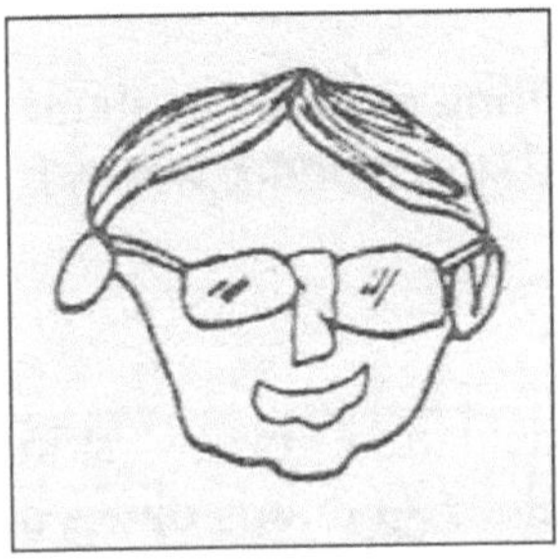

Eye protection mandatory

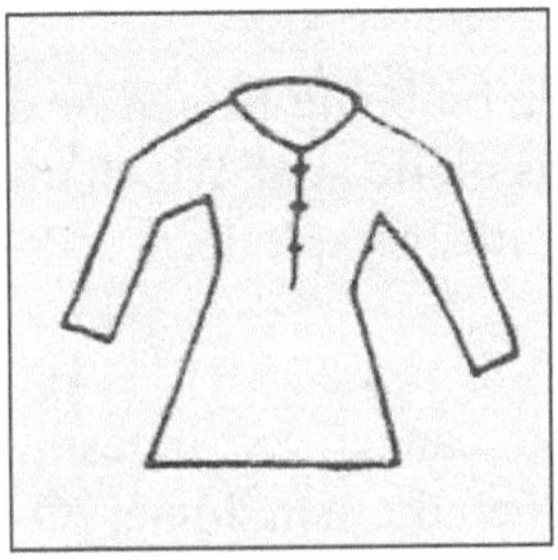

Lab. coat mandatory

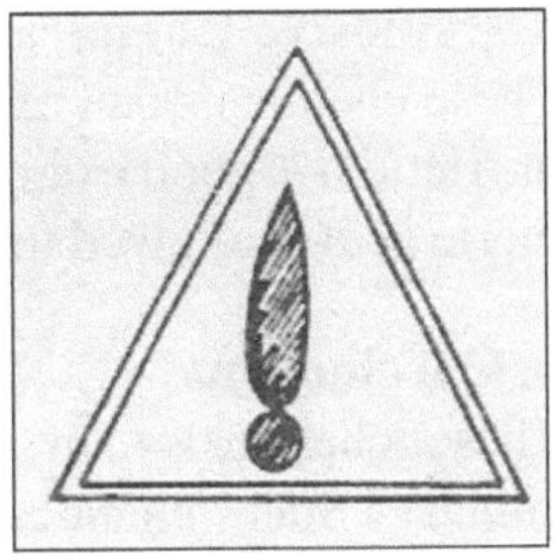

Risk of danger

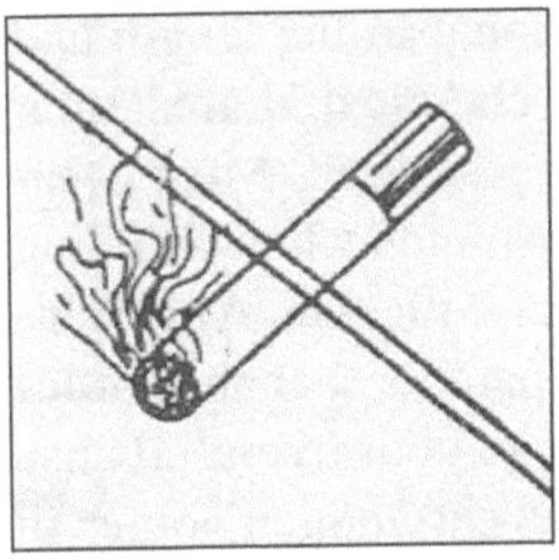

No smoking

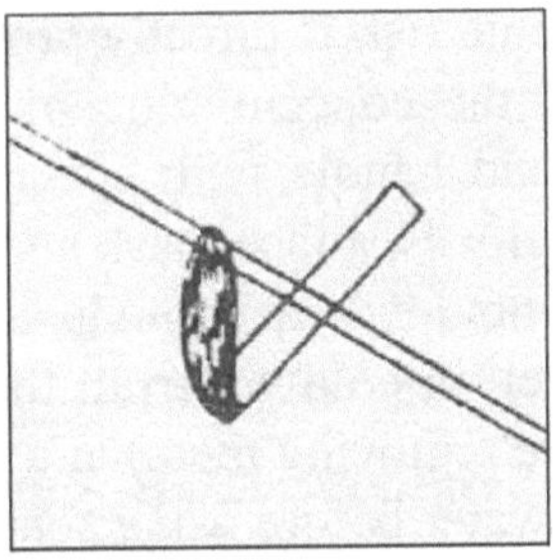

Naked flames prohibited

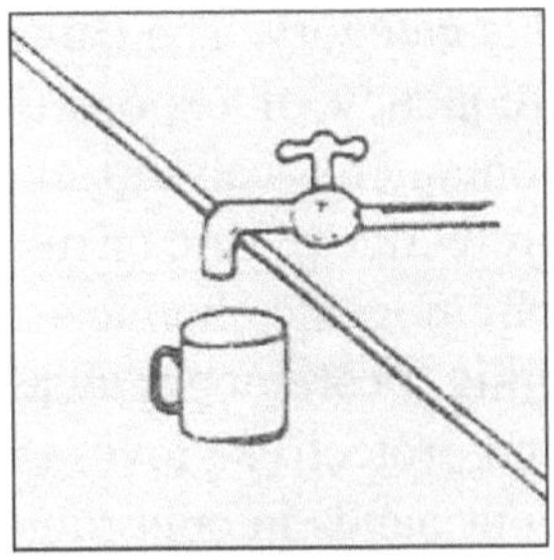

Not drinking water

3. Toxic, harmful, and Irritating Chemicals

These are chemicals that can cause death or serious ill-health if swallowed or inhaled or if they come in contact with skin. Examples are potassium cyanide, mercuric nitrate, sodium azide, sodium nitroprusside, formaldehyde solution, chloroform, barium chloride, methanol, iodine and sulphanic acid. Skin and mucous membrane irritants are xylene, formaldehyde and ammonia vapours. Store highly toxic chemicals *e.g.*, potassium cyanide in a locked cupboard. Stock solutions should also be stored safely in a cupboard, not on an open shelf. Always wear protective gloves and after working with them immediately lock them up. Always wash your hands after using a toxic or harmful chemical. Keep fume forming chemicals in a fume cupboard. Never mouth pipette them.

4. Oxidising Chemicals

These include chlorates, perchlorates, strong peroxides, potassium dichromate and chromic acid. Keep these away from organic materials and reducing agents. They can produce much heat when in contact with other chemicals, especially flammable chemicals. Handle them with utmost care. Most of them are dangerous to skin and eyes and when in contact with reducing agents.

5. Explosive Chemicals

These chemicals can explode on being heated or on getting exposed to flame or friction. A good example is picric acid, which must be stored under water. If picric acid is allowed to dry, it can explode.

6. Carcinogens

These chemicals can cause cancer by ingestion, inhalation, or by skin contact. Such chemicals include benzidine, O-tolidine, O-dianisidine, a and b naphthylamine, nitrosamines, nitrosophenols, nitronaphthalenes, and selenite. All substrates used in ELISA like OPD, DAB, etc. also fall under this category. The carcinogenic risk is directly proportional to the length and frequency of exposure and the concentration of the chemical. Label their containers "carcinogenic" and handle with special precautions. Must wear protective plastic or rubber gloves, a face mask and eyeshields when handling carcinogenic chemicals. Do not let them come in contact with skin. After handling a carcinogen, wash well in cold water all the apparatus, bench, bottles and protective gloves (before removing them) and change your overall. Rinse your hands in cold running water before using soap. If a carcinogen comes in contact with skin, wash the affected part in cold running water for 5 minutes.

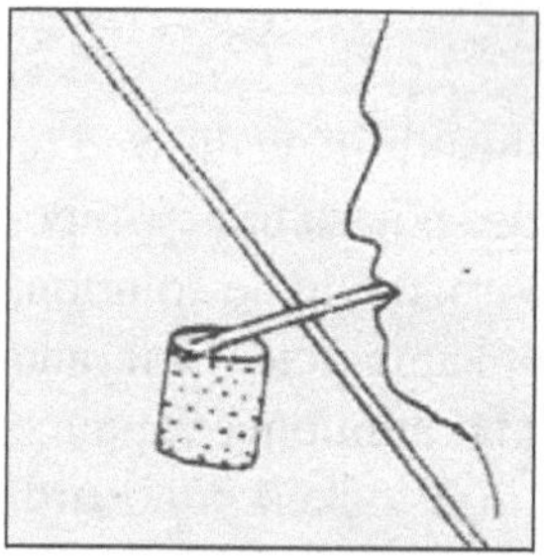

No mouth pipetting

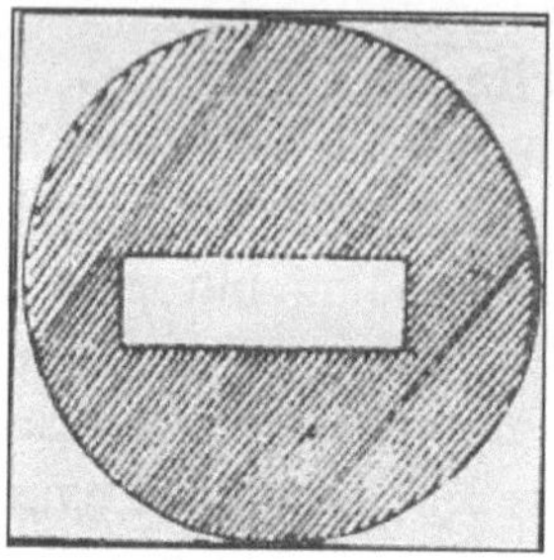

No entry

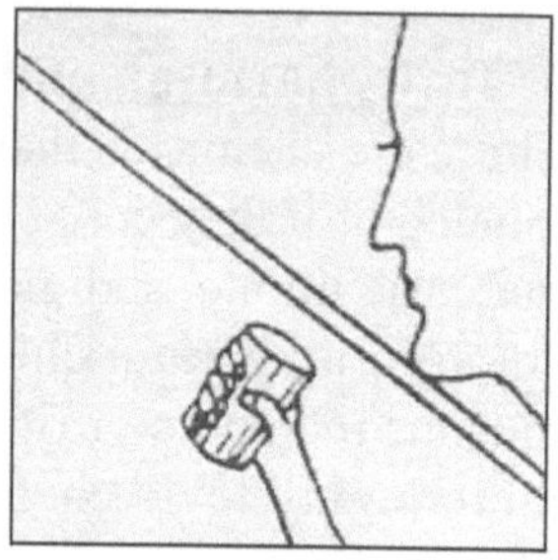

Drinking prohibited

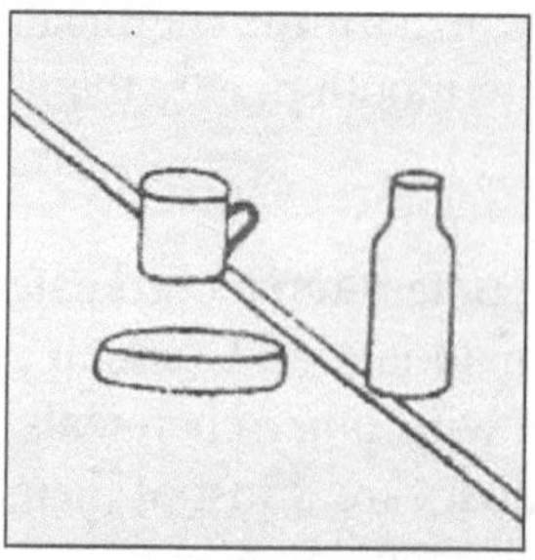

Drinking, eating prohibited

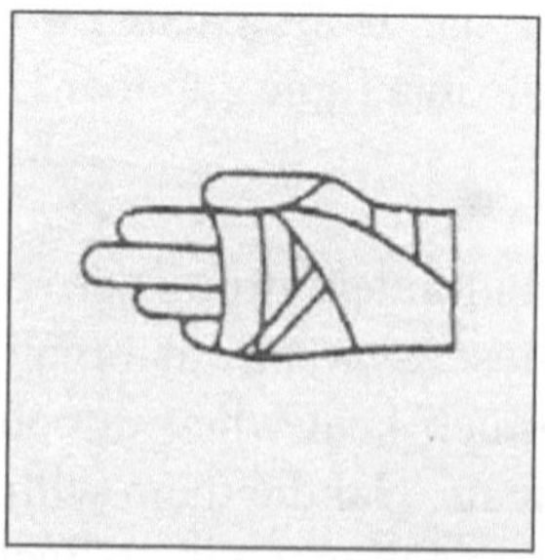

Chemical burn

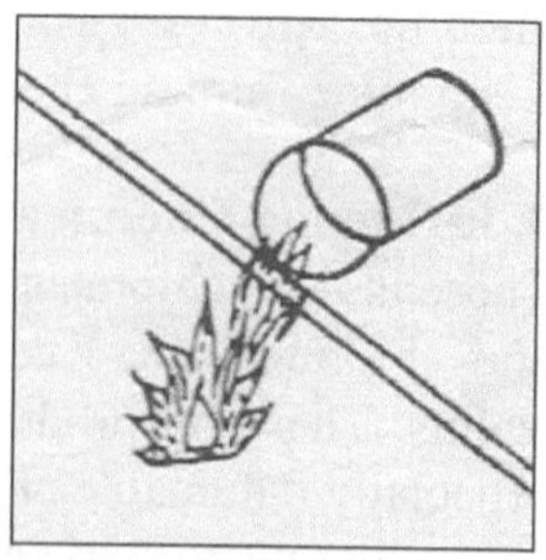

Not to be extinguished with water

Accidents

Accidents in the laboratory may be caused by:

(1) Acids	-	splashes on the skin
or	-	splashes in the eye
(2) Alkalis	-	swallowing
(3) Toxic substances	-	contact, swallowing, splashing
(4) Heat	-	open flames
	-	hot liquids
	-	inflammable liquids
	-	explosions
(5) Broken glass	-	physical injury
(6) Contamination by	-	contact, damage due to needle/ syringe infected material
(7) Electric shock	-	damaged electric switches, naked/ corroded wires
(8) Fire	-	spirit lamps, gas burners, electric appliances, flammable chemicals

First Aid

Requirements

Suggested list of first aid materials for laboratory

1. 5% aqueous sodium carbonate
2. 2% aqueous sodium bicarbonate in an eyedrop bottle
3. 5% acetic acid
4. Saturated solution of boric acid in an eyedrop bottle
5. Soap powder solution (5 g per litre of water)
6. Acriflavine ointment
7. 2% Mercurochrome
8. Antiseptic lotion
9. Cotton wool
10. Gauze

11. Roller bandage
12. Adhesive tape
13. Scissors

First aid materials should be readily available at the time of need and these should not be kept under lock.

(1) Acid burns

I. Acid splashes on the skin:

   (a) Wash the affected part thoroughly and repeatedly with large quantity of water.

   (b) Bathe the affected skin with cotton wool soaked in 5% aqueous sodium carbonate.

II. Acid splashes in the eye:

   (a) Wash the eye immediately with large quantities of water sprayed from a wash bottle or rubber bulb. Squirt the water into the corner of the eye near the nose.

   (b) After washing, put 4 drops of 2% aqueous sodium bicarbonate into the eye.

   (c) Refer the patient to a physician. Continue to apply bicarbonate solution to the eye while waiting for the doctor. Alternatively hold the eye under the running tap.

III. Swallowing acids (accidental swallowing while using a pipette):

   (a) Call a physician/ send the person to the hospital.

   (b) Drink some 5% soap solution immediately. Alternatively, give him/her two whites of egg mixed with 500 ml of water or milk. If neither of these is available, he/she should drink ordinary water.

   (c) Make him/her gargle with the soap solution.

   (d) Give him/her 3 or 4 glasses of ordinary water.

   (e) If the lips and tongue are burned by the acid:

      - rinse thoroughly with water
      - bathe with 2% aqueous sodium bicarbonate.

(2) Alkali burns

Wash immediately with large quantities of water. Alkali burns are as serious as, and often more serious than, acid burns.

I. Alkali splashes on the skin:

(a) Wash thoroughly and repeatedly with water.

(b) Bathe the affected skin with cotton soaked in 5% acetic acid (or undiluted vinegar).

II. Alkali splashes in the eye:

(a) Wash immediately with large quantities of water sprayed from a wash bottle or rubber bulb. Allow the water into the corner of the eye near the nose.

(b) After washing with water, wash the eye with a saturated solution of boric acid (apply drops repeatedly).

(c) Refer to a physician at once.

III. Swallowing alkalis (accidental swallowing while using a pipette):

(a) Call a physician/ send the person to hospital.

(b) Make the patient drink at once

- a 5% solution of acetic acid or lemon juice or dilute vinegar (1 part vinegar to 3 parts water).

(c) Make him gargle with the same acid solution.

(d) Give him 3 or 4 glasses of ordinary water.

(e) If the lips and tongue are burned by the alkali

- rinse thoroughly with water
- bathe with 5% acetic acid

(3) Poisoning

Poisoning can be caused by inhaling toxic vapours or gases (*e.g.* chloroform) and/or accidental swallowing while pipetting a poisonous solution. Call a physician or qualified nurse, specifying the toxic substance involved. Till then place the victim in the open air while waiting for the doctor.

(4) Burns caused by heat

A. Severe burns affecting large areas of skin, *e.g.* burns caused when boiling water or hot solution is spilled over the victim.

(a) If the victim is on fire, *e.g.* if splashed with burning ether or other inflammable solvent, roll him in a blanket or overall to smother the flames.

(b) Inform the physician on duty immediately.

(c) Lay the victim on the ground. Do not remove his clothing. Cover him if he is cold.

(d) Do not apply any treatment to the burns. This must be left to the physician.

(e) Never tear off the blisters that form over the burns.

B. Minor burns affecting a small area of skin, *e.g.* burns caused by hot glassware or a Bunsen flame.

(a) Plunge the affected part into cold water or ice-water to soothe the pain.

(b) Apply mercurochrome or acriflavine ointment to the burn.

(c) Apply a dry gauze dressing loosely.

(d) If the burn becomes infected or does not heal, refer the patient to a physician.

(e) Never tear off the blisters that form over the burns.

(5) Injuries caused by broken glass

These are caused by broken test tubes, syringes, petridishes, pipettes, flasks or other glassware.

(a) Wash the wound immediately to remove any glass pieces.

(b) Apply mercurochrome or acriflavine ointment to the wound.

(c) Cover with gauze and adhesive tape.

(d) If the cut bleeds profusely, stop the bleeding by pressing down on it with a compress. Refer the patient to a physician.

(e) If the cut bleeds heavily with the blood spurting out at intervals, try to stop the bleeding with a compress and call a physician or qualified nurse.

(f) Continue to press on the wound while awaiting the physician's or nurse's arrival. He or she will decide whether a tourniquet should be applied.

(6) Contamination by infected material

I. Wounds caused by broken glassware containing stools, pus, infectious material, etc.:

(a) Wash the wound immediately.

(b) Check whether the cut is bleeding. If not, squeeze hard to make it bleed for several minutes.

(c) Bathe the whole area, *i.e.* the edges of the cut and inside the cut, with antiseptic lotion.

(d) Wash thoroughly with soapy water.

(e) Bathe again with antiseptic lotion.

(f) Refer the patient to a physician if the material involved is known to be very infective, *e.g.* pus.

II. If infected material (Broth culture) is accidentally sucked into the mouth:

(a) Spit it out immediately.

(b) Wash out the mouth with diluted antiseptic lotion.

(c) Wash out the mouth thoroughly with large amounts of clean water.

(7) Bodily damage by electric shock

A low-voltage alternating electric current (220 V) is usually used in the laboratory and electric shocks are rare. They may occur when faulty equipment is being handled, particularly with wet hands. The symptoms are fainting and asphyxia.

(a) Before doing anything else, put off the main switch.

(b) Call a physician or send the affected person to nearby hospital.

(c) Begin giving mouth-to-mouth respiration immediately.

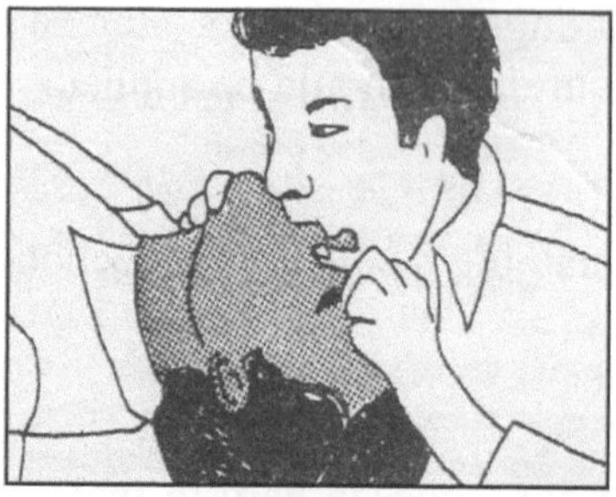

2. Precautions for the Avoidance of Accidents

(i) Handling acids and alkalis

(a) Always add the acid to the water drop by drop, stirring the mixture after each drop for making dilution of acid. Do this preferably in a sink. Never pour water into concentrated acid because of the danger of splashing.

(b) Keep the bottles of acids and alkalis on the lower shelves of the cupboards. When you take one out, hold it firmly upright with a dry hand. Do not keep acids and alkalis in bottles with ground glass stoppers as they may get stuck.

(c) Where possible, use small measuring cylinders for measuring acids and alkalis. If more accurate measurement is required, use a pipette plugged with non-absorbent cotton wool or with a rubber tube attached. Pipette slowly, watching the level of the liquid.

(ii) Heating glassware and liquids

(a) Test tubes: Never heat the bottom of a test tube. The liquid inside might sputter. Heat the middle of the tube, shaking gently. The mouth of the tube should be facing away from the worker and any other person, towards an empty space or a sink.

(b) Ordinary glass and Pyrex: Only Pyrex glassware and porcelain pots can be heated over a Bunsen flame. Ordinary glass will break.

(c) Inflammable liquids: Only small quantities of inflammable liquids such as ether, ethanol, acetone, benzene, toluene and carbon disulphide should be kept in the laboratory. *Warning*: Ether will ignite at a distance of several metres from a flame. Never place a bottle of ether on a workbench where there is an open flame (Bunsen burner, spirit lamp, etc.). Carbon disulphide is even more dangerous.

(iii) Do not use broken, cracked or chipped laboratory glassware.

(iv) Put clear labels on poisons. Keep them in a locked cupboard.

(v) Do not use nylon clothes while working as these are easily inflammable. Always use a laboratory apron.

(vi) Always ensure that electrical wiring and electrical appliances are in good condition.

Precautionary Measures

1. Care and cleanliness must be practiced by the entire laboratory personnel at all times. Always wear lab aprons and Hand gloves during work in the laboratory. After work leave the apron in the laboratory premises and discard the hand gloves.
2. Keep finger nails short.
3. After removing the gloves, hands should be washed with detergent solution and water.
4. Smoking, eating, drinking and using snuff are not desirable in a laboratory
5. Care should be taken to ensure that all gas taps work efficiently and that no gas escapes when the taps are turned off. Do not attempt to find gas leaks by using a lighted match
6. Care should also be taken to ensure that all water taps are working efficiently. There should no leakage in the tap and tap connections. Also make sure to close all the taps, when leaving the lab.
7. Electric switches and connections should be repeatedly inspected and kept free from corrosion, so that no danger shall arise from short circuiting or due to the exposure of naked wire from which the insulation has been broken or corroded away
8. When a laboratory is to be left unattended for any length of time all electrical switches except refrigerator, incubator, BOD, deep freezer, etc. should be turned off
9. The main taps for gas and water and the electrical switches should also be located so that these services can be turned off in emergency.
10. Laboratory personnels must also know the meanings of safety signs.

11. Eyes are specially vulnerable to splashes from reagents and safety spectacles should always be worn when carrying out any procedure when there is risk.
12. Always make sure that during centrifugation all tubes are firmly capped to avoid formation and inhalation of aerosols, containing microorganisms, which may be highly dangerous.
13. Infection can also occur when working with tissue, body fluids and whole animals. Animals can also cause allergies in some individuals. All experiments should therefore be performed with the greatest care and strict precautions taken.
14. No work with pathogenic material should be carried out by any body, having an open cut, skin lesion and injury.
15. Proper disposal of waste from a laboratory is a problem of a considerable importance. There should be an ample supply of bins of suitable size for disposal of solid materials such as broken glass, porcelain, filter papers, match sticks, etc. Lighted matches or smoldering materials should never be thrown into these bins. The bins should be cleared often, at least daily.
16. Dispose all infected material properly. Can put such material in hypochlorite solution or in an acidic solution *e.g.* diluted sulphuric acid (25%). Burn off all dried contaminated articles *e.g.*, filter papers.
17. For disposal of waste from bio-origin, a different covered bin should be used which should be sterilized periodically.
18. Breakable items should be kept in proper racks and never at the edge of the working table.
19. All wastes of liquids and solids must be separated and stored in separate containers
20. Petri plates should not be discarded directly after experiments. They should properly treated to kill pathogens/ microorganisms before their disposal preferably through autoclaving.
21. Paper should never be used to carry light from one burner to another. Insoluble waste should not be thrown into the sink.
22. If corrosive, Poisonous, or radioactive liquids are thrown down the sink, they should be accompanied by a generous supply of water to ensure

that by the time they reach the main drain they will be too dilute to be dangerous.

23. When working in a laboratory it is better to wear some sort of protective coat, apron or overall.
24. All bottles and containers should be carefully and distinctly labeled so that no confusion or possible error can arise when several containers are being filled with different chemicals.
25. Poisonous and dangerous chemicals should be stored separately and in a locked cupboard. Explosive chemicals are kept in a lead lined rectangular box fitted with a good lock, outside the building but close to the lab and readily accessible to the attendant but not to the public (Br_2, PCl_5 and PCl_3 etc.)
26. Greatest care should be taken when handling radioactive materials. Special precautions are given under radioisotope methodology.
27. Always wear protective aprons, hand gloves, cap to avoid direct physical contact with the radio active substance.
28. All the radioactive work should be carried out preferably in a fume hood. Polythene sheet must be spread in the fume hood or working bench before starting to help in rapid clean up.
29. All radioactive materials must be stored sealed and labeled properly, with date and person's name written on it.
30. A film badge or a Thermo Luminescent Dosimeter (TLD) for personnel monitoring of radiation exposure must be worn by the person while working with radioactive material.
31. Many accidents occur in transporting bulky containers from room to room or from one part of the laboratory to another. Bottles should never be carried by the neck. Trays or polythene buckets or suitable trolley should be used.
32. Adequate and conveniently accessible storage of both apparatus and chemicals are essential to the laboratory safety. Bottles containing liquids will be kept on the lower shelves whilst solids are kept on the higher ones.
33. The floor space should be kept perfectly free from spillage, broken glass, straw, paper etc. as their presence may lead to accidents.

34. When dealing with volatile inflammable liquids no flames should be allowed in the vicinity and care should be taken to avoid inhalation of vapours.
35. Cylinders of gases under pressure are best kept upright in a suitable stand well away from any source of heat.
36. When pouring liquids from one container into another keep both vessels well away from the body so that any spillage shall not fall upon the person. When corrosive chemicals are involved it is a good plan to carry out the operation over a sink so that any spillage can be easily flushed away.
37. It is often an advantage to use a glass rod to direct the liquid stream when pouring from one bottle to another.
38. When diluting concentrated sulphuric acid always add the acid to the water kept in ice and not vice versa; add the acid slowly, preferably down a glass rod with stirring to reduce the violence of the reaction.
39. When NaOH is dissolved in water great heat is evolved. Use cold water and add NaOH to it little by little. Do not handle NaOH with unprotected hands.
40. When corrosive, poisonous, volatile and offensive chemicals are being used carry out the operations in a fume hood.
41. Ether or any other volatile inflammable solvents should not be heated directly over a naked flame. Use water baths or heating mantles.
42. When pushing a glass tube or rod through a hole in rubber cork lubricate well with water
43. Poisonous, radioactive and offensive reagents should never be pipetted directly by mouth, use pipetting devices
44. It is not advisable to use glass stoppers in bottles containing KOH and NaOH. The stoppers are apt to stick and their removal involve breaking the neck of the bottle. Use rubber stopper or store them in polythene containers.
45. Workers in a veterinary diagnostic laboratory are in frequent contact with microbes. Whenever pathogenic microorganisms are handled the work should be done in an area having controlled ventilation and safety cabinets. The person should have prior vaccination.

46. There should always be available in easily accessible places fire buckets, containing sand and water. Fire extinguisher should be kept at readily accessible points. A fire extinguisher should always be handy, and be placed in such a location that can be easily taken up for use in emergency. They should be sent for filling immediately after being used.

47. In case of emergency, Medical attention should be quickly obtained. Meanwhile first-aid should be given to the person. A First-aid cabinet should be readily accessible and be placed in the charge of a staff member capable of dealing with an emergency. One should learn where to find the following even in the dark; cold water, telephones, fire alarm, exits, first-aid box and fire extinguishers. In an emergency, a fire blanket, antidotes, chart about poison antidotes, chart explaining artificial respiration and emergency battery operated lamp etc. should be available.

48. Many accidents are caused by failure to seek advice or, information. Never attempt to use equipment that you do not fully understand.

49. The person incharge of a lab should of course point out where the safety equipments is located and also draw attention to any specific hazards to be found in a particular experiment.

23

Biosafety in Veterinary Clinical Pathology Laboratories

- General considerations
- Biosafety levels-1 and -2
- Biosafety level-3
- Biosafety level-4

General Considerations

Biosafety is a combination of laboratory practices, techniques, equipments and other facilities appropriate for the protection of hazards posed by infectious agents handled in the laboratory. There are guidelines for maintaining the biosafety in laboratory at various levels described as under:

Biosafety levels-1 and -2 (BSL-1&2)

The basic laboratories working with Risk Group I and II microorganisms posing low or moderate risk to the laboratory worker and have low or limited risk to the community require BSL-1 and 2 facilities. Although some of the precautions may appear to be unnecessary for some organisms, they are desirable for training purposes to promote good microbiological techniques (GMT) safe for handlers and others.

Guidelines for biosafety Levels 1 and 2 described here are comprehensive and detailed, as they are fundamental to all biosafety laboratories. The guidelines for biosafety level-3 and biosafety level-4 are modifications and additions to these guidelines, designed for work with the more dangerous pathogens. Each laboratory should adopt a safety or operations manual that identifies known and potential hazards, and specifies practices and procedures to eliminate or minimize such hazards. Good management practice is fundamental to laboratory safety. The most important concepts are listed below:

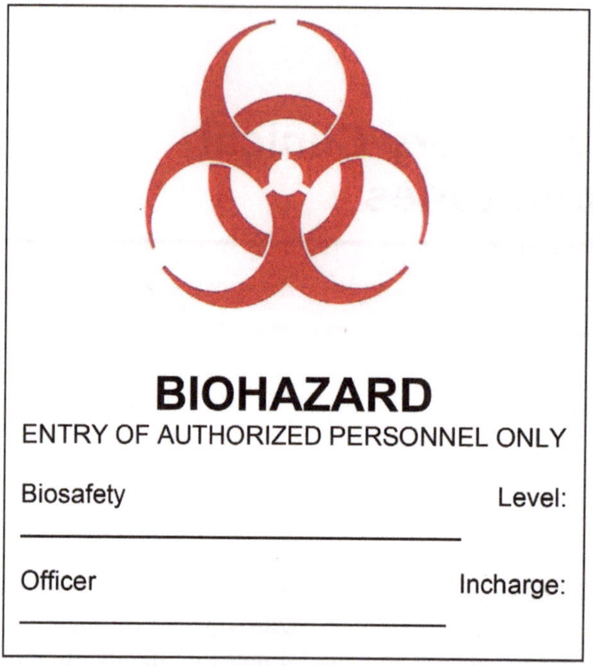
BIOHAZARD
ENTRY OF AUTHORIZED PERSONNEL ONLY
Biosafety Level:
Officer Incharge:

Access in the Laboratory

- The international biohazard warning symbol and sign must be displayed at the entrance where microorganisms of Risk Group 2 or higher risk groups are handled.
- Laboratory doors should be kept closed. Only authorized persons should be allowed to enter the laboratory working areas.
- Children under the age of 16 years should not be allowed to enter laboratory working areas.
- Access to animal houses should be available to authorized personnels only. No unwanted person should be permitted to visit laboratory animal house.
- Animals not involved in the work of the laboratory should not be kept in the laboratory.
- Authorization for entrance must be obtained from the Officer Incharge of the laboratory.

Personnel Protective Clothing/ Equipment

- Laboratory aprons, gowns or uniforms must be worn always at work place.
- Appropriate gloves must be worn for all procedures and after use, gloves should be removed aseptically and hands must then be washed.
- Person must wash his hands after handling of infectious materials and animals before leaving the laboratory.
- Safety glasses, face shields and other protective devices must be worn to protect the eyes and face from splashes, impacting objects and sources of artificial ultraviolet radiation.
- Protective laboratory clothing should not be worn outside the laboratory, e.g. in canteens, coffee rooms, offices, libraries, staff rooms and toilets.
- Open-toed footwear should not be permitted in laboratories.
- Eating, drinking, applying cosmetics and handling contact lenses should not be permitted in the laboratory. Storing human foods or drinks anywhere in the laboratory working areas should not be permitted.
- Protective laboratory clothing used in the laboratory should not be kept with other street clothing in the same lockers or cupboards.

Safety Procedures

- Pipetting by mouth must be strictly forbidden. Materials must not be placed in the mouth. Labels must not be licked.
- There should be minimum formation of aerosols and droplets in all technical procedures.
- The hypodermic needles and syringes must not be used as substitutes for pipetting devices.
- Any spills, accident or potential exposures to dangerous materials must be taken in the notice to the laboratory supervisor and a written record of such accidents and incidents must be maintained.
- For cleaning of all spills, a written procedure must be developed and adopted.
- Contaminated liquid must be decontaminated before discharge to the sanitary sewage.

- Written document to be removed from the laboratory should be protected from contamination.
- All reagent and solvent bottles should be labeled properly alongwith date of preparation.

Laboratory Working Areas

- The laboratory should be neat, clean and free from non-pertinent materials.
- Work surfaces must be decontaminated at the end of the every working day.
- All contaminated materials, specimens and cultures must be decontaminated before disposal or cleaning for reuse.
- Packing and transportation must follow national and international regulations.
- Windows should be fitted with insect proof screens.

Biosafety Management

- It is the responsibility of the laboratory incharge to ensure the development and adoption of a biosafety management plan and a safety or operations manual.
- The laboratory supervisor (reporting to the laboratory incharge) should ensure that regular training in laboratory safety is provided to other working persons in laboratory.
- Personnel should be advised to read the safety or operations manual and follow standard practices and procedures. The laboratory supervisor should make sure that all personnel understand these. A copy of the safety or operations manual should be available in the laboratory.
- Laboratory should be insect and rodent proof and facilities for control of these also be available.
- Medical facilities should be available for all personable at the time of need and its record should also be maintained.
- Baseline serum samples may be collected from laboratory staff and other persons at risk. These should be stored appropriately according to national or local guidelines. Additional specimens may be collected periodically depending on the organisms handled and the function of the laboratory.

Laboratory Design and Facilities

In designing a laboratory, special attention should be paid to conditions posing safety problems. These are: formation of aerosols, working with large volumes and/or high concentrations of microorganisms, overcrowding of persons and equipments, infestation of rodents and arthropods, unauthorized entrance, working instructions regarding samples and reagents.

- Sufficient space must be provided to conduct laboratory work satisfactorily and for cleaning and maintenance.
- Walls, ceilings and floors should be smooth, easy to clean, impermeable to liquids and resistant to the chemicals and disinfectants normally used in the laboratory. Floors should be slip-resistant. Exposed pipes and ducting should be avoided where possible.
- Bench tops should be sealed to the walls, impervious to water and resistant to disinfectants, acids, alkalis, organic solvents and moderate heat.
- Light should be sufficient and free from reflection and glare.
- Open spaces between and under benches, cabinets and equipment should be accessible for cleaning.
- Storage space must be adequate to hold supplies for immediate use.
- Space and facilities for safe handling and storage of solvents, radioactive materials, and compressed and liquefied gases should be provided.
- Facilities for storing outer garments and personal items should be provided outside the laboratory working areas.
- Facilities for eating and drinking and for rest should be provided outside the laboratory working areas.
- Wash basins, should be provided in each laboratory room, preferably near the exit door.
- Doors should have vision panels and self-closing.
- An autoclave should be available in the same building in the proximity to the laboratory.
- Safety systems should cover fire, electrical emergencies, emergency shower and eyewash facilities.
- Suitably equipped and readily accessible first-aid should be available.

- There are no specific ventilation requirements for laboratories handling Risk Group 1 and 2 microorganisms. However, in the planning of new facilities, consideration should be given to the provision of mechanical ventilation systems that provide an inward flow of air without recirculation. If there is no mechanical ventilation, windows should be able to opened and should be fitted with insect proof screens.
- A dependable supply of good quality water is essential. An anti-backflow device should protect the public water system.
- There should be a reliable and adequate electricity supply and emergency lighting arrangement like stand-by generator is desirable to run equipment and maintain system.
- There should be a reliable and adequate supply of gas with good maintenance.
- Waste disposal needs special attention to meet performance and pollution-control requirements. These are- autoclaves for the treatment of solid waste need specially designed accommodation and services, incinerators should be of special design, equipped with afterburners and smoke-consuming devices, contaminated wastewater must be decontaminated.
- Laboratories and animal houses are occasionally the targets of mischievous element. Physical and fire security must be considered. Strong doors, screened windows, and restricted issue of keys are compulsory.

LaboratoryEquipment

The use of safety equipment will help to reduce risks when dealing with biosafety hazards for laboratories of all biosafety levels. The laboratory director should, after consultation with the biosafety officer and safety committee, ensure that adequate equipment is provided and that it is used properly. Equipment should be selected to take account of certain general principles, i.e. it should be:

- designed to prevent contact between the operator and the infectious material
- constructed of materials that are impermeable to liquids, resistant to corrosion and meet structural requirements
- free of burrs, sharp edges and unguarded moving parts

- designed, constructed and installed to facilitate simple operation and provide for ease of maintenance, cleaning, decontamination and certification testing; glassware and other breakable materials should be avoided, whenever possible.

1. Pipetting aids– to avoid mouth pipetting.
2. Biological safety cabinets for handling of infectious materials and such materials should be handled in a biological safety cabinet.
3. There is an increased risk of airborne infection in procedures viz., centrifugation, grinding, blending, vigorous shaking or mixing, sonic disruption, opening of containers of infectious materials whose internal pressure may be different from the ambient pressure, intranasal inoculation of animals, and harvesting of infectious tissues from animals and eggs. Therefore, procedures should be adopted to minimize aerosols and droplets of infectious materials.
4. Plastic disposable transfer loops. Alternatively, electric transfer loop incinerators may be used inside the biological safety cabinet (BSC) to reduce aerosol production.
5. Screw-capped tubes and bottles.
6. Autoclaves to decontaminate infectious materials.
7. Plastic disposable Pasteur pipettes, whenever available, to avoid glass.
8. Equipment such as autoclaves and biological safety cabinets must be validated before being taken into use. Recertification is also needed.

Health and Medical Surveillance

The employing authority, through the laboratory Incharge, is responsible for ensuring the adequate health surveillance of laboratory staff. Under this activity includes, to provide active or passive immunization, to facilitate the early detection of laboratory-acquired infections, to exclude highly susceptible individuals (such as pregnant women) from highly hazardous laboratory work, to provide effective personal protective equipment and procedures.

Guidelines for the Surveillance of Laboratory Workers Handling Microorganisms at Biosafety Level-1

The microorganisms are unlikely to cause human or animal disease. All laboratory workers should undergo a pre employment health check up at which their medical history is recorded. Prompt reporting of illnesses or laboratory accidents is desirable and all staff members should be made aware of the importance of maintaining good microbiological techniques.

Guidelines for the Surveillance of Laboratory Workers Handling Microorganisms at Biosafety Level-2

1. Same as for biosafety level-1 and records of illness and absence should be maintained by the laboratory management.
2. Women of childbearing age should be made aware of the risk to an unborn child of occupational exposure to certain microorganisms, e.g. rubella virus and *Toxoplasma gondi*.

Training

Human error and poor technique can harm the laboratory worker. Thus, a safety-conscious staff, well informed about the recognition and control of laboratory hazards, is key to the prevention of laboratory-acquired infections, incidents and accidents. For this reason, training at regular interval in safety measures is essential. An effective safety programme begins with the laboratory managers, who should ensure that safe laboratory practices and procedures are integrated into the basic training of employees. Training in safety measures should be an integral part of new employees' introduction to the laboratory. Employees should be introduced to the code of practice and to local guidelines. Measures to assure that employees have read and understood the guidelines, such as signature pages, should be adopted. Laboratory supervisors play the key role in training their immediate staff in good laboratory techniques. The biosafety officer can assist in training and with the development of training aids and documentation. Common laboratory hazards are-

1. Inhalation risks (i.e. aerosol production), such as using loops, streaking agar plates, pipetting, making smears, opening cultures, taking blood/ serum samples, centrifugation
2. Ingestion risks, such as handling specimens, smears and cultures
3. Risks of percutaneous exposures, through the use of syringe and needle techniques
4. Animal handling that may result in bites and scratches
5. Handling of blood and other potentially hazardous pathological materials
6. Decontamination and disposal of infectious material.

Waste Handling

Most glassware, instruments and laboratory clothing can be reused or recycled. The overriding principle is that all infectious materials should be decontaminated, autoclaved or incinerated within the laboratory.

The principal questions to be asked before discharge of any objects or materials from laboratories that deal with potentially infectious microorganisms or animal tissues are as follows:

1. Have the objects or materials been effectively decontaminated or disinfected by an approved procedure?
2. If not, have they been packaged in an approved manner for immediate on-site incineration or transfer to another facility with incineration capacity?
3. Does the disposal of the decontaminated objects or materials involve any additional potential hazards, biological or otherwise, to those who carry out the immediate disposal procedures or who might come into contact with discarded items outside the facility?

Decontamination

Steam autoclaving is the preferred method for all decontamination processes. Materials for decontamination and disposal should be placed in containers, e.g. autoclavable plastic bags that are colour-coded according to whether the contents are to be autoclaved and/or incinerated.

Disinfectants and chemicals

The safety or operations manual should include a written policy stating which disinfectants are to be used for what purposes, and the manufacturer's recommended dilution for each disinfectant. The manufacturer should be able to provide relevant documentation. Make sure each disinfectant has been validated for its indicated use in the laboratory. Sodium hypochlorite and phenolic compounds are the disinfectants recommended for general laboratory use. For special purposes, various surface-active or lipid-destroying agents, including alcohols, iodine, iodophors and other oxidizing agents, as well as a very high or extremely low pH, can be effective, provided that it has been established that the agent to be destroyed is not resistant to the procedure.

Disposal Procedures

An identification and separation system for infectious materials and their containers should be adopted Indian Govt. has notified Bio-medical Waste

Management Rules 1998 for bio-medical waste. Defaulters for this liable to be prosecuted or fined Rs. 1 lakh/ 5 years imprisonment. Categories includes:

1. Non-contaminated (non-infectious) waste that can be reused or recycled or disposed of as general, "household" waste putting in black bag or black container.
2. Contaminated (infectious) "sharps"– hypodermic needles, scalpels, knives and broken glass; these should always be collected in puncture-proof containers fitted with covers and treated as infectious. The hypodermic needles should not be recapped or removed from disposable syringes. The complete assembly should be placed in a sharps container. These materials should be incinerated. Sharps containers must not be disposed of in landfills.
3. Contaminated material for decontamination by autoclaving and thereafter washing and reuse or recycling. No precleaning should be attempted of any contaminated (infectious).
4. Contaminated (infectious) materials for disposal should be autoclaved in leakproof containers, e.g. autoclavable, colour-coded plastic bags, before disposal. After autoclaving, the material may be placed in transfer containers for transport to the incinerator. If possible, materials deriving from health care activities should not be discarded in landfills even after decontamination. If an incinerator is available on the laboratory site, autoclaving may be omitted: the contaminated waste should be placed in designated containers e.g. colour-coded bags (yellow bag for animal waste and tissues, red bag for microbiological, biotechnological waste and soiled cotton swab, blue bag for infected plastic and polythene) and transported directly to the autoclave or incinerator.
5. Contaminated material for direct incineration. Incineration is the method of choice for the final disposal of contaminated waste, including carcasses of laboratory animals. Incineration of contaminated waste must meet with the approval of the public health and air pollution authorities, as well as that of the laboratory biosafety officer.

Reusable transfer containers should be leakproof and have tightfitting covers. They should be disinfected and cleaned before they are returned to the laboratory for further use. Discard pots, pans or jars, preferably unbreakable (e.g. plastic), and containing a suitable disinfectant, freshly prepared each day, should be placed at every work station. Waste materials should remain in intimate contact with the disinfectant for the appropriate time, according to the disinfectant used. The disinfectant should then be poured into a container for autoclaving or incineration. The discard pots should be autoclaved and washed before reuse.

Chemical, Fire, Electrical and Radiation Safety

A breakdown in the containment of pathogenic organisms may be the indirect result of chemical, fire, electrical or radiation accidents. It is therefore essential to maintain high standards of safety in these fields in any microbiological laboratory. Statutory rules and regulations for each of these will normally be laid down by the competent national or local authority, whose assistance should be sought if necessary. Knowledge of chemical, fire, electrical and radiation hazards is essential.

Biosafety Level-3

Containment laboratory is designed and provided for work with Risk Group 3 microorganisms and with large volumes or high concentrations of Risk Group 2 microorganisms that pose an increased risk of aerosol spread. Biosafety Level-3 containment requires the strengthening of the operational and safety programmes above those for basic laboratories– Biosafety Levels 1 and 2. The guidelines described are the additions to those for basic laboratories. Laboratories in this category should be registered or listed with the national or other appropriate health authorities.

- The international biohazard warning symbol and sign displayed on laboratory access doors must identify the microorganism(s) handled and the name of the laboratory supervisor who controls access, and indicate any special conditions for entry into the area, e.g. immunization.
- Laboratory protective clothing must be of the type with solid-front or wrap-around gowns, scrub suits, coveralls, head covering and, where appropriate, shoe covers or dedicated shoes. Front-buttoned standard laboratory coats are unsuitable. Laboratory protective clothing must not be worn outside the laboratory, and it must be decontaminated before it is given to laundry.
- Manipulations of all potentially infectious material must be conducted within a biological safety cabinet.

Laboratory Design and Facilities

The laboratory design and facilities for basic laboratories– Biosafety Levels 1 and 2 will also apply except some modification as follows:

- The laboratory should be separated from the areas that are open to unrestricted traffic flow within the building. Additional separation may be achieved by placing the laboratory at the blind end of a corridor, or constructing a partition and door or access through a basic laboratory–Biosafety Level-2.
- Entry for personnel must be through a double-door entry.
- Access to the laboratory area must be designed to prevent entrance of arthropods and other worm.
- Access doors must be self-closing and interlockable. A break-through panel may be provided for emergency exit use.
- The surfaces of walls, floors and ceilings should be water-resistant and easy to clean. Openings in these surfaces (e.g. for service pipes) should be sealed to facilitate decontamination of the room(s).
- The laboratory room must be sealable for decontamination. Air-ducting systems must be constructed to permit gaseous decontamination.
- Windows must be closed, sealed and break-resistant.
- A foot- or elbow-operated or automatically controlled water source at the hand-wash basin should be provided near to each exit door.
- There must be a ventilation system that establishes a directional air flow from access spaces into the laboratory room. Staff must at all times ensure that proper directional air flow into the laboratory room is maintained.
- The building ventilation system must be so constructed that air from the containment laboratory– Biosafety Level-3 is not recirculated to other areas within the building. Air may be HEPA filtered, reconditioned and recirculated within that laboratory. Exhaust air from the laboratory (other than from biological safety cabinets) must be discharged to the outside of the building, so that it is dispersed away from occupied buildings and air intakes. It is recommended that this air is discharged through high-efficiency particulate air (HEPA) filters.
- Biological safety cabinets should be sited away from walking areas and out of cross-currents from doors and ventilation systems.
- The exhaust air from Class I or Class II biological safety cabinets, which will have been passed through HEPA filters, must be discharged in such

a way as to avoid interference with the air balance of the cabinet or the building exhaust system. All HEPA filters must be installed in a manner that permits gaseous decontamination and testing.

- An autoclave for the decontamination of contaminated waste material should be available in the containment laboratory. If infectious wastes have to be transported out of the containment laboratory for disposal, they must be transported in sealed, unbreakable and leakproof containers according to national or international regulations, as appropriate.
- Anti-backflow devices must be fitted to the water supply.
- Effluents should be decontaminated before being discharged to the sanitary sewer.
- Design and operational procedures of Biosafety level-3 should be documented.

Laboratory Equipment

The principles for the selection of equipment, including biological safety cabinets, are the same as for the basic laboratory– Biosafety Level-2, except that activities involving infectious materials are conducted in biological safety cabinets whenever possible, together with other physical containment devices, or special personal protective equipment. While Class I or Class II biological safety cabinets are normally used in the containment laboratory– Biosafety Level-3, a Class III biological safety cabinet may be needed for high-risk procedures involving Risk Group 3 microorganisms, in accordance with local national rules.

Health and Medical Surveillance

Additional health and medical surveillance are -

1. Medical examination of all laboratory personnel who work in Biosafety Level-3 containment laboratories is mandatory. This should include recording of a detailed medical history and a physical examination.
2. A baseline serum sample should be obtained and stored for future reference.
3. Individuals who are immunocompromised should not be employed in Biosafety Level-3 containment laboratories.
4. After a satisfactory clinical assessment, the examinee should be provided with a medical contact card stating that he or she is employed in a facility

with a containment laboratory– Biosafety Level-3. This card should include a picture of the card holder, should be walletsized and should always be carried by the holder. The name(s) of the contact persons to be entered will need to be agreed locally but might include the laboratory director, medical adviser and/or biosafety officer.

A. Front of card

ILLNESS SURVEILLANCE NOTICE

Name ____

____

TO THE EMPLOYEE

Keep this card in your possession. In case of unexplained febrile illness, present the card to your physician and notify one of the following in the order listed.

Dr. ______________________ Tel (Work): ______________________

______________________ Tel (Home): ______________________

Dr. ______________________ Tel (Work): ______________________

______________________ Tel (Home): ______________________

B. Back of card

TO THE PHYSICIAN

The holder of this card works in an area at ______________________ in which pathogenic viruses, rickettsia, bacteria, protozoa or helminths are present. In the event of an unexplained febrile illness, please call the employer for information on agents to which this employee may have been exposed.

Name of laboratory:

Address: ____

____

____

Tel: ____

Biosafety Level-4

The maximum containment laboratory– Biosafety Level-4 is designed for work with Risk Group 4 microorganisms. Before such a laboratory is constructed and put into operation, intensive consultations should be held with institutions that have had experience of operating a similar facility. Operational maximum containment laboratories– Biosafety Level-4 should be under the control of national or other appropriate health authorities. Additional code of practices are:

1. The two person rule should apply, whereby no individual ever works alone. This is particularly important if working in a Biosafety Level-4 suit facility.
2. A complete change of clothing and shoes is required prior to entering and upon exiting the laboratory.
3. Personnel must be trained in emergency extraction procedures in the event of personnel injury or illness.
4. A method of communication for routine and emergency contacts between persons working within Biosafety Level-4 and support personnel outside the laboratory.

Laboratory Design and Facilities

The features of a containment laboratory– Biosafety Level-3 also apply to a maximum containment laboratory– Biosafety Level-4 with the addition of the following:

1. **Primary containment:** An efficient primary containment system must be in place, consisting of one or a combination of the following:
    - *Class III cabinet laboratory:* Passage through a minimum of two doors prior to entering the rooms containing the Class III biological safety cabinet (cabinet room) is required. In this laboratory configuration the Class III biological safety cabinet provides the primary containment. A personnel shower with inner and outer changing rooms is necessary. Supplies and materials that are not brought into the cabinet room through the changing area are introduced through a double-door autoclave or fumigation chamber. Once the outer door is securely closed, staff inside the laboratory can open the inner door to retrieve the materials. The doors of the autoclave or fumigation chamber are interlocked in such a way that the outer door cannot open unless the autoclave has been operated through a sterilization cycle or the fumigation chamber has been decontaminated.
    - *Suit laboratory:* A protective suit laboratory with self-contained breathing apparatus differs significantly in design and facility requirements from a Biosafety Level-4 laboratory with Class III biological safety cabinets. The rooms in the protective suit laboratory are arranged to direct personnel through the changing

and decontamination areas prior to entering areas where infectious materials are manipulated. In this laboratory configuration, the suit area itself is considered to constitute the primary containment. The suit area is designed and maintained to provide personnel protection equivalent to that provided by Class III biological safety cabinets. A suit decontamination shower must be provided for personnel leaving the containment laboratory area. A separate personnel shower with inner and outer changing rooms is also provided. Personnel who enter the suit area are required to don a one-piece, positively pressurized, HEPA filter- supplied air suit. Air to the suit must be provided by a system that has a 100% redundant capability with an independent source of air, for use in the event of an emergency. Entry into the suit laboratory is through an airlock fitted with airtight doors. An appropriate warning system for personnel working in the suit laboratory must be provided for use in the event of mechanical system or air failure.

2. **Controlled access:** The maximum containment laboratory– Biosafety Level-4 must be located in a separate building or in a clearly delineated zone within a secure building. Entry and exit of personnel and supplies must be through an airlock or pass-through system. On entering, personnel must put on a complete change of clothing; before leaving, they should shower before putting on their street clothing.

3. **Controlled air system:** Negative pressure must be maintained in the facility. Both supply and exhaust air must be HEPA-filtered. There are significant differences in the ventilating systems of the Class III cabinet laboratory and suit laboratory:

   - *Class III cabinet laboratory:* The supply air to the Class III biological safety cabinet(s) may be drawn from within the room through a HEPA filter mounted on the cabinet or supplied directly through the supply air system. Exhaust air from the Class III biological safety cabinet must pass through two HEPA filters prior to release outdoors. The cabinet must be operated at negative pressure to the surrounding laboratory at all times. A dedicated non-recirculating ventilating system for the cabinet laboratory is required.

   - *Suit laboratory:* Dedicated room air supply and exhaust systems are required. The supply and exhaust components of the ventilating system are balanced to provide directional air flow within the suit area from the area of least hazard to the area(s) of greatest potential hazard.

Redundant exhaust fans are required to ensure that the facility remains under negative pressure at all times. The differential pressures within the suit laboratory and between the suit laboratory and adjacent areas must be monitored. Air flow in the supply and exhaust components of the ventilating system must be monitored and an appropriate system of controls must be used to prevent pressurization of the suit laboratory. HEPA-filtered supply air must be provided to the suit area, decontamination shower and decontamination airlocks or chambers. Exhaust air from the suit laboratory must be passed through a series of two HEPA filters prior to release outdoors. Alternatively, after double HEPA filtration, exhaust air may be recirculated but only within the suit laboratory. Under no circumstances shall the exhaust air from the Biosafety Level-4 suit laboratory be recirculated to other areas. Extreme caution must be exercised if recirculation of air within the suit laboratory is elected. Consideration must be given to the types of research conducted, equipment, chemicals and other materials used in the suit laboratory, as well as animal species that may be involved in the research.

All HEPA filters need to be tested and certified annually. The HEPA filter housings are designed to allow for in situ decontamination of the filter prior to removal. Alternatively, the filter can be removed in a sealed, gas-tight primary container for subsequent decontamination and/or destruction by incineration.

4. **Decontamination of effluents:** All effluents from the suit area, decontamination chamber, decontamination shower, or Class III biological safety cabinet must be decontaminated before final discharge. Heat treatment (autoclaving) is the preferred method. Effluents may also require correction to a neutral pH prior to discharge. Water from the personnel shower and toilet may be discharged directly to the sanitary sewer without treatment.

5. **Sterilization of waste and materials:** A double-door, pass-through autoclave must be available in the laboratory area. Other methods of decontamination must be available for equipment and items that cannot withstand steam sterilization.

6. **Airlock entry ports** for specimens, materials and animals must be provided.

7. **Emergency power** and dedicated power supply line(s) must be provided.
8. **Containment drain**(s) must be installed.

Because of the great complexity of the work in the Biosafety Level-4 laboratory, a separate detailed work manual should be developed and tested in training exercises. In addition, an emergency programme must be devised. In the preparation of this programme, active cooperation with national and local health authorities should be established. Other emergency services, e.g. fire, police and receiving hospitals, should also be involved.

24

Quality Management System (ISO 9001: 2008) in Veterinary Clinical Pathology Laboratory

- General considerations
- Quality management principles
- Objectives of 9001:2008
    1. Scope
    2. Normative reference
    3. Terms and definitions
- Main clauses and sections of ISO 9001:2008
    4. Quality management system
    5. Management responsibility
    6. Resource management
    7. Product realization
    8. Measurement, analysis and Improvement

General Considerations

The livestock sector is one of the most important components of Indian economy occupy an important place in the social fabric of rural India. The country has large population of various species of livestock, majority of which get inadequate nutrition and health care. Animal husbandry sector contribute about 8 per cent to National gross domestic product (GDP) and this accounts for 27 percent of the value of the agricultural output. The livestock sector currently employs about 8 percent of the India's work force and has been growing for last 2 decades at an annual growth of 4.5%. It is a well-recognized fact that the livestock and poultry production is having vast potential in income generation, providing employment and gender empowerment. The diseases cause enormous economic losses by way of morbidity and mortality. The losses due to diseases can be drastically reduced by adopting appropriate and timely measures for prevention, control and eradication, besides treatment.

During liberalized regime of international trade of animal products particularly after the year 2005, we have to be extra vigilant to improve our professional competence in disease diagnosis. A correct diagnosis provides way to early containment of disease in animals. It has been estimated that if an appropriate diagnosis is timely provided by a Veterinarian, it can save money and manpower and may enhance the National GDP by 1 percent as it will save veterinary costs, save the man days, increase the production of animals, reduce the mental tension of owner and his/her family and animal is put to work or production early.

Diagnosis is an art of precisely knowing the cause of a disease; the diagnosis is based on history, careful clinical examination of animal, collection of material for laboratory examination and correlation and interpretation of findings. The importance of clinical, physical and laboratory diagnosis has been recognized equally as each of these is necessary to arrive on any conclusion. According to a well known diagnostician ***"A Veterinarian who does not need a laboratory is uninformed and a Veterinarian who is totally dependent upon the laboratory findings is inexperienced and in either case the animal is in danger"***.

Laboratory diagnosis also provides information of introduction of a new disease among the animals of a particular area or the presence of the disease at its endemic levels. It is necessary for confirmation of the clinical diagnosis and to evaluate the therapeutic approach so that the animal can be saved and put to work/ production at the earliest. Laboratory diagnosis includes the following:

1. Blood examination
2. Faeces examination
3. Urine examination
4. Serological/ immunological tests including tuberculin, Johnin and Mallein tests
5. Skin scrapings examination
6. Milk examination
7. Examination of body fluids such as synovial, CSF and peritoneal
8. Histopathology including immunohistochemistry
9. Microbiological examination including antibacterial drug sensitivity

The above said laboratory diagnostic tests are performed through the management of various laboratories including:

1. Pathology Laboratory
2. Virology Laboratory
3. Bacteriology Laboratory
4. Toxicology Laboratory
5. Parasitology Laboratory
6. Epidemiology Laboratory
7. Networking and Disease Control Laboratory

The quality management of these laboratories may result in accurate and valid diagnosis acceptable internationally. Total quality management evolved from a wide range of management practices and productivity movement efforts. Total quality management has its roots in the quality focused on product, performance and customer satisfaction.

International Organization for Standardization (ISO) was established in 1947 to promote the development of standardization and related activities in the world with a view to facilitating the international exchange of goods and services. ISO published ISO 9000 series of standards in 1987 and revised them further and again published in the year 1994 and 2008. Now these standards are known as ISO 9000: 2008 family of standards. The ISO 9000: 2008 family of standards are developed to assist organizations, of all types and sizes, to implement and operate quality management system. The standards are based on a process model that uses eight quality management principles which reflect best practices and are designed to facilitate continual improvement in order to improve customer satisfaction. The following standards are included in ISO 9000: 2008 family:

1. **ISO 9001: 2008-** specifies requirements for quality management systems for use where an organization's capability to provide products that meets customer's satisfaction and applicable regulatory requirements needs to be demonstrated.
2. **ISO 9004: 2008-** provides guidance on quality management systems including the process for continual improvement for customer satisfaction.
3. **ISO 9009: 2008-** describes fundamentals of quality management systems and specifies the terminology for the same.

4. **ISO 17025-** describes general requirement for the competence of testing and calibration laboratories.
5. **ISO 19011-** provides guidance on managing and conducting environmental and quality system audits. It includes earlier ISO 10011, 14010, 14011 and 14012.

Quality Management Principles

Eight quality management principles have been identified and that can be used by Executive managers in order to lead the organization towards improved process and performance:

1. *Customer focus*: Organizations depend on their customers and therefore should understand current and future needs of the customers and should meet the customer requirements and strive to exceed customer expectations, *viz.*, Rapid diagnosis, Reliable diagnosis upto the satisfaction of animal owners.
2. *Leadership*: Leaders establish the direction of the organization. They should create and maintain the internal environment in which people should be involved in achieving the organizations objective, *viz.*, Facilities to scientists, facilities in laboratories, behaviour of RMPs, understanding the problems of each other, encouraging Technicians/ Scientists, motivation.
3. *Involvement of people:* People at all levels are the essence of an organization and their full involvement enables their ability to be used for the benefit of the organization, *viz.*, Distribution of work, meeting for discussion on key points, Advice to all concerned, Share of information.
4. *Process approach:* A desired result is achieved more effectively when activities and related resources are managed in a standardize process, *viz.*, A set of protocols, SOPs, defined procedures, Availability of SOPs at the point of use.
5. *System approach to Management:* Identifying, understanding and managing interrelated processes as a system contributes to the organization's effectiveness and efficiency in achieving its objectives, *viz.*, Integrated process- less paper work, purchases, reporting, compilation.
6. *Continual improvement:* Continual improvement of the organization's overall performance should be a permanent objective of the organization,

viz., Development of quick diagnostic test, rapidness, reporting of results- decrease time.

7. *Factual approach to decision making:* Effective decisions are based on the analysis of data and information, *viz.*, Analysis of back data, find out the problems, try to remove/ reduce them, decision should be shown practically enforceable, make data accessible to those who need it.
8. *Mutually beneficial supplier relationship:* An organization and its suppliers are interdependent, and a mutually beneficial relationship enhances the ability of both to create value, *viz.*, Document requirement of suppliers, commitment to customer's satisfaction, short and long term gains, sharing information and future plans, customized antibodies for different diagnostic tests.

Objectives of ISO 9001: 2008

The main objectives of quality management system (QMS) in ISO 9001: 2008 are:

1. Performance
2. Customer satisfaction
3. Continual improvement

1. Scope

1.1. General

This International Standard specifies requirements for a quality management system where an organization

a) needs to demonstrate its ability to consistently provide product that meets customer and applicable regulatory requirements, and

b) aims to enhance customer satisfaction through the effective application of the system, including processes for continual improvement of the system and the assurance of conformity to customer and applicable regulatory requirements.

Note: In this International Standard, the term "product" applies only to the product intended for, or required by, a customer.

1.2. Application

All requirements of this International Standard are generic and are intended to be applicable to all organizations, regardless of type, size and product provided. Where any requirement(s) of this International Standard cannot be applied due to the nature of an organization and its product, this can be considered for exclusion. Where exclusions are made, claims of conformity to this International Standard are not acceptable unless these exclusions are limited to requirements within clause 7, and such exclusions do not affect the organization's ability, or responsibility, to provide product that meets customer and applicable regulatory requirements.

2. Normative Reference

The following normative document contains provisions which, through reference in this text, constitute provisions of this International Standard. For dated references, subsequent amendments to, or revisions of, any of these publications do not apply. However, parties to agreements based on this International Standard are encouraged to investigate the possibility of applying the most recent edition of the normative document indicated below. For undated references, the latest edition of the normative document referred to applies. Members of ISO and IEC maintain registers of currently valid International Standards.

ISO 9000:2008, *Quality management systems - Fundamentals and vocabulary.*

3. Terms and Definitions

For the purposes of this International Standard, the terms and definitions given in ISO 9000 apply.

The following terms, used in this edition of ISO 9001 to describe the supply chain, have been changed to reflect the vocabulary currently used:

Supplier à Organization à Customer

The term "organization" replaces the term "supplier" used in ISO 9001: 1994, and refers to the unit to which this International Standard applies. Also, the term "supplier" now replaces the term "subcontractor".

Throughout the text of this International Standard, wherever the term "product" occurs, it can also mean "service".

Main Clauses and Sections of ISO 9001: 2008

4. Quality Management System

4.1 General Requirements

The organization shall establish, document, implement and maintain a quality management system and continually improve its effectiveness in accordance with the requirements of this International Standard.

The organization shall

a) identify the processes needed for the quality management system and their application throughout the organization,

b) determine the sequence and interaction of these processes,

c) determine criteria and methods needed to ensure that both the operation and control of these processes are effective,

d) ensure the availability of resources and information necessary to support the operation and monitoring of these processes,

e) monitor, measure and analyse these processes, and

f) implement actions necessary to achieve planned results and continual improvement of these processes.

These processes shall be managed by the organization in accordance with the requirements of this International Standard. Where an organization chooses to outsource any process that affects product conformity with requirements, the organization shall ensure control over such processes. Control of such outsourced processes shall be identified within the quality management system.

Note: Processes needed for the quality management system referred to above should include processes for management activities, provision of resources, product realization and measurement.

4.2. Documentation Requirements

4.2.1. General

The quality management system documentation shall include

a) documented statements of a quality policy and quality objectives,

b) a quality manual,

c) documented procedures required by this International Standard,

d) documents needed by the organization to ensure the effective planning operation and control of its processes, and

e) records required by this International Standard.

Note

1. Where the term "documented procedure" appears within this International Standard, this means that the procedure is established, documented, implemented and maintained.

2. The extent of the quality management system documentation can differ from one organization to another due to
   a. the size of organization and type of activities,
   b. the complexity of processes and their interactions, and
   c. the competence of personnel.
3. The documentation can be in any form or type of medium.

4.2.2. Quality Manual

The organization shall establish and maintain a quality manual that includes

a) the scope of the quality management system, including details of and justification for any exclusions (See 1.2),

b) the documented procedures established for the quality management system, or reference to them, and

c) a description of the interaction between the processes of the quality management system.

4.2.3. Control of Documents

Documents required by the quality management system shall be controlled. Records are a special type of document and shall be controlled according to the requirements given in 4.2.4.

A documented procedure shall be established to define the controls needed

a) to approve documents for adequacy prior to issue,

b) to review and update as necessary and re-approve documents,

c) to ensure that changes and the current revision status of documents are identified,

d) to ensure that relevant versions of applicable documents are available at points of use,

e) to ensure that documents remain legible and readily identifiable,

f) to ensure that documents of external origin are identified and their distribution controlled, and

g) to prevent the unintended use of obsolete documents, and to apply suitable identification to them if they are retained for any purpose.

4.2.4. Control of Records

Records shall be established and maintained to provide evidence of conformity to requirements and of the effective operation of the quality management system. Records shall remain legible, readily identifiable and retrievable. A documented procedure shall be established to define the controls needed for the identification, storage, protection, retrieval, retention time and disposition of records.

5. Management Responsibility

5.1. Management Commitment

Top management shall provide evidence of its commitment to the development and implementation of the quality management system and continually improving its effectiveness by

a) communicating to the organization the importance of meeting customer as well as statutory and regulatory requirements,

b) establishing the quality policy,

c) ensuring that quality objectives are established,

d) conducting management reviews, and

e) ensuring the availability of resources.

5.2. Customer Focus

Top management shall ensure that customer requirements are determined and are met with the aim of enhancing customer satisfaction.

5.3. Quality Policy

Top management shall ensure that the quality policy

a) is appropriate to the purpose of the organization,

b) includes a commitment to comply with requirements and continually improve the effectiveness of the quality management system,

c) provides a framework for establishing and reviewing quality objectives,

d) is communicated and understood within the organization, and

e) is reviewed for continuing suitability.

5.4. Quality Management System Planning

5.4.1. Quality objectives

Top management shall ensure that quality objectives, including those needed to meet requirements for product (See 7.1a) are established at relevant functions and levels within the organization. The quality objectives shall be measurable and consistent with the quality policy.

5.4.2. Quality Management System Planning

Top management shall ensure that

a) the planning of the quality management system is carried out in order to meet the requirements given in 4.1, as well as the quality objectives, and

b) the integrity of the quality management system is maintained when changes to the quality management system are planned and implemented.

5.5. Responsibility, Authority and Communication

5.5.1. Responsibility and Authority

Top management shall ensure that responsibilities and authorities are defined and communicated within the organization.

5.5.2. Management Representative

Top management shall appoint a member of management who, irrespective other responsibilities, shall have responsibility and authority that includes

a) ensuring that processes needed for the quality management system are established, implemented and maintained,

b) reporting to top management on the performance of the quality management system and any need for improvement, and

c) ensuring the promotion of awareness of customer requirements throughout the organization.

Note: The responsibility of a management representative can include liaison with external parties on matters relating to the quality management system.

5.5.3. Internal Communication

Top management shall ensure that appropriate communication 'processes are established within the organization and that communication takes place regarding the effectiveness of the quality management system.

5.6. Management Review

5.6.1. General

Top management shall review the organization's quality management system, at planned intervals, to ensure its continuing suitability, adequacy and effectiveness. This review shall include assessing opportunities for improvement and the need for changes to the quality management system, including the quality policy and quality objectives. Records from management reviews shall be maintained (See 4.2.4).

5.6.2. Review Input

The input to management review shall include information on

a) results of audits,

b) customer feedback,

c) process performance and product conformity,

d) status of preventive and corrective actions,

e) follow-up actions from previous management reviews,

f) changes that could affect the quality management system, and

g) recommendations for improvement.

5.6.3. Review Output

The output from the management review shall include any decisions and actions related to

a) improvement of the effectiveness of the quality management system and its processes,

b) improvement of product related to customer requirements, and

c) resource needs.

6. Resource Management

6.1. Provision of Resources

The organization shall determine and provide the resources needed

a) to implement and maintain the quality management system and continually improve its effectiveness, and

b) to enhance customer satisfaction by meeting customer requirements.

6.2. Human Resources

6.2.1. General

Personnel performing work affecting product quality shall be competent on the basis of appropriate education, training, skills and experience.

6.2.2. Competence, Awareness and Training

The organization shall

a) determine the necessary competence for personnel performing work affecting product quality,

b) provide training or take other actions to satisfy these needs,

c) evaluate the effectiveness of the actions taken,

d) ensure that its personnel are aware of the relevance and importance of their activities and how they contribute to the achievement of the quality objectives, and

e) maintain appropriate records of education, training, skills and experience (See 4.2.4).

6.3. Infrastructure

The organization shall determine, provide and maintain the infrastructure needed to achieve conformity to product requirements. Infrastructure includes, as applicable

a) buildings, workspace and associated utilities,

b) process equipment (both hardware and software), and

c) supporting services (such as transport or communication).

6.4. Work environment

The organization shall determine and manage the work environment needed to achieve conformity to product requirements.

7. Product Realization

7.1. Planning of product realization

The organization shall plan and develop the processes needed for product realization. Planning of product realization shall be consistent with the requirements of the other processes of the quality management system (See 4.1).

In planning product realization, the organization shall determine the following, appropriate:

a) quality objectives and requirements for the product;

b) the need to establish processes, documents, and provide resources specific to the product;

c) required verification, validation, monitoring, inspection and test activities specific to the product and the criteria for product acceptance;

d) records needed to provide evidence that the realization processes and resulting product meet requirements (See 4.2.4)

The output of this planning shall be in a form suitable for the organization's method of operations.

Note

1. A document specifying the processes of the quality management system (including the product realization processes) and the resources to be applied to a specific product, project or contract, can be referred to as a quality plan.
2. The organization may also apply the requirements given in 7.3 to the development of product realization processes.

7.2. Customer-related Processes

7.2.1. Determination of requirements related to the product

The organization shall determine

a) requirements specified by the customer, including the requirements for delivery and post-delivery activities,

b) requirements not stated by the customer but necessary for specified or intended use, where known,

c) statutory and regulatory requirements related to the product, and

d) any additional requirements determined by the organization.

7.2.2. Review of Requirements Related to the Product

The organization shall review the requirements related to the product. This review shall be conducted prior to the organization's commitment to supply a product to the customer (e.g. submission of tenders, acceptance of contracts or orders, acceptance of changes to contracts or orders) and shall ensure that

a) product requirements are defined,

b) contract or order requirements differing from those previously expressed are resolved, and

c) the organization has the ability to meet the defined requirements.

Records of the results of the review and actions arising from the review shall be maintained (See 4.2.4). Where the customer provides no documented statement of requirement, the customer requirements shall be confirmed by the organization before acceptance. Where product requirements are changed, the organization shall ensure that relevant documents are amended and that relevant personnel are made aware of the changed requirements.

Note: In some situations, such as internet sales, a formal review is impractical for each order. Instead the review can cover relevant product information such as catalogues or advertising material.

7.2.3. Customer Communication

The organization shall determine and implement effective arrangements for communicating with customers in relation to

a) product information,

b) enquiries, contracts or order, handling, including amendments, and

c) customer feedback, including customer complaints.

7.3. Design and Development

7.3.1. Design and Development Planning

The organization shall plan and control the design and development of product. During the design and development planning, the organization shall determine-

a) the design and development stages,

b) the review, verification and validation that are appropriate to each design and development stage, and

c) the responsibilities and authorities for design and development.

The organization shall manage the interfaces between different groups involved in design and development to ensure effective communication and clear assignment of responsibility. Planning output shall be updated, as appropriate, as the design and development progresses.

7.3.2. Design and Development Inputs

Inputs relating to product requirements shall be determined and records maintained (See 4.2.4). These inputs shall include

a) functional and performance requirements,

b) applicable statutory and regulatory requirements,

c) where applicable, information derived from previous similar designs, and

d) other requirements essential for design and development.

These inputs shall be reviewed for adequacy. Requirements shall be complete, unambiguous and not in conflict with each other.

7.3.3. Design and Development Outputs

The outputs of design and development shall be provided in a form that enables verification against the design and development input and shall be approved prior to release.

Design and development outputs shall

a) meet the input requirements for design and development,

b) provide appropriate information for purchasing, production and for service provision,

c) contain or reference product acceptance criteria, and

d) specify the characteristics of the product that are essential for its safe and proper use.

7.3.4. Design and Development Review

At suitable stages, systematic reviews of design and development shall be performed in accordance with planned arrangements (See 7.3.1).

a) to evaluate the ability of the results of design and development to meet requirements, and

b) to identify any problems and propose necessary actions.

Participants in such reviews shall include representatives of functions concerned with the design and development stage(s) being reviewed. Records of the results of the reviews and any necessary actions shall be maintained (See 4.2.4).

7.3.5. Design and Development Verification

Verification shall be performed in accordance with planned arrangements (See 7.3.1) to ensure that the design and development outputs have met the design and development input requirements. Records of the results of the verification and any necessary actions shall be maintained (See 4.2.4).

7.3.6. Design and Development Validation

Design and development validation shall be performed in accordance with planned arrangements (See 7.3.1) to ensure that the resulting product is capable of meeting the requirements for the specified application or intended use, where known. Wherever practicable, validation shall be completed prior to the delivery or implementation of the product. Records of the results of validation and any necessary actions shall be maintained (See 4.2.4).

7.3.7. Control of Design and Development Changes

Design and development changes shall be identified and records maintained. The changes shall be reviewed, verified and validated, as appropriate, and approved before implementation. The review of design and development changes shall include evaluation of the effect of the changes on constituent parts and product already delivered. Records of the results of the review of changes and any necessary actions shall be maintained (See 4.2.4).

7.4. Purchasing

7.4.1. Purchasing Process

The organization shall ensure that purchased product conforms to specified purchase requirements. The type and extent of control applied to the supplier and the purchased product shall be dependent upon the effect of the purchased product on subsequent product realization or the final product. The organization shall evaluate and select suppliers based on their ability to supply product in accordance with the organization's requirements. Criteria for selection, evaluation and re-evaluation shall be established. Records of the results of evaluations and any necessary actions arising from the evaluation shall be maintained (See 4.2.4).

7.4.2. Purchasing Information

Purchasing information shall describe the product to be purchased, including where appropriate

a) requirements for approval of product, procedures, processes and equipment,

b) requirements for qualification of personnel, and

c) quality management system requirements.

The organization shall ensure the adequacy of specified purchase requirements prior to their communication to the supplier.

7.4.3. Verification of Purchased Product

The organization shall establish and implement the inspection or other activities necessary for ensuring that purchased product meets specified purchase requirements. Where the organization or its customer intends to perform verification at the supplier's premises, the organization shall state the intended verification arrangements and method of product release in the purchasing information.

7.5. Production and Service Provision

7.5.1. Control of Production and Service Provision

The organization shall plan and carry out production and service provision under controlled conditions. Controlled conditions shall include, as applicable

a) the availability of information that describes the characteristics of the product,

b) the availability of work instructions, as necessary,

c) the use of suitable equipment,

d) the availability and use of monitoring and measuring devices,

e) the implementation of monitoring and measurement, and

f) the implementation of release, delivery and post-delivery activities.

7.5.2. Validation of Processes for Production and Service Provision

The organization shall validate any processes for production and service provision where the resulting output cannot be verified by subsequent monitoring or measurement. This includes any processes where deficiencies become apparent only after the product is in use or the service has been delivered. Validation shall demonstrate the ability of these processes to achieve planned results.

The organization shall establish arrangements for these processes including, as applicable

a) defined criteria for review and approval of the processes,

b) approval of equipment and qualification of personnel,

c) use of specific methods and procedures,

d) requirements for records, (See 4.2.4) and

e) revalidation.

7.5.3. Identification and Traceability

Where appropriate, the organization shall identify the product by suitable means throughout product realization. The organization shall identify the product status with respect to monitoring and measurement requirements. Where traceability is a requirement, the organization shall control and record the unique identification of the product (See 4.2.4).

Note: In some industry sectors, configuration management is a means by which identification and traceability are maintained.

7.5.4. Customer Property

The organization shall exercise care with customer property while it is under the organization's control or being used by the organization. The organization shall identify, verify, protect and safeguard customer property provided for use or incorporation into the product. If any customer property is lost, damaged or otherwise found to be unsuitable for use, this shall be reported to the customer and records maintained (See 4.2.4).

Note: Customer property can include intellectual property.

7.5.5. Preservation of Product

The organization shall preserve the conformity of product during internal processing and delivery to the intended destination. This preservation shall include identification, handling, packaging, storage and protection. Preservation shall also apply to the constituent parts of a product.

7.6. Control of Monitoring and Measuring Devices

The organization shall determine the monitoring and measurement to be undertaken and the monitoring and measuring devices needed to provide evidence of conformity of product to determined requirements (See 7.2.1). The organization shall establish processes to ensure that monitoring and measurement can be carried out and are carried out in a manner that is consistent with the monitoring and measurement requirements.

Where necessary to ensure valid results, measuring equipment shall

a) be calibrated or verified at specified intervals, or prior to use, against measurement standards traceable to international or national measurement standards; where no such standards exist, the basis used for calibration or verification shall be recorded;

b) be adjusted or re-adjusted as necessary;

c) be identified to enable the calibration status to be determined;

d) be safeguarded from adjustments that would invalidate the measurement result;

e) be protected from damage and deterioration during handling, maintenance and storage.

In addition, the organization shall assess and record the validity of the previous measuring results when the equipment is found not to conform to requirements. The organization shall take appropriate action on the equipment and any product affected. Records of the results of calibration and verification shall be maintained (See 4.2.4). When used in the monitoring and measurement of specified requirements, the ability of computer software to satisfy the intended application shall be confirmed. This shall be undertaken prior to initial use and reconfirmed as necessary.

8. Measurement, Analysis and Improvement

8.1. General

The organization shall plan and implement the monitoring, measurement, analysis and improvement processes needed

a) to demonstrate conformity of the product,

b) to ensure conformity of the quality management system, and

c) to continually improve the effectiveness of the quality management system.

This shall include determination of applicable methods, including statistical techniques, and the extent of their use.

8.2. Monitoring and Measurement

8.2.1. Customer Satisfaction

As one of the measurements of the performance of the quality management system, the organization shall monitor information relating to customer perception as to whether the organization has met customer requirements. The methods for obtaining and using this information shall be determined.

8.2.2. Internal Audit

The organization shall conduct internal audits at planned intervals to determine whether the quality management system

a) conforms to the planned arrangements (See 7.1) to the requirements of this International Standard and to the quality management system requirements established by the organization, and

b) is effectively implemented and maintained.

An audit programme shall be planned, taking into consideration the status and importance of the processes and areas to be audited, as well as the results of previous audits. The audit criteria, scope, frequency and methods shall be defined. Selection of auditors and conduct of audits shall ensure objectivity and impartiality of the audit process. Auditors shall not audit their own work. The responsibilities and requirements for planning and conducting audits, and for reporting results and maintaining records (See 4.2.4) shall be defined in a documented procedure. The management responsible for the area being audited shall ensure that actions are taken without undue delay to eliminate detected nonconformities and their causes. Follow-up activities shall include the verification of the actions taken and the reporting of verification results (See 8.5.2).

8.2.3. Monitoring and Measurement of Processes

The organization shall apply suitable methods for monitoring and, where applicable, measurement of the quality management system processes. These methods shall demonstrate the ability of the processes to achieve planned results. When planned results are not achieved, correction and corrective action shall be taken, as appropriate, to ensure conformity of the product.

8.2.4. Monitoring and Measurement of Product

The organization shall monitor and measure the characteristics of the product to verify that product requirements have been met. This shall be carried out at appropriate stages of the product realization process in accordance with the planned arrangements (See 7.1). Evidence of conformity with the acceptance criteria shall be maintained. Records shall indicate the person(s) authorizing release of product (See 4.2.4). Product release and service delivery shall not proceed until the planned arrangements (See 7.1) have been satisfactorily completed, unless otherwise approved by a relevant authority and, where applicable, by the customer.

8.3. Control of Nonconforming Product

The organization shall ensure that product which does not conform to product requirements is identified and controlled to prevent its unintended use or delivery. The controls and related responsibilities and authorities for dealing with nonconforming product shall be defined in a documented procedure.

The organization shall deal with nonconforming product by on or more of the following ways:

a) by taking action to eliminate the detected nonconformity;

b) by authorizing its use, release or acceptance under concession by a relevant, authority and where applicable, by the customer;

c) by taking action to preclude its original intended use or application,

Records of the nature of nonconformities and any subsequent actions taken. including concessions obtained; shall be maintained (See 4.2.4). When nonconforming product is corrected it shall be subject to re-verification to demonstrate conformity to the requirements. When nonconforming product is detected after delivery or use has started, the organization shall take action appropriate to the effects, or potential effects, of the nonconformity.

8.4. Analysis of Data

The organization shall determine, collect and analyze appropriate data to demonstrate the suitability and effectiveness of the quality management system and to evaluate where continual improvement of the effectiveness of the quality management system can be made. This shall include data generated as a result of monitoring and measurement and from other relevant sources.

The analysis of data shall provide information relating to

a) customer satisfaction (See 8.2.1),

b) conformity to product requirements (See 7.2.1),

c) characteristics and trends of processes and products including opportunities for preventive action, and

d) suppliers.

8.5. Improvement

8.5.1. Continual Improvement

The organization shall continually improve the effectiveness of the quality management system through the use of the quality policy, quality objectives, audit results, analysis of data, corrective and' preventive actions and management review.

8.5.2. Corrective Action

The organization shall take action to eliminate the cause of nonconformities in order to prevent recurrence. Corrective actions shall be appropriate to the effects of the nonconformities encountered.

A documented procedure shall be established to define requirements for

a) reviewing nonconformities (including customer complaints),

b) determining the causes of non-conformities,

c) evaluating the need for action to ensure that nonconformities do not recur,

d) determining and implementing action needed,

e) records of the results of action taken (See 4.2.4), and

f) reviewing corrective action taker.

8.5.3. Preventive Action

The organization shall determine action to eliminate the causes of potential nonconformities in order to prevent their occurrence. Preventive actions shall be appropriate to the effects of the potential problems.

A documented procedure shall be established to define requirements for

a) determining potential non-conformities and their causes,

b) evaluating the need for action to prevent occurrence of nonconformities,

c) determining and implementing action needed,

d) records of results of action taken (See 4.2.4), and

e) reviewing preventive action taken.

The organization shall establish, document, implement and maintain a quality management system and continually improve its effectiveness in accordance with the requirements of this International Standard.

If things are managed as per ISO standards of quality management system, certainly the importance of Veterinary Laboratory Diagnosis will be enhanced and recognized. ISO standards seem difficult to be implemented initially but if there is a firm determination to achieve total quality in laboratory diagnosis, these can be easily implemented. Certainly, it will enhance the reputation of the Veterinary Science profession, particularly diagnosticians working in this area. Moreover, we have to make ourselves competitive in this global market, if at all we have to survive and in my opinion, ISO is one of the best system to achieve the quality as it is based on the principles of *Bhagawat Gita* "Do your jobs, and let the results left on God. If you do good job through Quality Management System, certainly you will get good results as per your Karmas".

25

Competence Accreditation (ISO 17025) of Veterinary Clinical Pathology Laboratory

- General considerations
- Purpose and goals of laboratory
- Standards, guides and references
- Accreditation for competence
- Identification of scope
- Test methods
- Benefits of ISO17025 accreditation
- Processing of application

General Considerations

In India, animal husbandry is considered as one of the important enterprises providing 8% to national GDP with a growth rate of 4.5% per annum. It also provides jobs to 8% rural youths. The income from animal husbandry can be increased substantially by way of promotion of healthy animals or their products for international trade. It has been observed that the good health of animals can be managed through proper and quick diagnosis of animal diseases and their control using appropriate methods. For the purpose of animal disease diagnosis, Govt. of India and the State Govts. has set up a chain of diagnostic laboratories in the country.

Central Disease Diagnostic Laboratory
CADRAD, IVRI, Izatnagar
↓
Regional Disease Diagnostic Laboratories
↓

NERDDL Guwahati	ERDDL Kolkata	WRDDL Pune	NRDDL Jalandhar	SRDDL Bangalore
↓	↓	↓	↓	↓
Area of Jurisdiction				
1. Assam	1. West Bengal	1. Maharashtra	1. Jammu & Kashmir	1. Karanatka
2. Sikkim	2. Bihar	2. Gujarat	2. Punjab	2. Andhra Pradesh
3. Arunachal Pradesh	3. Orissa	3. Madhya Pradesh	3. Haryana	3. Tamilnadu
4. Tripura	4. Jharkhand	4. Chattishgarh	4. Himachal Pradesh	4. Kerala
5. Manipur	5. Andaman & Nicobar Islands	5. Goa	5. Rajasthan	5. Pondicherry
6. Meghalaya		6. Daman & Div	6. Chandigarh	
7. Nagaland			7. Delhi	

However, these diagnostic laboratories require strengthening as per the international standards.

1. Purpose and Goals of Laboratory

The following points should be considered for developing a disease diagnostic laboratory:

i) The type of testing undertaken for diagnosis of various diseases of animals.

ii) The purpose of the diagnosis and its use in prevention and control of disease.

iii) The impact of false positive or false negative results.

iv) Financial inputs.

v) The need of the owner of animal including costs etc.

vi) Fulfilling of legal and regulatory requirements.

vii) Inter-laboratory comparisons/ assessment, mutual recognition of test/ results.

viii) Income generation vis-à-vis business goals.

ix) Requirement of accreditation as per International standards for quality management system and competence (ISO 9001: 2000 and ISO 17025).

x) Infrastructure development and deployment of competent personnels.

2. Standards, Guides and References

It is recommended that the laboratory choose reputed and accepted standards and guides to assist in designing the quality management programme. For laboratories seeking accreditation, the use of ISO 17025 is essential. Further information on standards may be obtained from NABL which has its accreditation with the International Laboratory Accreditation Cooperation (ILAC). Technical and international organizations such as the AOAC International and the ISO publish useful references, guides, and/or standards that supplement the general requirements of ISO 17025. International Standard ISO 9001: 2000 is a general standard for quality management systems and one of the many standards in the group commonly termed the 'ISO 9000 series'. For technical matters, standard books written by Indian and foreign authors on the subject matter must be consulted. Laboratory should also develop its own SOP's based on the available technical information because in biological system, there are several variations while conducting a test on clinical specimens. ***The basic principle and methodology will remain same but their optimization and standardization in a particular laboratory is necessary before adopting any diagnostic test and/or kits.***

3. Accreditation for Competence

If the laboratory has determined that it needs formal recognition of its quality management programme, then third party verification of its conformity with the selected standard(s) is necessary. The NABL accreditation body will provide recognition to a laboratory for its competence to carry out specific tests. The use of *competence* is significant; it means much more than having and following the documented procedures. Having competence also means that the laboratory:

i) Has technically valid and validated test methods, procedures, and specifications that are documented in accordance with the requirements of ISO 17025.

ii) Has adequate qualified personnel(s) who understand the science behind the procedures.

iii) Has correct and adequate equipments.

iv) Has adequate facilities and environmental control.

v) Has procedures and specifications that ensure accurate and reliable results.

vi) Can foresee technical needs and problems.

vii) Can cope with and prevent technical problems that may arise.

viii) Can accurately estimate and control the uncertainty in testing.

ix) Can demonstrate proficiency to conduct the test methods used.

4. Identification of Scope

Laboratory should determine its scope which ideally cover all areas of activity affecting all testing that is done at the laboratory. However, for the purpose of accreditation, the laboratory should determine the scope of testing to be included in the accreditation. Factors that might affect the laboratory's choice of scope of accreditation include:

i) The availability and cost of necessary personnel(s), facilities and equipment(s).

ii) The cost of environmental monitoring against the possibility of cross contamination(s).

iii) The deadline for accreditation.

iv) The impact of the test results.

v) The number of tests done.

vi) Frequency of testing (no. of test samples handled).

vii) Out sourcing of a particular test(s).

viii) The quality assurance of materials, reagents and media.

ix) The availability of reference standards *e.g.* standardized reagents, internal quality control samples, reference cultures, manuals, guidelines, etc..

x) The availability of proficiency testing.

xi) The availability, from reputable sources, of standard and/or fully validated test methods.

xii) The evaluation and validation of test methods to be done.

xiii) The technical complexity of the method (s).

5. Test Methods

ISO 17025 requires the use of appropriate test methods and has requirements for selection, development, and validation. Test methods of following sources can be adopted:

(a) OIE terrestrial animal health code

(b) International/ National journals of repute

(c) Textbooks, practical manuals

(d) National standards

(e) AOAC methods

In veterinary diagnostic laboratories, even with the use of standard methods, some in-house evaluation, optimization, and/or validation generally must be done to ensure valid results. Clients and laboratory staff must have a clear understanding of what performance can be expected from a test. Many veterinary diagnostic laboratories will, therefore, need to demonstrate competence in the development, adaptation, and validation of test methods.

Valid results begin with the selection of an appropriate test method for the diagnosis. Following criteria can be used to select a method for testing laboratory:

i) It should have international acceptance.

ii) It should have scientific acceptance.

iii) It should not be outdated.

iv) It should show promising performance characteristics (*e.g.* diagnostic sensitivity and specificity, repeatability, reproducibility, lower limit of detection and uncertainty).

v) Test method should be applicable to various species/ population of interest.

vi) Resources and time required for development, adaptation, and/or evaluation.

vii) Performance time and turnaround time.

viii) Type of sample (*e.g.* serum, tissue) and its expected quality on arrival at the laboratory (preservation).

ix) Analyte (*e.g.* antibody, antigen, toxin level, causative agent, etc.).

x) Nature of the intended use (*e.g.* export, import, surveillance, screening, confirmatory, individual animal use, herd use).

xi) Client expectations (time, cost, validity, etc.).

xii) Safety factors.

xiii) Number of tests to be done.

xiv) Cost of test, per sample.

xv) Existence of reference standards, including reference materials.

xvi) Availability of proficiency testing schemes in particular area.

Optimization and Standardization of the Test Method

Once the method has been selected, it must be set up at the laboratory. Whether the method was developed in-house or imported from an outside source, generally some additional optimization is necessary. *Optimization* is a series of experiments and subsequent data analysis. Optimization establishes critical specifications and performance standards for the test process and for use in monitoring the correct performance of the test. Optimization should ensure that a method is brought under statistical control. Optimization should also determine:

i) Critical specifications for equipment and instruments.

ii) Critical specifications for reagents (*e.g.* chemicals, biologicals).

iii) Critical specifications for reference standards, reference materials, and internal controls.

iv) The quality control activities necessary to monitor critical control points.

v) The type test controls needed.

vi) The level of technical competence required of those who carry out and/or interpret the test.

Validation of a Diagnostic Rest

Validation further evaluates the test for its fitness for a given use, such as sensitivity, specificity, positive/negative cut-off, and titre of interest or significance. Validation should be done using an optimized, documented, and fixed procedure. Validation may include:

a) Field data analysis.

b) Epidemiological studies.

c) Comparison with other methods, preferably standard methods.

d) Comparison with reference standards.

e) Collaborative studies with other laboratories.

f) Reproduction of data from an accepted standard method, or from a reputable publication.

g) Experimental infection studies.

h) Analysis of internal quality control data.

ISO 17025 recognizes that ***Validation is always a balance between costs, risks, and technical possibilities***. A valid, highly sensitive, highly specific, rapid, cost effective, easily to perform test method for diagnosis of disease is considered good for use in a veterinary diagnostic laboratory.

Continuous improvement in laboratory working is essential. It is always advisable that the scientists/ technicians working in laboratory should be knowledgeable with current standard methods used to demonstrate laboratory competence. It can be achieved through continual educational programmes like:

1. Participation in conferences, symposia, seminars, etc.
2. Participation in training programmes.
3. Consultation of publications: Books, journals, internet searching.
4. Visits to other standard laboratories.
5. Conducting research.
6. Participation in cooperative/ collaborative programmes.
7. Exchange of procedures, test methods, reagents, samples, personnels, and/or ideas.
8. Third party accreditation.
9. Presenting papers using laboratory generated data in conferences/ symposia/ meetings, etc.
10. Publishing papers using laboratory generated data in journals of repute.

Benefits of ISO 17025 Accreditation

1. National and international recognition.
2. Public and industry acceptance.
3. Assurance to clients of good laboratory practice.
4. Provides global equivalence.
5. Provides comparability in measurements.
6. Decision makers can rely on test results.
7. Improves staff motivation.
8. Ensures better support in the event of legal challenge.
9. Saves money by getting it right at first time.

Processing of Application

There should be a commitment of top management of the laboratory who will decide for accreditation of the laboratory from NABL. It is very important because without firm determination and commitment one may not be able to provide requisite support and generate interest in the staff. The management of the laboratory should make a definite plan of action for getting accreditation and nominate a responsible person to coordinate all activity; such person should be familiar with laboratory's working, and quality system. This person will be known as Management Representative (MR)/ Technical Manager. There are a number of formalities to be done before making an application to NABL for accreditation; these include:

1. Understanding of ISO 17025
2. Documentation
    - Preparation of quality policy
    - Preparation of quality manual
3. Successful participation in proficiency testing or in inter laboratory comparison
4. Internal audit
    - At least one internal audit should be done before making application to NABL.
5. Management review

The applicant laboratory must comply with all clauses of "General requirements for the competence of testing and calibration laboratories" (ISO 17025) and with the relevant NABL specific criteria.

The applicant laboratory must have participated satisfactorily in the proficiency testing programme conducted by NABL or any other international body. The minimum stipulated participation for testing laboratories is one parameter/ type of test per discipline prior to grant of accreditation. The applicant laboratory must have conducted at least one internal audit and a management review before the submission of application.

After completing all above mentioned formalities, a request may be made to NABL secretariat for procurement of relevant documents. One should carefully study the documents and in case of any query or clarification may contact NABL on phone or in person. There should be a clear understanding on procedure and methodology of making application for accreditation.

It is necessary to ascertain the status of the existing quality system and technical competence of the laboratory with regards to the requirements for NABL accreditation. Practically, the system of veterinary diagnostic laboratory should be properly documented and effective and in any case if it is not effective modifications, can be done at this stage. Even if some modifications/ alterations are not able to make the system effective, then start to build the quality system from beginning. It must be remembered that quality manual is a policy document which has to be supplemented by a set of other documents like procedural manuals, work instructions, etc. to align the quality system in accordance with ISO 17025. The relevant requirements for NABL accreditation should be discussed amongst concerned staff of the laboratory to enable them to understand their weakness and strengths. The management must ensure that the procedures described in the quality manual and other documents are really being implemented.

Take the application form number NABL-151 meant for accreditation of testing laboratories from NABL Secretariat or download from their website. Here, one should take care that as far as the Veterinary Diagnostic Laboratories are concerned they fall under two sub-areas *viz.*, clinical lab. and forensic lab. Submit the five copies of application along with 5 copies of quality manual and requisite application fee (Revised from time to time) to NABL and get customer reference number.

The application will be checked at NABL secretariat for its correctness and adequacy of quality manual and in case of any difference of opinion, it will be sent back to veterinary diagnostic laboratory or else secretariat may ask for additional information/ clarification. If there are gross inadequacies, quality manual is returned back for rewriting. It will be processed further for appointment of a lead assessor who will further take about 45 days to go through quality manual and other aspects of laboratory. Lead assessor will make a visit to laboratory for pre-assessment and if there is any non-conformity, he/she will direct the laboratory to close it within 90 days.

The pre-assessment of the laboratory is conducted to:

- have a better understanding of the documentation.
- familiarize with the facilities, sites/ location, circumstances and to have better knowledge of operations.
- make the methodology to be adopted for the assessment.
- check the preparedness of the laboratory to undergo assessment.
- review the scope of accreditation and to ascertain the requirement of the number of assessors/ experts and the duration of assessment.

The lead assessor shall submit a pre-assessment report to NABL Secretariat with a copy to the laboratory within 10 days of completion of pre-assessment. The laboratory shall comply with the inadequacies of the documented quality system and its implementation and submit a corrective action report to NABL Secretariat.

After the laboratory confirms removal of inadequacies, NABL shall propose constitution of an assessment team. The team shall include the lead assessor (already appointed), the assessor(s)/ technical expert(s) in order to cover various disciplines within the scope of accreditation sought. Thereafter, NABL shall fix up dates for on-site assessment of the laboratory in consultation with the laboratory, the lead assessor and assessor(s).

The assessment team reviews the laboratory's documented quality system and verifies its compliance with the requirements of ISO 17025 and specific criteria. The documented quality system, SOPs, work instructions, test methods, etc. are assessed for its implementation and effectiveness. The laboratory's technical competence to perform specific tests is also adjudged. The non-compliances, if identified are reported in the assessment report.

The assessment report shall contain the evaluation of technical manpower, all relevant material examined, test witnessed; compliance to ISO 17025 and relevant specific criteria and the non-conformances, if any.

The assessment report shall be examined by NABL, who shall communicate the outcome of the assessment to the laboratory and shall ensure that the non-conformances raised by the assessment team, which were not closed during the assessment, are well understood by the laboratory.

Laboratory shall take necessary corrective action on the remaining non-conformance(s)/ other concerns and shall submit a report to NABL Secretariat within a maximum period of 3 months. NABL shall monitor the progress of closing of non-conformances. When there are significant non-conformance(s) identified during the onsite assessment, NABL may arrange for a verification visit for the closure of the non-conformance(s).

After satisfactory corrective action by the laboratory, the Accreditation Committee examines the assessment report, additional information received from the laboratory and the consequent verifications.

In case the Accreditation Committee finds deficiencies in the assessment report to arrive at the decision, the Secretariat obtains clarification from the Lead Assessor/ Assessor/ Laboratory concerned. In case everything is in order, the Accreditation Committee shall make appropriate recommendations regarding accreditation of a laboratory to the Chairman, NABL.

Only after approval of the chairman, a certificate will be issued to laboratory. The following things are important on NABL accreditation:

1. Veterinary diagnostic laboratory can use NABL logo for its defined scope.
2. The accreditation, once granted, is valid for 3 years with annual surveillance by NABL lead assessors for compliance of the ISO 17025.
3. At the end of 3 years, there will be reassessment through similar procedure which should be initiated 6 months in advance *i.e.* on completion of 2½ years of accreditation.
4. During this period, veterinary diagnostic laboratory should participate in the proficiency testing programme at least once or twice.

26

Good Laboratory Practice in Veterinary Clinical Pathology Laboratory

- General considerations
- Purpose
- Scope
- Five pillars of GLP
- Good laboratory practice principles
  - Test facility organization and personnel
  - Quality assurance programme
  - Facilities
  - Apparatus, materials and reagents
  - Test systems
  - Test and reference items
  - Standard operating procedures
  - Performance of the study
  - Reporting of study results
  - Storage and retention of records and materials
- Comparison with laboratory accreditation ISO17025 (NABL)

General Considerations

Good laboratory practice is a quality system concerned with the organizational process and conditions under which non-clinical health and environmental safety studies are planned performed, monitored, recorded, reported and archived.

In 1979 and 1980, an international group of experts established under the special programme on control of chemicals developed "the principles of good laboratory practice (GLP)". These principles of GLP were adopted by Organization for Economic Cooperation and Development (OECD) council in 1981. Subsequently, in 1995 and 1996, a new group of experts was formed to revise and update the principles of GLP, which are applicable now a days.

Purpose

The purpose of Good Laboratory Practice is to promote the development of quality test data. Comparable quality of test data forms the basis for the mutual acceptance of data among countries. If individual country can confidently rely on test data developed in other countries, duplicative testing can be avoided, thereby saving time and resources. The application of GLP principles should help to avoid the creation of technical barriers to trade and further improve the protection of human health and the environment.

Scope

The GLP principles should be applied to the non-clinical safety testing items contained in pharmaceutical products, pesticide products, cosmetic products, veterinary drugs/ biologicals, food/feed additives, industrial chemicals, etc. These test items may include synthetic chemicals, natural products, biological products, living organisms etc. The purpose of testing is to obtain data on their properties and/or their safety with respect to human health and/or environment.

Non-clinical health and environment safety studies covered by GLP principles include work conducted in the laboratory, in green houses and in the field. Unless specifically exempted by national legislation, these principles of GLP apply to all non-clinical health and environmental safety studies required by regulations for the purpose of registering or licensing pharmaceuticals, pesticides, food/ feed additives, cosmetics products, veterinary drugs/ biologicals and other similar products and for the regulation of industrial chemicals.

Five pillars of GLP

There are 5 pillars of basic components of Good Laboratory Practice:

1. **Resources-** Facilities, personnels, equipments, Infrastructural facilities, etc.
2. **Rules-** Guidelines, procedures, protocols, study plans, etc.
3. **Organization-** Test article, identification of quality test system.
4. **Documentation-** Raw data, draft report, final report, archive.
5. **Quality assurance-** Audit/ implementation, training, advice, etc.

The application of GLP principles in any organization requires a firm commitment of the management to provide all resources, facilities and freedom of work for quality assurance of its products. Organization(s), once complied with the principles of GLP for testing their products, may approach National GLP Compliance Monitoring Authority for Certification.

Good Laboratory Practice Principles

There are ten principles of GLP, which have to be completed by any organization/ test facilities to get certificate.

1. Test Facility Organization and Personnel

1.1 Test Facility Management's Responsibilities

1. Each test facility management should ensure that these Principles of Good Laboratory Practice are complied with, in its test facility.
2. At a minimum it should:
    a) ensure that a statement exists which identifies the individual(s) within a test facility who fulfil the responsibilities of management as defined by these Principles of Good Laboratory Practice;

    b) ensure that a sufficient number of qualified personnel, appropriate facilities, equipment, and materials are available for the timely and proper conduct of the study;

    c) ensure the maintenance of a record of the qualifications, training, experience and job description for each professional and technical individual;

    d) ensure that personnel clearly understand the functions they have to perform and where necessary, provide training for these functions;

    e) ensure that appropriate and technically valid Standard Operating Procedures are established and followed, and approve all original and revised Standard Operating Procedures;

    f) ensure that there is a Quality Assurance Programme with designated personnel and assure that the quality assurance responsibility is being performed in accordance with these Principles of Good Laboratory Practice;

    g) ensure that for each study an individual with the appropriate qualifications, training, and experience is designated by the management as the Study Director before the study is initiated.

Replacement of a Study Director should be done according to established procedures, and should be documented.

h) ensure, in the event of a multi-site study, that, if needed, a Principal Investigator is designated, who is appropriately trained, qualified and experienced to supervise the delegated phase(s) of the study. Replacement of a Principal Investigator should be done according to established procedures, and should be documented.

i) ensure documented approval of the study plan by the Study Director;

j) ensure that the Study Director has made the approved study plan available to the Quality Assurance personnel;

k) ensure the maintenance of an historical file of all Standard Operating Procedures;

l) ensure that an individual is identified as responsible for the management of the archive(s);

m) ensure the maintenance of a master schedule;

n) ensure that test facility supplies meet requirements appropriate to their use in a study;

o) ensure for a multi-site study that clear lines of communication exist between the Study Director, Principal Investigator(s), the Quality Assurance Programme(s) and study personnel;

p) ensure that test and reference items are appropriately characterized;

q) establish procedures to ensure that computerized systems are suitable for their intended purpose, and are validated, operated and maintained in accordance with these Principles of Good Laboratory Practice.

3. When a phase(s) of a study is conducted at a test site, test site management (if appointed) will have the responsibilities as defined above with the following exceptions: 1.1.2 g), i), j) and o).

1.2 Study Director's Responsibilities

1. The Study Director is the single point of study control and has the responsibility for the overall conduct of the study and for its final report.
2. These responsibilities should include, but not be limited to, the following functions. The Study Director should:

a) approve the study plan and any amendments to the study plan by dated signature;

b) ensure that the Quality Assurance personnel have a copy of the study plan and any amendments in a timely manner and communicate effectively with the Quality Assurance personnel as required during the conduct of the study;

c) ensure that study plans and amendments and Standard Operating Procedures are available to study personnel;

d) ensure that the study plan and the final report for a multi-site study identify and define the role of any Principal Investigator(s) and any test facilities and test sites involved in the conduct of the study;

e) ensure that the procedures specified in the study plan are followed, and assess and document the impact of any deviations from the study plan on the quality and integrity of the study, and take appropriate corrective action if necessary; acknowledge deviations from Standard Operating Procedures during the conduct of the study;

f) ensure that all raw data generated are fully documented and recorded;

g) ensure that computerized systems used in the study have been validated;

h) sign and date the final report to indicate acceptance of responsibility for the validity of the data and to indicate the extent to which the study complies with these Principles of Good Laboratory Practice;

i) ensure that after completion (including termination) of the study, the study plan, the final report, raw data and supporting material are archived.

1.3 Principal Investigator's Responsibilities

The Principal Investigator will ensure that the delegated phases of the study are conducted in accordance with the applicable Principles of Good Laboratory Practice.

1.4 Study Personnel's Responsibilities

1. All personnel involved in the conduct of the study must be knowledgeable in those parts of the Principles of Good Laboratory Practice which are applicable to their involvement in the study.

2. Study personnel will have access to the study plan and appropriate Standard Operating Procedures applicable to their involvement in the

study. It is their responsibility to comply with the instructions given in these documents. Any deviation from these instructions should be documented and communicated directly to the Study Director, and/or if appropriate, the Principal Investigator(s).

3. All study personnel are responsible for recording raw data promptly and accurately and in compliance with these Principles of Good Laboratory Practice, and are responsible for the quality of their data.
4. Study personnel should exercise health precautions to minimize risk to themselves and to ensure the integrity of the study. They should communicate to the appropriate person any relevant known health or medical condition in order that they can be excluded from operations that may affect the study.

2. Quality Assurance Programme

2.1 General

1. The test facility should have a documented Quality Assurance Programme to assure that studies performed are in compliance with these Principles of Good Laboratory Practice.
2. The Quality Assurance Programme should be carried out by an individual or by individuals designated by and directly responsible to management and who are familiar with the test procedures.
3. This individual(s) should not be involved in the conduct of the study being assured.

2.2 Responsibilities of the Quality Assurance Personnel

1. The responsibilities of the Quality Assurance personnel include, but are not limited to, the following functions. They should:
   a) maintain copies of all approved study plans and Standard Operating Procedures in use in the test facility and have access to an up-to-date copy of the master schedule;
   b) verify that the study plan contains the information required for compliance with these Principles of Good Laboratory Practice. This verification should be documented;
   c) conduct inspections to determine if all studies are conducted in accordance with these Principles of Good Laboratory Practice. Inspections should also determine that study plans and Standard

Operating Procedures have been made available to study personnel and are being followed.

Inspections can be of three types as specified by Quality Assurance Programme Standard Operating Procedures:

- Study- based inspections,
- Facility- based inspections,
- Process- based inspections.

Records of such inspections should be retained.

d) inspect the final reports to confirm that the methods, procedures, and observations are accurately and completely described, and that the reported results accurately and completely reflect the raw data of the studies;

e) promptly report any inspection results in writing to management and to the Study Director, and to the Principal Investigator(s) and the respective management, when applicable;

f) prepare and sign a statement, to be included with the final report, which specifies types of inspections and their dates, including the phase(s) of the study inspected, and the dates inspection results were reported to management and the Study Director and Principal Investigator(s), if applicable. This statement would also serve to confirm that the final report reflects the raw data.

3. Facilities

3.1 General

1. The test facility should be of suitable size, construction and location to meet the requirements of the study and to minimize disturbance that would interfere with the validity of the study.
2. The design of the test facility should provide an adequate degree of separation of the different activities to assure the proper conduct of each study.

3.2 Test System Facilities

1. The test facility should have a sufficient number of rooms or areas to assure the isolation of test systems and the isolation of individual projects, involving substances or organisms known to be or suspected of being biohazardous.

2. Suitable rooms or areas should be available for the diagnosis, treatment and control of diseases, in order to ensure that there is no unacceptable degree of deterioration of test systems.

3. There should be storage rooms or areas as needed for supplies and equipment. Storage rooms or areas should be separated from rooms or areas housing the test systems and should provide adequate protection against infestation, contamination, and/or deterioration.

3.3 Facilities for Handling Test and Reference Items

1. To prevent contamination or mix-ups, there should be separate rooms or areas for receipt and storage of the test and reference items, and mixing of the test items with a vehicle.

2. Storage rooms or areas for the test items should be separate from rooms or areas containing the test systems. They should be adequate to preserve identity, concentration, purity, and stability, and ensure safe storage for hazardous substances.

3.4 Archive Facilities

Archive facilities should be provided for the secure storage and retrieval of study plans, raw data, final reports, samples of test items and specimens. Archive design and archive conditions should protect contents from untimely deterioration.

3.5 Waste Disposal

Handling and disposal of wastes should be carried out in such a way as not to jeopardise the integrity of studies. This includes provision for appropriate collection, storage and disposal facilities, and decontamination and transportation procedures.

4. Apparatus, Material and Reagents

1. Apparatus, including validated computerized systems, used for the generation, storage and retrieval of data, and for controlling environmental factors relevant to the study should be suitably located and of appropriate design and adequate capacity.

2. Apparatus used in a study should be periodically inspected, cleaned, maintained and calibrated according to Standard Operating Procedures. Records of these activities should be maintained. Calibration should, where appropriate, be traceable to national or international standards of measurements.

3. Apparatus and materials used in a study should not interfere adversely with the test systems.

4. Chemicals, reagents, and solutions should be labelled to indicate identity (with concentration if appropriate), expiry date and specific storage instructions. Information concerning source, preparation date and stability should be available. The expiry date may be extended on the basis of documented evaluation or analysis.

5. Test Systems

5.1 Physical/Chemical

1. Apparatus used for the generation of physical/chemical data should be suitably located and of appropriate design and adequate capacity.

2. The integrity of the physical/chemical test system should be ensured.

5.2 Biological

1. Proper conditions should be established and maintained for the storage, housing, handling and care of biological test systems, in order to ensure the quality of the data.

2. Newly received animal and plant test systems should be isolated until their health status has been evaluated. If any unusual mortality or morbidity occurs, this lot should not be used in studies and, when appropriate, should be humanely destroyed. At the experimental starting date of a study, test systems should be free of any disease or condition that might interfere with the purpose or conduct of the study. Test systems that become diseased or injured during the course of a study be isolated and treated, if necessary to maintain the integrity of the study. Any diagnosis and treatment of any disease before or during a study should be recorded.

3. Records of source, date of arrival, and arrival condition of test systems should be maintained.

4. Biological test systems should be acclimatized to the test environment for an adequate period before the first administration/application of the test or reference item.

5. All information needed to properly identify the test systems should appear on their housing or containers. Individual test systems that are to be removed from their housing or containers during the conduct of the study should bear appropriate identification, wherever possible.

6. During use, housing or containers for test systems should be cleaned and sanitized at appropriate intervals. Any material that comes into contact with the test system should be free of contaminants at levels that would interfere with the study. Bedding for animals should be changed as required by sound husbandry practice. Use of pest control agents should be documented.

7. Test systems used in field studies should be located so as to avoid interference in the study from spray from past usage of pesticides.

6. Test and Reference Items

6.1 Receipt, Handling, Sampling and Storage

1. Records including test item and reference item characterization, date of receipt, expiry date, quantities received and used in studies should be maintained.

2. Handling, sampling and storage procedures should be identified in order that the homogeneity and stability are assured to the degree possible and contamination or mix-up are precluded.

3. Storage container(s) should carry identification information, expiry date, and specific storage instructions.

6.2 Characterization

1. Each test and reference item should be appropriately identified (e.g., code, Chemical Abstracts Service Registry Number [CAS number], name, biological parameters).

2. For each study, the identity, including batch number, purity, composition, concentrations, or other characteristics to appropriately define each batch of the test or reference items should be known.

3. In cases where the test item is supplied by the sponsor, there should be a mechanism, developed in co-operation between the sponsor and the test facility, to verify the identity of the test item subject to the study.

4. The stability of test and reference items under storage and test conditions should be known for all studies.

5. If the test item is administered or applied in a vehicle, the homogeneity, concentration and stability of the test item in that vehicle should be determined. For test items used in field studies (e.g., tank mixes), these may be determined through separate laboratory experiments.

6. A sample for analytical purposes from each batch of test item should be retained for all studies except short-term studies.

7. Standard Operating Procedures

7.1 A test facility should have written Standard Operating Procedures approved by test facility management that are intended to ensure the quality and integrity of the data generated by that test facility. Revisions to Standard Operating Procedures should be approved by test facility management.

7.2 Each separate test facility unit or area should have immediately available current Standard Operating Procedures relevant to the activities being performed therein. Published test books, analytical methods, articles and manuals may be used as supplements to these Standard Operating Procedures.

7.3 Deviations from Standard Operating Procedures related to the study should be documented and should be acknowledged by the Study Director and the Principal Investigator(s), as applicable.

7.4 Standard Operating Procedures should be available for, but not be limited to, the following categories of test facility activities. The details given under each heading are to be considered as illustrative examples.

1. Test and Reference Items

   Receipt, identification, labelling, sampling and storage

2. Apparatus, Materials and Reagents

   a) Apparatus

      Use, maintenance, cleaning and calibration.

   b) Computerized Systems

      Validation, operation, maintenance, security, change control and back-up.

   c) Materials, Reagents and Solutions

      Preparation and labelling.

3. Record Keeping, Reporting, Storage and Retrieval

   Coding of studies, data collection, preparation of reports, indexing systems, handling of data, including the use of computerized systems.

4. Test System (where appropriate)

a) Room preparation and environmental room conditions for the test system.

b) Procedures for receipt, transfer, proper placement, characterization, identification and care of the test system.

c) Test system preparation, observations and examinations, before, during and at the conclusion of the study.

d) Handling of test system individuals found moribund or dead during the study.

e) Collection, identification and handling of specimens including necropsy and histopathology.

f) Sitting and placement of test systems in test plots.

5. Quality Assurance Procedures

Operation of Quality Assurance personnel in planning, scheduling, performing documenting and reporting inspections.

8. Performance of the Study

8.1 Study Plan

1. For each study, a written plan should exist prior to the initiation of the study. The study plan should be approved by dated signature of the Study Director and verified for GLP compliance by Quality Assurance personnel as specified in Section 2.2.1.b., above. The study plan should also be approved by the test facility management and the sponsor, if required by national regulation or legislation in the country where the study is being performed.

2. a)Amendments to the study plan should be justified and approved by dated signature of the Study Director and maintained with the study plan.

b) Deviations from the study plan should be described, explained acknowledged and dated in a timely fashion by the Study Director and / or Principal Investigator(s) and maintained with the study raw data.

3. For short term studies, a general study plan accompanied by a study specific supplement may be used.

8.2 Content of the Study Plan

The study plan should contain, but not be limited to the following information:

1. Identification of the Study, the Test Item and Reference Item
   a) A descriptive title;
   b) A statement which reveals the nature and purpose of the study;
   c) Identification of the test item by code or name (IUPAC; CAS number, biological parameters, etc.);
   d) The reference item to be used.
2. Information Concerning the Sponsor and the Test Facility
   a) Name and address of the sponsor;
   b) Name and address of any test facilities and test sites involved;
   c) Name and address of the Study Director;
   d) Name and address of the Principal Investigator(s), and the phase(s) of the study delegated by the Study Director and under the responsibility of the Principal Investigator(s).
3. Dates
   a) The date of approval of the study plan by signature of the Study Director. The date of approval of the study plan by signature of the test facility management and sponsor if required by national regulation or legislation in the country where the study is being performed.
   b) The proposed experimental starting and completion dates.
4. Test Methods

   Reference to the OECD Test Guideline or other test guideline or method to be used.
5. Issues (where applicable)
   a. The justification for the selection of the test system;
   b. Characterization of the test system, such as the species, strain, substrain, source of supply, number, body weight range, sex, age and other pertinent information;
   c. The method of administration and the reason for its choice;

d. The dose levels and/or concentration(s), frequency, and duration of administration/ application;

e. Detailed information on the experimental design, including a description of the chronological procedure of study, all methods, materials and conditions, type and frequency of analysis, measurements, observations and examinations to be performed, and statistical methods to be used (if any).

6. Records

A list of records to be retained.

8.3 Conduct of Study

1. A unique identification should be given to each study. All items concerning this study should carry this identification. Specimens from study should be identified to confirm their origin. Such identification should enable their traceability, as appropriate for the specimen and study.
2. The study should be conducted in accordance with the study plan.
3. All data generated during the conduct of the study should be recorded directly, promptly, accurately, and legibly by the individual entering the data. These entries should be signed or initialed and dated.
4. Any change in raw data should be made so as not to obscure the previous entry, should indicate the reason for change and should be dated and signed or initialed by the individual making the change.
5. Data generated as a direct computer input should be identified at the time of data input by the individual(s) responsible for direct data entries. Computerized system design should always provide for the retention of full audit trails to show all changes to the data without obscuring the original data. It should be possible to associate all changes to data with the persons having made those changes, for example, by use of timed and dated (electronic) signatures. Reason for changes should be given.

9. Reporting of Study Results

9.1 General

1. A final report should be prepared for each study. In case of the short term studies, a standardized final report accompanied by a study specific extension may be prepared.

2. Reports of principal investigator or scientists involved in the study should be signed and dated by them.
3. The final report should be signed and dated by study Director to indicate acceptance of responsibility for the validity of the data. The extent of compliance with these Principles of Good Laboratory Practice should be indicated.
4. Corrections and additions to a final report should be in the form of amendments. Amendments should clearly specify the reason for the corrections or additions and should be signed and dated by the study Director.
5. Reformatting of the final report to comply with the submission requirements of a national registration or regulatory authority does not constitute a correction, addition or amendment to the final report.

9.2 Content of the Final report

The final report should include, but not be limited to the following information:

2. Reports of principal investigator or scientists involved in the study should be signed and dated by them.

1. Identification of the study, the Test Item and reference Item
   a. A descriptive title;
   b. Identification of the test item by code or name (IUPAC, CAS number, biological parameters, etc.);
   c. Identification of the reference item by name;
   d. Characterization of the test item including purity, stability and homogeneity.
2. Information Concerning the Sponsor and the Test Facility
   a. Name and address of the sponsor;
   b. Name and address of any test facilities and test sites involved;
   c. Name and address of the study Director;
   d. Name and address of the Principal investigator(s) and the phase(s) of the study delegated, if applicable;
   e. Name and address of scientists having contributed reports to the final report.

3. Dates

   Experimental starting and completion dates.

4. Statement

   A Quality Assurance Programme statement listing the types of inspections made and their dates, including the phase(s) inspected, and the dates any inspection results were reported to management and to study Director and Principal Investigator(s), if applicable. This statement would also serve to confirm that the final report reflects the raw data.

5. Description of Materials and Test Methods

   a. Description of methods and materials used;

   b. Reference to OECD Test Guideline or other test guideline or method.

6. Results

   a. A summary of results;

   b. All information and data required by the study plan;

   c. A presentation of the results, including calculations and determinations of statistical significance.

   d. An evaluation and discussion of the results and where appropriate, conclusions.

7. Storage

   The location(s) where the study plan, samples of test and reference items, specimens, raw data and final report are to be stored.

10. Storage and Retention of Records and Materials

10.1 The following should be retained in archives for the period specified by the appropriate authorities:

a. The study plan, raw data, samples of test and reference items, specimens and the final report of each study;

b. Records of all inspections performed by the Quality Assurance Programme, as well as master schedules;

c. Records of qualifications, trainings, experience and job description of personnel;

d. Records and reports of the maintenance and calibrations of apparatus;

e. Validation documentation for the computerized system;

f. The historical file of the all Standard Operating procedures;

g. Environmental monitoring records.

In the absence of a required retention period, the final deposition of any study materials should be documented. When samples of test and reference items and specimens are disposed of before the expiry of the required retention period for any reason, this should be justified and documented. Samples of test and reference items and specimens should be retained only as long as the quality of preparation permits evaluation.

10.2 Material retained in the archives should be indexed so as to facilitate orderly storage and retrieval.

10.3 Only personnel authorized by management should have success to archives. Movement of materials in and out of archives should be properly recorded.

10.4 If a test facility or an archive contracting facility goes out of business and has no legal successor, the archive should be transferred to the archives of sponsor(s) of the study(s).

Govt. of India has established National GLP compliance monitoring Authority under the chairmanship of Secretary, Department of Science and Technology. This authority accepted the OECD principles of GLP and its guidelines. The desirous test facilities/ organizations may further contact at the following address for certification and further information:

National GLP Compliance Monitoring Authority

Department of Science & Technology, Govt. of India,

Technology Bhawan, New Mahrauli Road,

New Delhi – 110 016

Comparison with laboratory accreditation ISO 17025 (NABL)

The testing and calibration laboratories are required to comply with the accreditation system ISO 17025 in NABL of QCI, which is specifically meant for clinical laboratories. There are, however, some common features of ISO 17025 and GLP principles mentioned as under:

GLP Principles	Common Subjects	ISO 17025
• Master Schedule • Study Director • Archivist • Quality Assurance Unit • Animal Care • Study Plan • Test Article System • Inspection Monitoring	• Management & Organization • Responsibilities • SOP's • Equipment • Training of Staff • Validation of Methods • Quality Control Procedure • Audits • Corrective Action • Reports • Sampling & Sample Receipt	• Processing of Complaints • Uncertainty Calculation • Service to Clients • Preventive Action • Inter Laboratory Comparisons • Proficiency Testing • Customer Review

Besides, ISO 9001: 200 is meant for Quality Management System to improve the system and document the procedures and maintenance of records.

All these principles are formulated to generate quality data out of the experimental studies or provide a quality biological/ diagnostic service to the customer. It needs the firm commitment of the top management for availability of sufficient funds and manpower to implement these quality principles in Veterinary Diagnostic Laboratories and Veterinary Biologicals Institutes.

27

Clinical Signs, Pathological Lesions and Samples Required for Laboratory Examinations

- Nutritional diseases
- Viral diseases
- Prion, Mycoplasmal, Rickettsial, Chlamydial, Spirochaetal and Bacterial diseases
- Fungal diseases
- Parasitic diseases
- Toxic conditions
- Miscellaneous conditions

A. Nutritional Diseases

1. Hypovitaminosis A. (vitamin A deficiency)

   Clinical signs and lesions: ***Night blindness*** (***nyctalopia***), dryness of eyes (xerophthalmia)- ***urolithiasis*** in males prolonged gestation in cattle; ***nutritional roup***, Anophthalmos, microphthalmos.

   Collection of material: Feed, liver and blood samples

2. Hypovitaminosis B

	Clinical signs and lesions	**Collection of material**
Thiamine deficiency (B1)	Weakness of limbs, ascending paralysis, ***star grazing*** in chick	Feed, liver and blood samples
Riboflavin deficiency (B2)	***Curled toe paralysis*** in chicks	
Nicotinic cid deficiency	Cyanosis of distal portion of tongue (***canine pellegra***), ulcer formation on its borders, petechiae on digestive canal, vomiting, diarrhoea, dysentery	

	Clinical signs and lesions	Collection of material
Deficiency of Pantothenic acid	Hemorrhages and necrotizing colitis, dermatitis in chicks, nodular hyperplasia cracks in skin, atrophy of spleen	
Deficiency of Pyridoxine (B6)	Encephalomalaia	
Folic acid	Deaths of embryos, distorted ribs & back paralysis of neck.	
Biotin deficiency	Dermatitis, distorted limbs, ***Perosis***	
Choline deficiency	Slipped tendon (***perosis***)	
B12 deficiency	Atrophy of leg muscles, stunted growth	

3. **Hypovitaminosis C (Vitamin C deficiency)**

   Clinical signs and lesions: Failure of ossification in long bones, sub periosteal hemorrhages, scurvy retardation of fibroplasia, delayed wound healing.

   Collection of material: Feed sample

4. **Hypovitaminois D (vitamin D deficiency)**

   Clinical signs and lesions: Leg weakness in chick, soft shoelled eggs, Rickets, osteomalacia.

   Collection of material: Feed sample

5. **Hypovitaminosis E (vitamin E Deficiency)**

   Clinical signs and lesions: Necrosis of skeletal and cardiac muscles, hepatic necrosis, anemia, steatitis in calves, dogs cats and pigs, white muscle disease, encephalomalacia in chicks. Stifflamb disease, Myoglobinuria, crazy chick disease.

   Collection of material: Muscle samples

6. **Hypovitaminosis K (vitamin K deficiency)**

   Clinical signs and lesions: Hypoprothrombinemia, hemorrhages. Blood coagulation time increases.

   Collection of material: Feed sample

7. **Hypervitaminosis A (vitamin A excess)**

   Clinical signs and lesions: Osteoporosis, retarded bone growth in cattle, pigs.

   Collection of material: Feed sample

8. **Hypervitaminosis D (vitamin D excess.)**

   Clinical signs and lesions: Metastatic calcification due to hypercalcemia in myocardium, lungs, gastric mucosa and kidneys.

   Collection of material: Feed sample

9. **Hypocalcemia (calcium deficiency)**

   Clinical signs and lesions: Milk fever in post-parturient dairy cattle, rickets in young ones.

   Collection of material: Serum sample

10. **Hypomagnesemia (magnesium deficiency)**

    Clinical signs and lesions: Hyperirritability, tetany, tonic or clonic convulsions, congestion of viscera, hemorrhages in heart, intestines and mesentry. Calcification of heart muscles and large blood vessels, incoordination of limbs, stunted birds.

    Collection of material: Serum sample

11. **Hyperphosphatemia (phosphorus deficiency)**

    Clinical signs and lesions: Pain in walking, rheumatism like syndrome, hemoglobinurea, pica, intestinal parasitism

    Collection of material: Serum sample, fecal sample

12. **Hypomagnesemia (Phosphorus excess)**

    Clinical signs and lesions: Bran disease in horses, adult rickets, osteomalacia, loosening of teeth.

    Collection of material: Serum sample

13. **Selenium deficiency**

    Clinical signs and lesions: Muscular dystrophy in lambs; Hepatic necrosis in swine

    Collection of material: Serum sample

14. **Selenium toxicity (excess of selenium)**

    Clinical signs and lesions: *Acute* Hemorrhagic enteritis, ***proctitis***, inflammation of gall bladder and urinary bladder

    Collection of material: Serum sample

15. **Zinc deficiency**

    Clinical signs and lesions: ***Parakeratosis***, acanthosis, loss of hair/ wool scaly limb, ***perosis***. Fascial eczema in cattle, Thymic hypoplasia in calves

    Collection of material: Serum sample

16. **Manganese deficiency**

    Clinical signs and lesions: Suppresssion of epiphyseal cartilage growth, reduced osteoblastic activity, rarefaction of bones, joint deformities, Tendon slippage; ***perosis*** or sliped tendon in chicken

    Collection of material: Serum sample

17. **Cobalt deficiency**

    Clinical signs and lesions: ***Anemia***; marked hemorrhages on liver, spleen, kidneys enzootic marasmus, cachexia, hemosiderosis.

    Collection of material: Serum sample

18. **Excessive cobalt**

    Clinical signs and lesions: Polycythemia

    Collection of material: Serum sample

19. **Iron deficiency**

    Clinical signs and lesions: Hypochromic,microcytic anemia

    Collection of material: Blood sample

20. **Copper deficiency**

    Clinical signs and lesions: Microcytic hypochromic anemia, ***sway back*** in sheep and goat, weakness and incoordination of limbs, blindness; Osteoporosis, ***steely wool*** in sheep, enzootic ataxia in goats.

    Collection of material: Serum sample; caudate lobe of liver in case of toxicity

21. **Iodine deficiency**

    Clinical signs and lesions: ***Goiter*** in calves, lambs, pigs; Hairless pig litter; Reproductive disorders.

    Collection of material: Plasma for estimation of TSH, thyroxin, etc.

22. **Iodism (excess iodine)**

Clinical signs and lesions: Lacrimation, exfoliation of epidermal scales, cutaneous eruptions, pharyngitis.

Collection of material: Plasma

23. **Hypoproteinemia (Deficiency of protein)**

Clinical signs and lesions: Anemia, poor growth, delayed healing of wounds, atrophy of thymus and lymphoid tissue, edema, ***immunosuppression***.

Collection of material: Serum sample

24. **Hyperglycemia (excess of glucose)**

Clinical signs and lesions: Polyuria, polydipsia, glycosuria, fibrosis, ketonuria, chronic pancreatitis.

Collection of material: Blood sample

25. **Diabetes insipidus (sodium chloride deficieiny)**

Clinical signs and lesions: Polyuria, polydipsia.

Collection of material: Blood in sodium fluoride

26. **Fluorosis (exces of fluoride)**

Clinical signs and lesions: Short and broad teeth motling.

Collection of material: Serum sample

27. **Ketosis (Acetonemia)**

Clinical signs and lesions: Anorexia, depresion, coma, ketone bodies in blood/ urine, hypoglycemia.

Collection of material: Urine for ketone bodies estimation

28. **Salt poisoning (NaCl)**

Clinical signs and lesions: *Ascites* in birds

Collection of material: Feed sample, brain sample in 10% FS

B. Viral Diseases

1. Foot and mouth disease (Picorna virus)

Clinical signs and lesions: Hypersalivation, painful eating, smacking of lips and tongue, gastroenteritis, myocarditis in young animals, ***vesicular lesions*** on oral mucosa i.e. over lips, dorsum of tongue and palate ruminal pillar, skin of coronary band near to the interdigital space; lesions on vulva, teat, udder, and other hairless parts of body; greyish necrotic foci in myocardium ***'Tiger heart'***.

Collection of material: Tongue epithelium, vesicular fluid, saliva, pancreas in 50% buffered glycerine, serum samples from affected and convalescent animals. Tonsils, spleen, lymphnode vesiculated epithelium, heart muscles

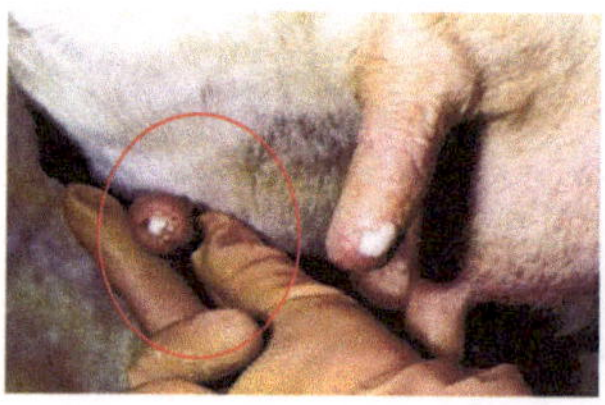
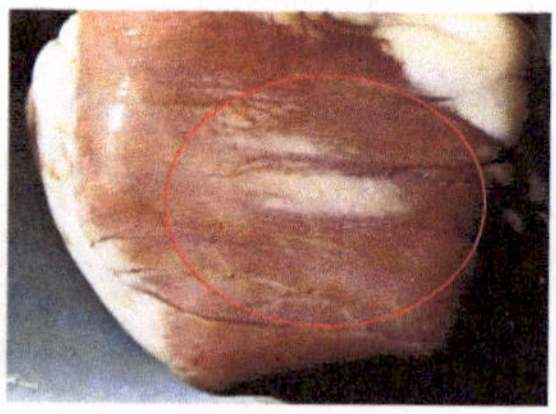
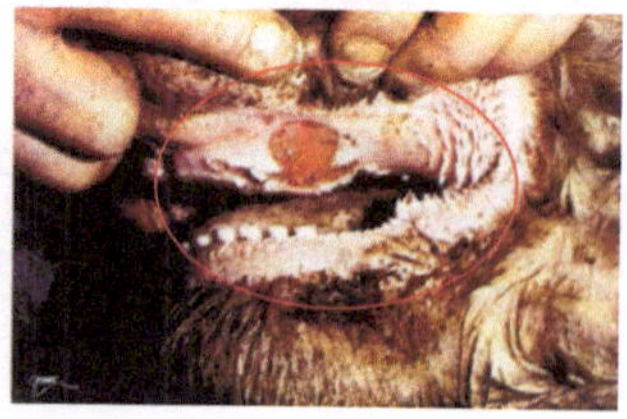

2. Vesicular stomatitis (Vesiculo virus)

Clinical signs and lesions: Vesicles in mouth cavity.

Collection of material: Vesicles and serum samples

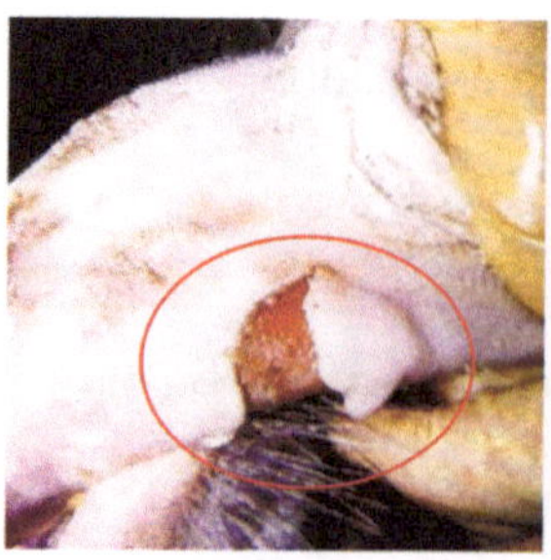
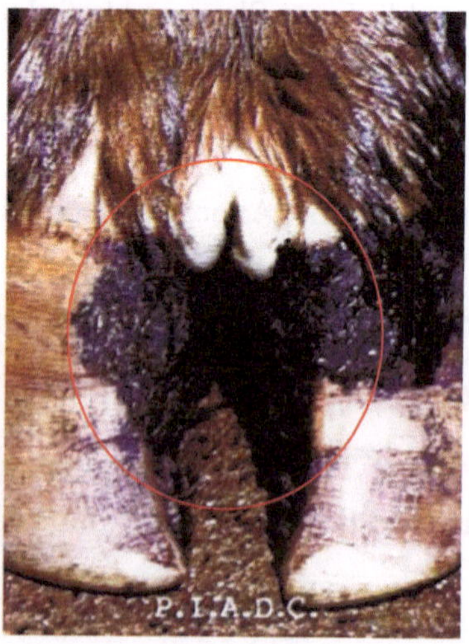

3. Vesicular exanthema (Calci virus)

Clinical signs and lesions: Fever, vesicles on snout, lips, nostrils, tongue, feet and mammary gland, between digits, around the coronary band, on the ball of foot; ulceration and pyogenic infection leads to lameness.

Collection of material: Vesicles and serum samples

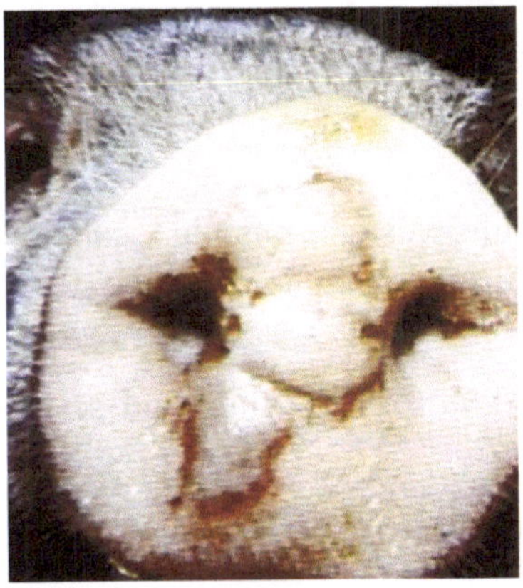

4. Cow Pox (Orthopox virus)

Clinical signs and lesions: Papule, vesicle, pustule and scab on hairless parts of body like teats, udder.

Collection of material: Scabs in ice and in 10% formol saline and serum samples

5. Pseudocow Pox (Parapox virus)

Clinical signs and lesions: Congestion, papules, vesicles on teat and udder.

Collection of material: Scabs in ice and in 10% formol saline and serum samples

6. Swine Pox (Sui pox virus)

Clinical signs and lesions: Erythema, papule, vesicles, pustules on inner portions of legs.

Collection of material: Scabs in ice and in 10% formol saline and serum samples

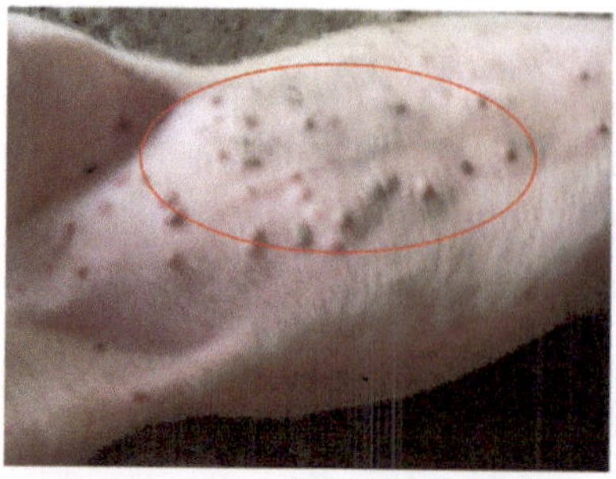

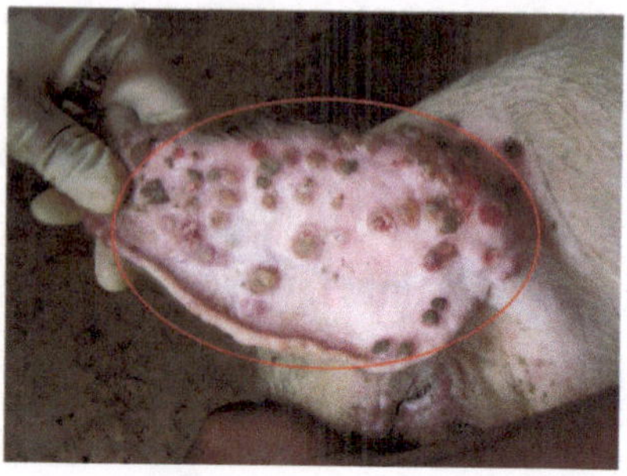

7. Sheep Pox (Capripox virus)

Clinical signs and lesions: Pock lesions (papule, vesicle, pustule, scab) on hairless parts of body, subcutaneous gelatinous edema, hemorrhage from vesicles.

Collection of material: Scabs in ice and in 10% formol saline and serum samples

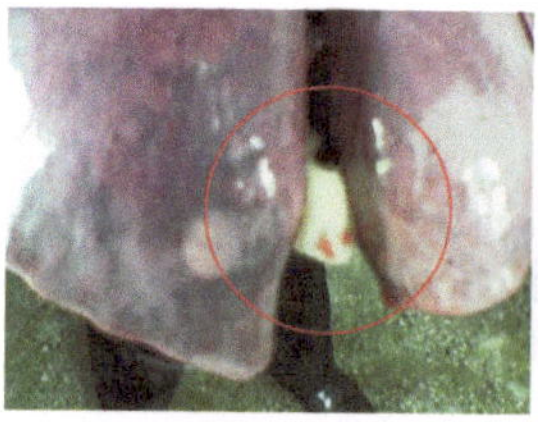

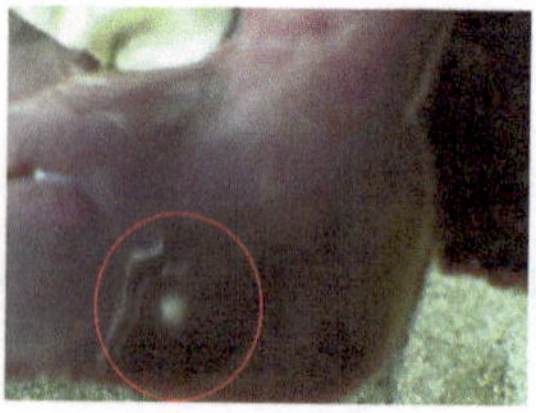

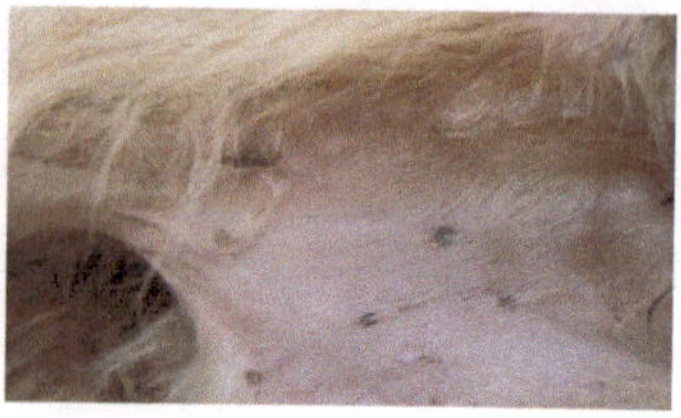

Presence of pock lesions (scabs) on Sheep skin

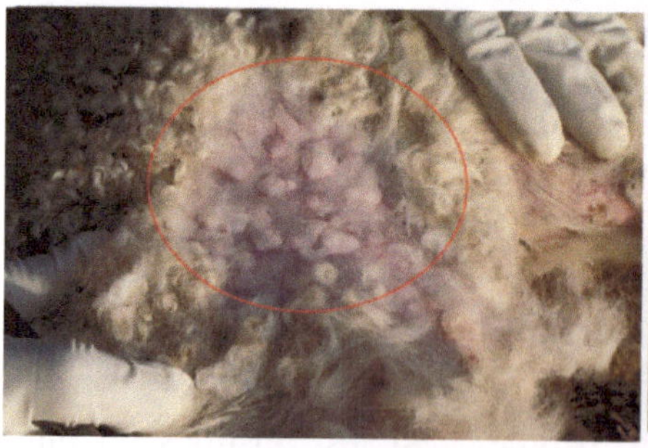

Presence of pock lesions (papules) on sheep skin

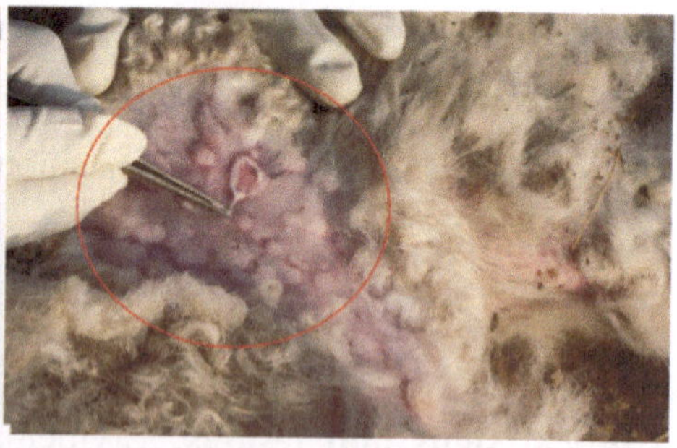

Presence of pock lesions (vesicles) on sheep skin

8. Goat Pox (Capripox virus)

Clinical signs and lesions: Less severe than sheep pox, skin lesions are smaller.

Collection of material: Scabs in ice and in 10% formol saline and serum samples

9. Fowl Pox (Avipox virus)

Clinical signs and lesions: Pock lesions in the form of small nodules on comb, wattles, and on face, cheese like material on mucosa of tongue, palate and laryngeal orifice, on removal leave the ulceration, coniunctivitis, cheesy material in eyelids.

Collection of material: Nodules and serum samples

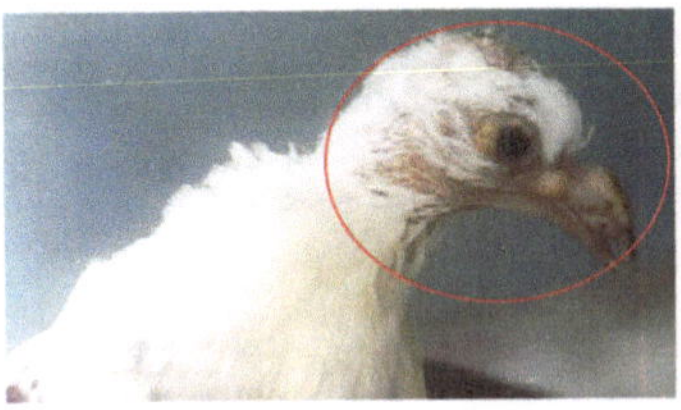

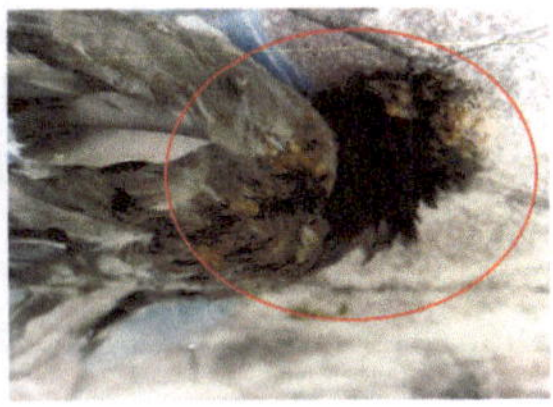

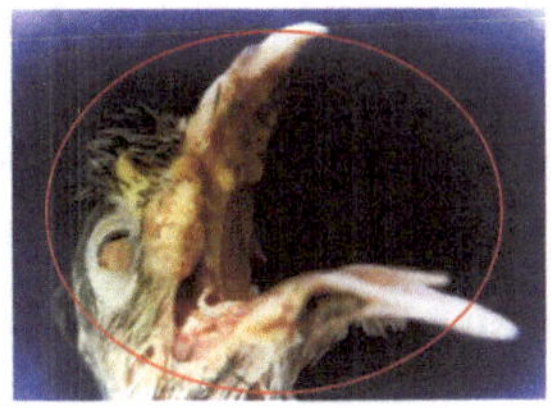

10. Lumpy skin disease (Capripox virus)

Clinical signs and lesions: Cutaneous eruptions as round, firm nodules on oral, nasal and genital mucosa, enlargement of superficial lymphnode.

Collection of material: Cutaneous lesions and serum samples

11. Contagious bovine ecthyma/ or (Parapox virus)

Clinical signs and lesions: Papular, vesicular and pustular lesions on lips, oral mucosa, udder, feet; necrosis and sloughing of affected area.

Collection of material: Skin lesion and serum samples

12. Bovine papular stomatitis (Parapox virus)

Clinical signs and lesions: Erythema, papule on lips, muzzle, nostrils, tongue, oral mucosa, esophagus, rumen, reticulum and abomasum; hyperplasia.

Collection of material: Skin lessions and serum samples

13. Equine influenza (Orthomyxo virus)

Clinical signs and lesions: Nasal discharge, cough, dyspnea, fever, depression, reluctance to move, non-fetal, mucopurulent exudate in trachea and bronchi.

Collection of material: Serum sample and nasal discharge.

14. Swine influenza (Orthomyxo virus)

Clinical signs and lesions: Fever, rhinitis, cough, dyspnoea, mucopurulent exudate in trachea, bronchi, plugging in bronchioles, consolidation of lungs, ***fibrinous pleuritis***.

Collection of material: Nasal discharge and serum samples

15. Parainfluenza-3 infection (Paramyxo virus)

Clinical signs and lesions: Pneumonia, upper respiratory tract infection.

Collection of material: Nasal discharge, lung's tissue, serum

16. Bovine malignant catarrh (Herpes virus)

Clinical signs and lesions: Mucopurulent inflammation of eyes, nostrils, erosions on oral mucosa and large intestine leading to ***zebra strippings***; enlargement of lymph nodes; emaciation, corneal opacity, obstruction of nasal passage by mucopurulent exudate, diarrhoea.

Collection of material: Nasal discharge, serum and tissue

17. Equine viral pneumonitis (equine viral abortions) (Herpes virus)

Clinical signs and lesions: Abortions in mare during 8-11th month gestation, death of fetus, rapid recovery, in young horses 1-4 years of age-fever, congestion of nasal and conjunctival mucosa, dry cough, pneumonia. In fetus-grey, subcapsular 2-5 mm dia, necrotic foci in liver.

Collection of material: Serum and tissues

18. Infectious canine hepatitis (Adeno virus)

Clinical signs and lesions: Clonic spasms of neck and extremities, paralysis of hindquarters, anaemic mucous membranes, petechiae on mucous membranes, cloudiness of cornea of one eye, albuminurea, neutropenia, lymphopenia followed by lymphocytosis, enlarged liver.

Collection of material: Blood and serum ; several pieces of liver, gall bladder and kidney in 10% formol saline and over ice

19. Feline Panleukemia/ feline distemper (Parvo virus)

Clinical signs and lesions: Diphasic fever, ***panleukopenia***, enteritis, dehydration, emaciation mucopurulent exudate in nasal and lacrimal mucosa, hemorrhage at the ileum; mesenteric lymph nodes edematous; bone marrow of longbones becomes greasy, yellowish, white.

Collection of material: Blood and lymphnode, tissue samples

20. Canine parvoviral infection (Parvo virus)

Clinical signs and lesions: Vomiting, diarrhoea, dehydration, fever, leukopenia, necrotizing enteritis myocarditis in pups.

Collection of material: Blood, serum and tissue samples

21. Bluetongue (Orbi virus)

Clinical signs and lesions: High fever, reddening of oral, nasal mucosa, edematous swelling on lips, tongue, ears, face and intermandibullar space, edema and ***cyanosis of tongue***, petechiae on oral and nasal mucosa, lesions on skin of hoof leading to ***pododermatitis***, hemorrhage in tongue.

Collection of material: Blood serum and tissue samples

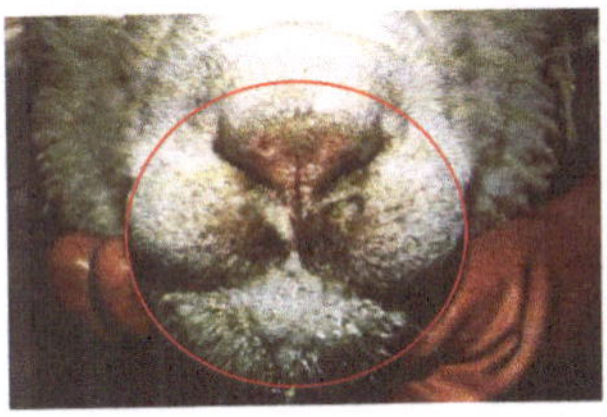
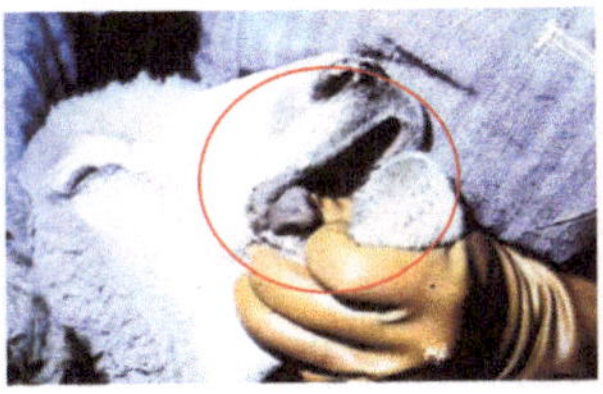
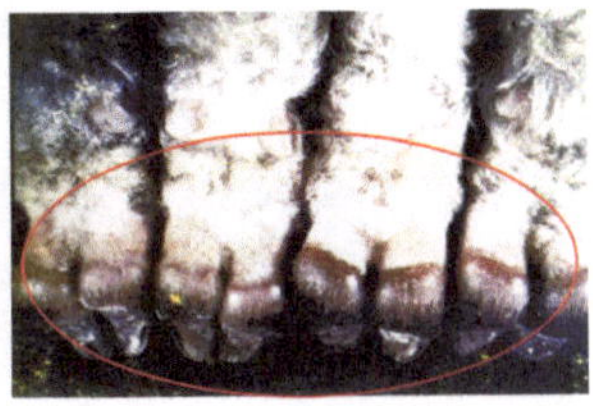

22. African horse sickness (Orbi virus)

Clinical signs and lesions: Fever, pulmonary edema, edema of head and neck, lips, eyelids, cheek, tongue and bulging of supraorbital fossa, petechiae on ventral tongue, paralysis of espohagus, hydrothorax edema, hydropericardiun, petechiae on endocardium, foci and myocardial necrosis.

Collection of material: Serum and tissue samples

23. Neonatal calf diarrhoea (Rotavirus)

Clinical signs and lesions: Yellowish watery diarrhoea, weakness, dehydration, congestion of intestines, enlargement of mesenteric lymph nodes.

Collection of material: Faecal sample, intestinal and other tissues in 10% formol saline and serum

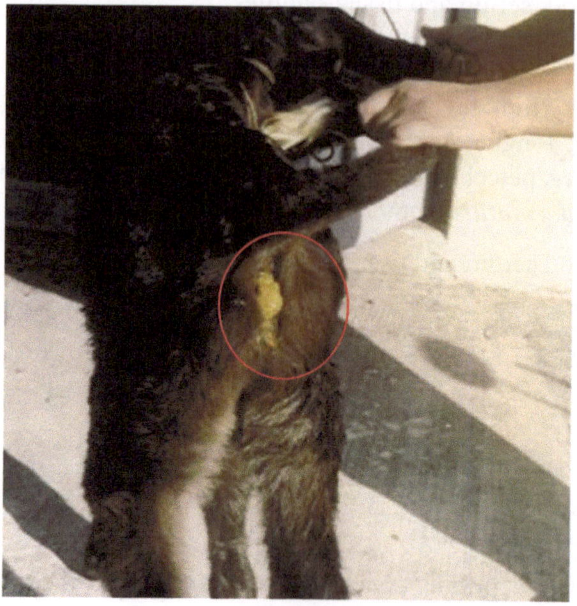

24. Swine fever/ Hog Cholera (Pestivirus)

Clinical signs and lesions: High fever, leukopenia, lethargyness, grinding of teeth, erythema of skin of abdomen herdling, ***glueing of eyes***, petechiae on kidneys, infarcts in spleen, hemorrhage in lymph nodes, ***button ulcers*** in colon.

Collection of material: Serum under refrigeration, spleen, liver, kidney in 50% glycerine/ ice, tissues from intestine, mesenteric lymph node and half of the brain stem in 10% formol saline.

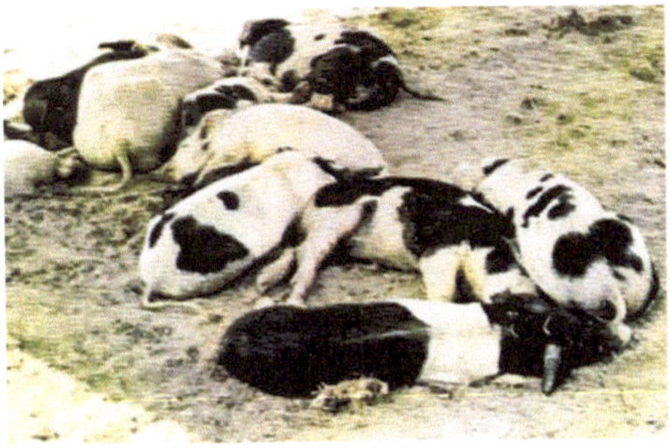

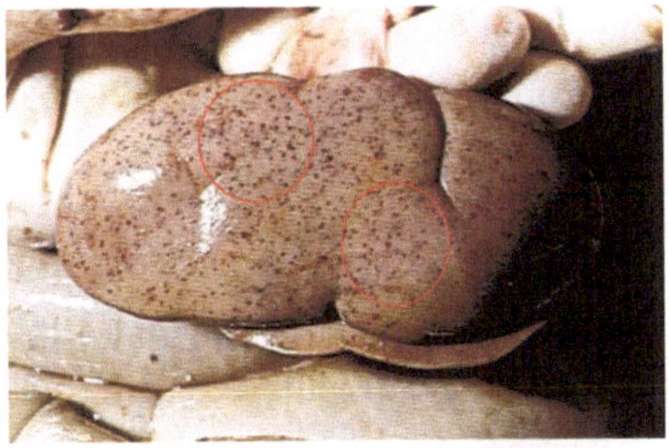

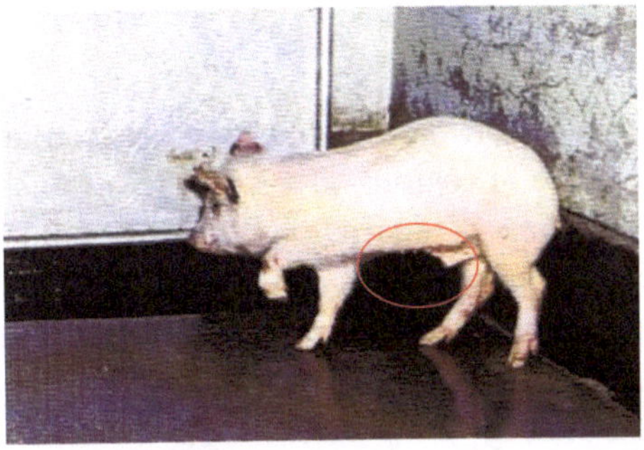

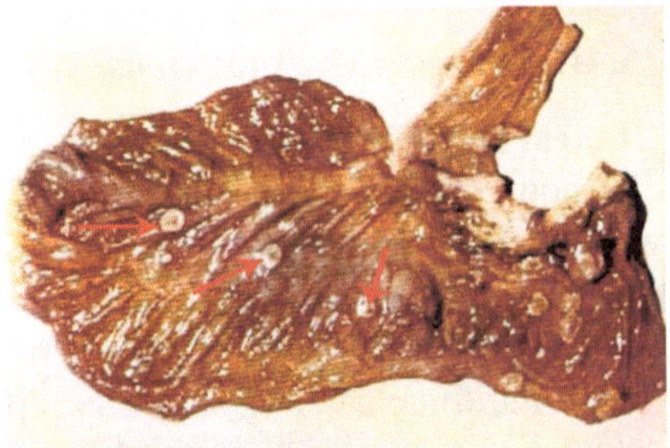

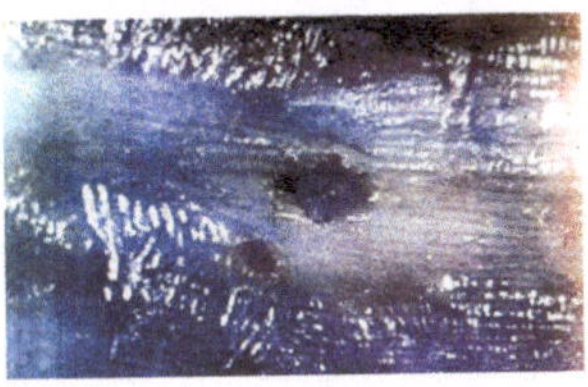

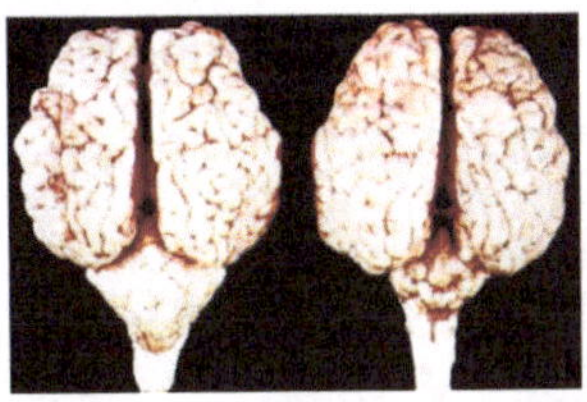

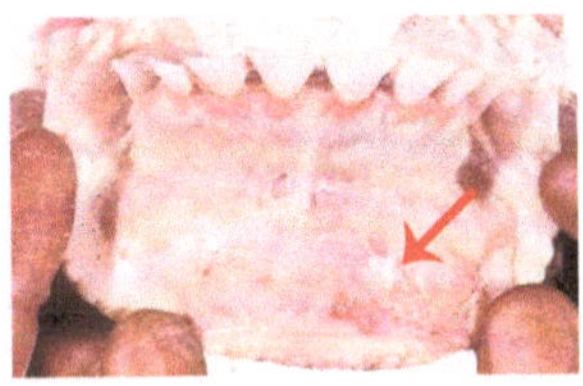

25. Bovine viral diarrhoea Mucosal disease (pesti virus)

Clinical signs and lesions: High fever, diarrhoea, leukopenia, ulcers in mouth, nose, muzzle, small and large intestine leading to ***zebra strippings*** congestion of nasal and oral mucosa, conjunctiva; abortions, still birth. In fetus, ulcers in oral cavity, esophagus, abomasum, congenital cerebral hypoplasia, cataract, retinal atrophy.

Collection of material: Blood, serum intestinal contents and tissue samples.

26. Equine viral arteritis (Arteri virus)

Clinical signs and lesions: Edematous swelling of legs, congestion on conjunctiva, palpebral edema, congestion of nasal mucosa, pharynx, and larynx, hydrothorax, enlargement of mediastinal lymph nodes, petichiae on endocardium and epicardium; Accumulation of fluid in peritoneal cavity, petechiae at ileo-cecal junction, sub mucosal edema in intestines, ***abortions, placentitis***.

Collection of material: Serum and tissue for samples

27. Canine distemper (Morbilli virus)

Clinical signs and lesions: Diphasic fever, coryza, purulent conjunctivitis, bronchitis, bronchopneumonia, vesiculopustular lesions on abdomen, diarrhoea, dehydration, emaciation, blindness, hyperkeratosis of the digital pads, eosinophilic ***intracytoplasmic and intranuclear inclusion bodies*** in nasal mucosa, gastrointestinal tract, in circulating neutrophils and lymphocytes

Collection of material: Skin lesion nasal swab, serum and tissue samples

28. Rinderpest (Morbilli virus)

Clinical signs and lesions: Fever, nasal and lacrimal discharges, leukopenia, diarrhoea, dysentry, erosions in oral mucosa. Erosions are shallow, greyish white with red and raw appearing floor, present on inside the lips, gums, cheeks ventral to the tongue, necrosis of lymphocytes in lymph nodes, spleen, Peyer patches of the intestines. ***Intracytoplasmic and intranuclear inclusions*** in the multinucleated giant cells, epithelial cells of the necrosed erosions, hemorrhagic streaks in large intestine simulating "***Zerba markings***"

Collection of material: Erosive mouth lesion in ice, serum and tissue samples.

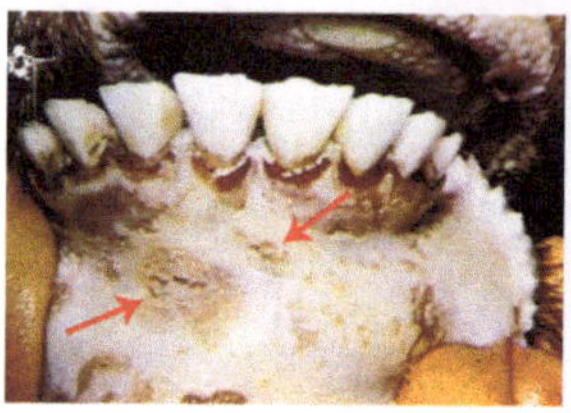

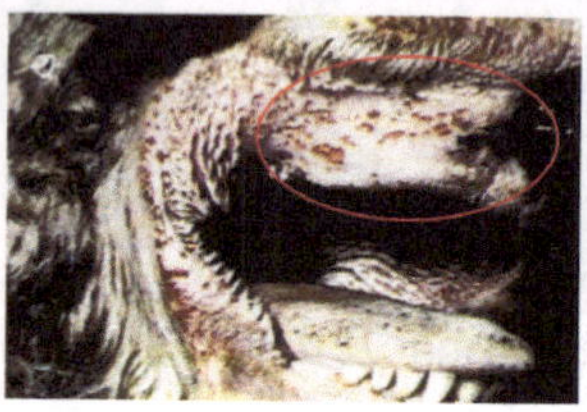

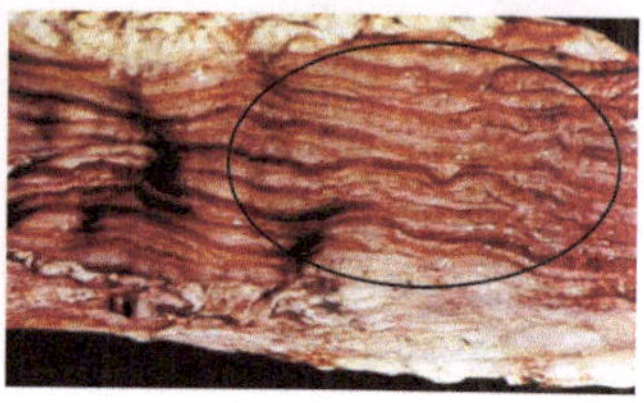

29. Bovine ephemeral fever (Rhabdovirus)

Clinical signs and lesions: Fever, mucopurulent nasal discharge, shivering, ***shifting lameness***, vascular engorgement, edema of lymph nodes, hydropericardium, hydrothorax, rhinitis, tracheitis, pulmonary emphysema, tendovaginitis, focal necrosis of muscles, cellulitis, hemosiderosis of spleen and lymph nodes.

Collection of material: Serum and tissues samples

30. Rabies (Lyssa virus)

Clinical signs and lesions: Biting of inanimate objects, furious champing of jaws, hypersalivation, paralysis, perivascular cuffing, neuronophagia in brain stem and hippocampus, eosinophilic ***intracytoplasmic inclusion bodies*** with clear hallo in the nerve cells, these are called ***"Negri bodies"***. On Seller's stain bright red or magenta colour inclusion bodies.

Collection of material: Intact head should be soaked in 1% carbolic acid, fracture the skull with hammer, remove skin and bones, take half brain in 10% formalin and half brain in 50% neutral glycerine.

31. Transmissible gastroenteritis

Clinical signs and lesions: Acute diarrhoea, vomition, dehydration, congestion of stomach and intestinal mucosa, atrophy of villi, mononuclear cell infiltration in lamina propria, hyperplasia of reticuloendothelial cells, depletion of lymphoid cells in spleen and lymph nodes.

Collection of material: Fecal, serum and tissue samples

32. Equine infectious anemia (Lenti virus)

Clinical signs and lesions: High fever, weakness, excessive thirst, edema of lower abdomen, sublingual or nasal hemorrhage, anemia, pallor of mucous membrane, increased erythrocyte sedimentation rate, icterus, hemorrhage, petechiae on pleura peritoneum, enlargement of lymph nodes, heart, spleen kidneys, hyperplasia of bone marrow.

Collection of material: Blood serum and tissue samples

33. Bovine immuno deficiency (Lenti virus)

Clinical signs and lesions: ***Lymphadenopathy***, leukopenia followed by lymphocytosis, progressive weakness, emaciation.

Collection of material: Blood serum and tissue samples

34. New castle disease/ Ranikhet disease (Paramyxo virus)

Clinical signs and lesions: Respiratory distress, greenish diarrhoea, paralysis of wings, legs, torticollis, ***hemorrhage around the orifice of glands in proventriculus***, hemorrhages at cecocolic junction, edema and lymphocytic infiltration in larynx and trachea; catarrhal inflammation of nasal and conjunctival mucosa, interstitial pneumonia, ***in intestines ulcers covered by bran like deposits***, encephalitis, ***pneumo-encephalitis***.

Collection of material: Liver, spleen in 50% neutral glycerine, proventriculus in 10% formalin, brain in ice, and serum

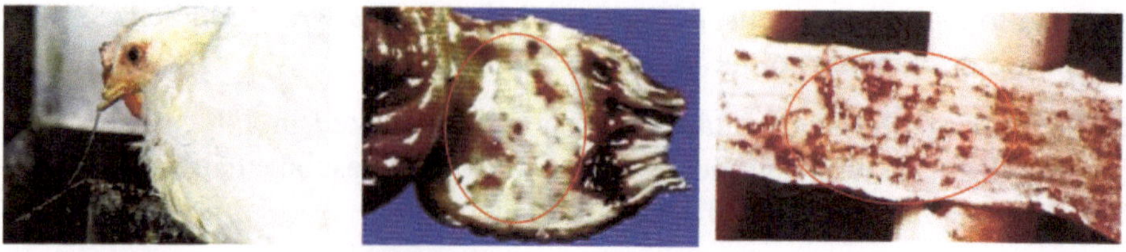

35. Infectious laryngotracheitis (Herpes virus)

Clinical signs and lesions: Respiratory distress, gasping, rales, coughing, bloody mucous from trachea, lacrimation, drop in egg production, beak soiled, tracheal and laryngeal mucosa covered with bloody tenacious exudate, hemorrhage in trachea, cheesy exudate in larynx.

Collection of material: Nasal swabs, trachea serum and tissue samples

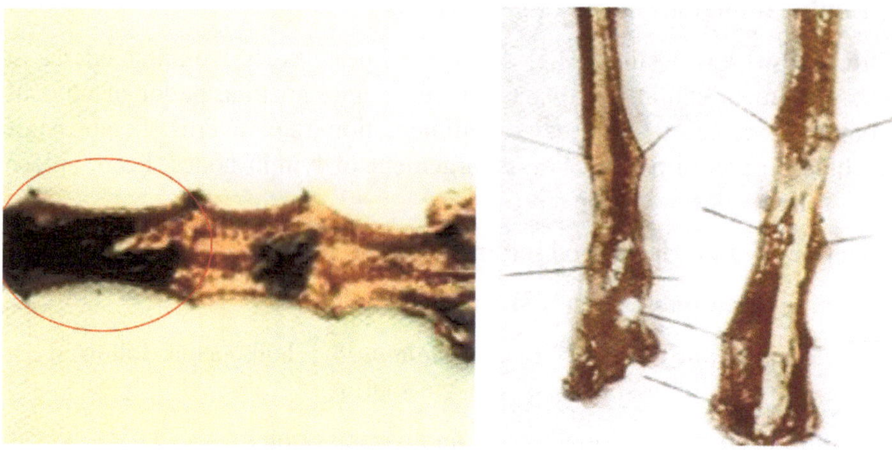

36. Infectious bronchitis (Corona virus)

Clinical signs and lesions: Nasal discharge, gasping, rales, coughing lacrimation, swelling of sinus, reduced egg production, ***mis-shapen eggs***, thin shelled eggs, watery yolk, catarrhal tracheitis, air sacs contain fibrinous exudate, yellow ***caseous material in bronchi specially at the point when enters in lungs***, catarrh of nasal passage, kidneys become pale and swollen deposition of ***urates on kidneys***.

Collection of material: Serum and bronchial tissue samples

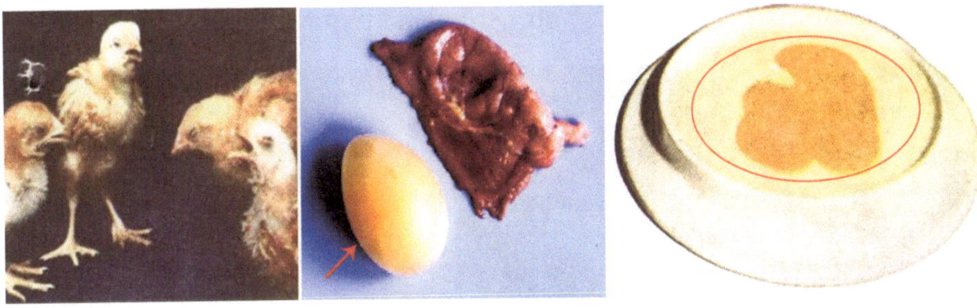

37. Avian encephalomyelitis/ epidemic tremor (Picorna virus)

Clinical signs and lesions: Dullness, disinclination to move, ataxia, ***tremors of head and neck***, bluish colouration of eyes, blindness.

Collection of material: Serum, brain and other tissues samples

38. Infectious bursal disease/ gumboro disease (Birna virus)

Clinical signs and lesions: Ruffled feathers, tremors of head and neck, discharge from eyes, diarrhoea, soild vent, ***enlarged bursa***, hemorrhage and contains gelatinous material, yellow caseous material in ***atrophied bursa***, nephrosis, mottling of kidneys due to urates deposition, ***intramuscular hemorrhages***, congestion and edema of bursa, depletion of lymphoid cells, cellular debris in tubes of kidneys, necrosis of cecal tonsils and thymus.

Collection of material: Bursa of Fabricious, kidney, muscles in 10% formol saline and in 50% buffered glycerine, serum

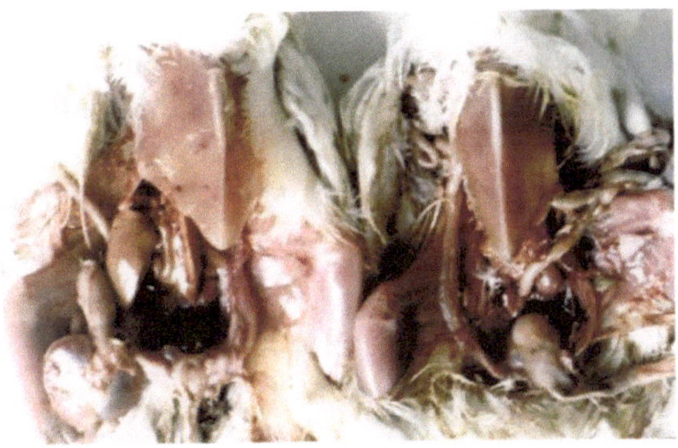

39. Avian influenza (Orthomyxo virus)

Clinical signs and lesions: ***Cyanosis of comb and wattles, edema of face,*** respiratory distress, reduced egg production, hemorrhage on epicardium, proventriculus, gizzard, necrotic foci on spleen, liver, lungs, kidneys, intestines and pancreas.

Collection of material: Nasal swab, serum and tissue samples

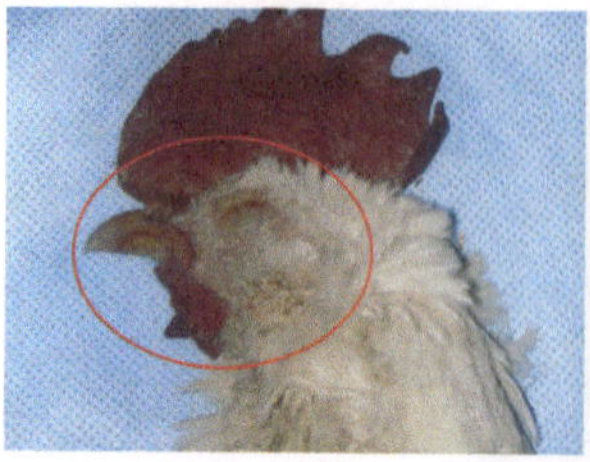

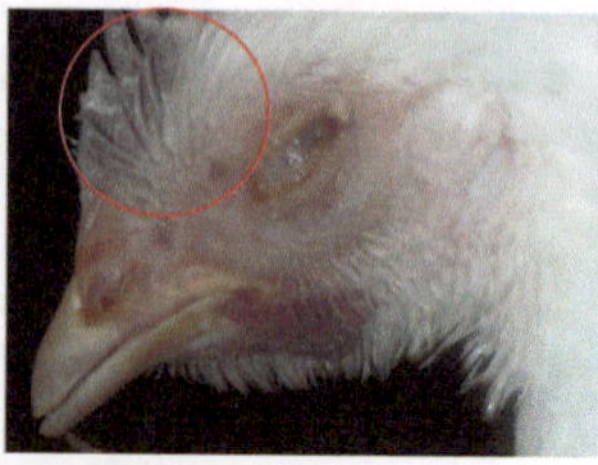

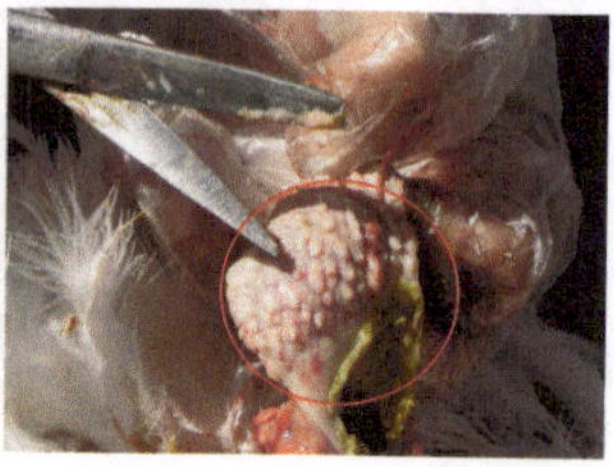

40. Avian leukosis complex (Retro virus)

Clinical signs and lesions: ***White tumours in liver***, spleen, lung, ovary and on other serosal surface; in ***osteopetrosis*** form long bones become thickened.

Collection of material: Tissue samples

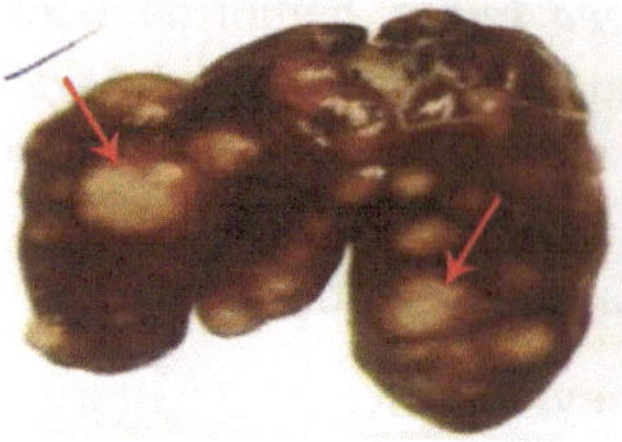

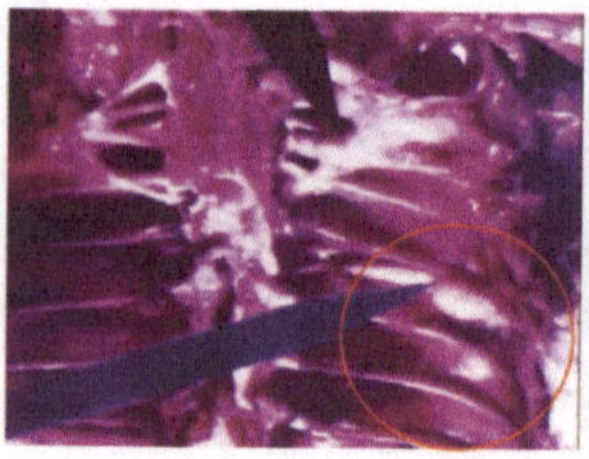

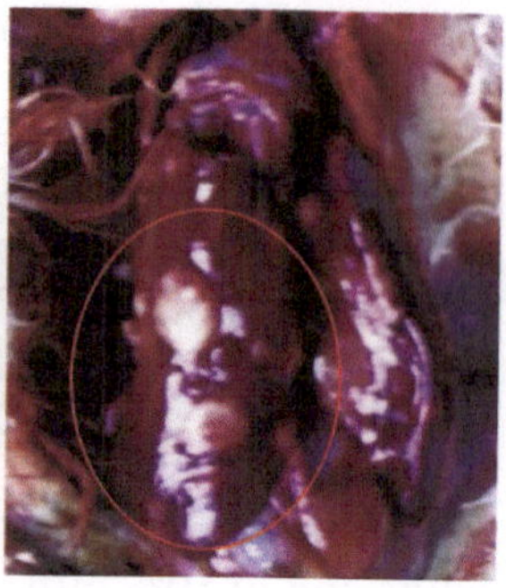

41. Marek's disease (Herpes virus)

Clinical signs and lesions: Sudden mortality, incoordination of legs, lameness, paralysis of wings, hanging of wings, torticollis, thickening of nerves, rounding, ***loss of striations in sciatic nerve***, brachial nerve, vagus nerve and mesenteric nerve. ***Tumours in gonads***, liver, spleen, lung, muscle, heart, kidneys proventriculus, intestines.

Collection of material: Feather follicles, serum and tissue samples

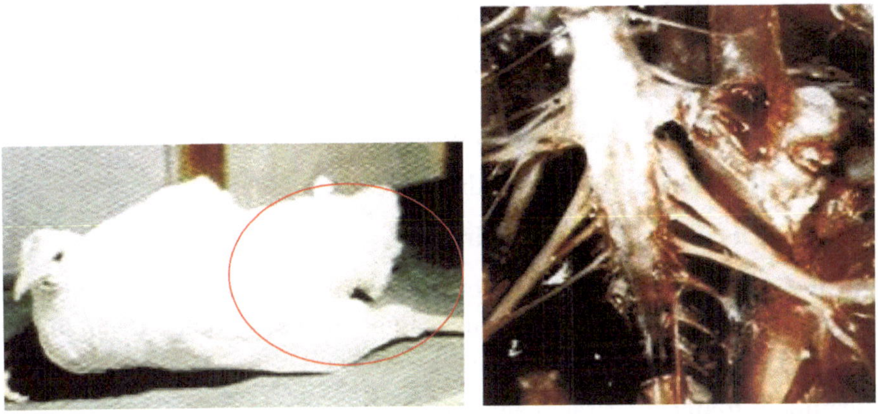

42. Avian reovirus infection (Reovirus)

Clinical signs and lesions: *Tenosynovitis:* ***Lameness***, swelling and congestion of synovial sheath of the tendon of hock joints and foot pads, Articular surface of tibia and metatarsal show erosions. *Stunting syndrome:* Poor feathering, poor shank pigmentation, undigested food material in intestines, distention of gall bladder, atrophy of bursa, ***atrophy*** of ***pancreas*** and fibrosis, catarrhal enteritis, ***pasty vent***.

Collection of material: Synovial fluid; Pancreas, intestine and tissue samples

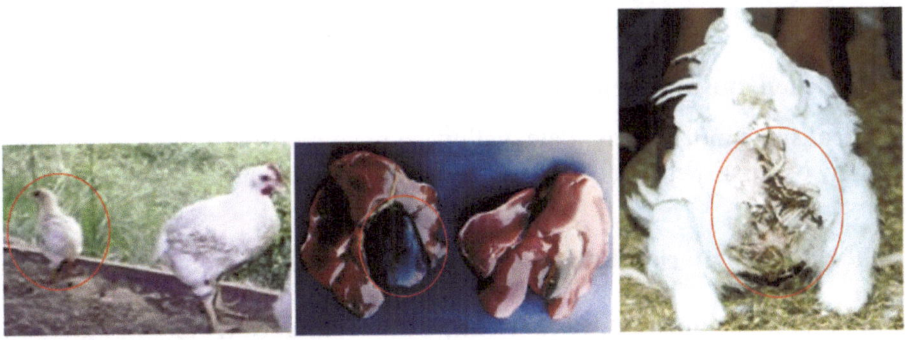

43. Avian rotavirus infection (Rota virus)

Clinical signs and lesions: Diarrhoea, mortality, dehydration, ***maldigestion***, ***malabsorption***, intestine and ceaca are filled with gases, congestion of intestines, ***cracking of feet*** and digits with dried fecal crusts.

Collection of material: Intestinal contents and tissue samples

44. Inclusion body hepatitis (Adenovirus)

Clinical signs and lesions: ***Pale muscles***, and bone marrow, swelling of liver with mottling, hemorrhage atrophy of bursa, petechiae on muscles, paleness and hemorrhage in kidneys, urates in ureters, icterus, ***hydropericardium***.

Collection of material: Liver and other tissue samples

45. Adenovirus infection (Adeno virus)

Clinical signs and lesions: Respiratory form: Ruffled feathers, tracheal rales, congestion and consolidation of lungs, Egg drop syndrome: ***Drop in egg production*** (30-40%), depigmented, craked or shell less eggs, diarrhoea.

Collection of material: Tissues and samples

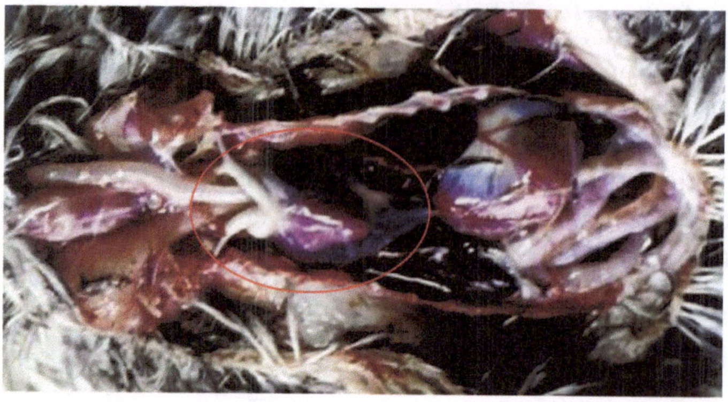

46. Chicken anemia agent infection (CAV)

Clinical signs and lesions: Pale, yellowish bone marrow, atrophy of thymus, atrophy of bursa, petechiae on breast muscles and proventriculus, enlargement of liver.

Collection of material: Bone marrow, serum and tissues sample

C. Prion, Mycoplasmal, Rickettsial, Chlamydial, Spirochetal and Bacterial Diseases

1. Scrapie (Prion proteins)

Clinical signs and lesions: Intense pruritus, scraping of skin against hard objects, incubation period long 1-5 years, stiffness of forelegs, grinding of teeth, epilepti form seizures.

Collection of material: Tissue samples

2. Bovine spongiform encephalopathy or mad cow disease (Prion proteins)

Clinical signs and lesions: Weight loss, hyperthesia, apprehensive behaviour, unmanagable behaviour of animal.

Collection of material: Tissue samples

3. Contagious bovine pleuropneumonia (CBPP) (*Mycopla mycoides*)

Clinical signs and lesions: Dyspnoea, mucopurulent nasal disccharge, edema of lower thorax, ***polyarthritis, abortions***, unilateral lesions, cut surface of lungs have ***marbled appearance***.

Collection of material: Nasal swabs, serum and tissue samples

4. Contagious caprine pleuropneumonia (CCPP) (*Mycoplasma mycoides* var. capri)

Clinical signs and lesions: Fever, nasal discharge, congestion and consolidation of lungs, ***fibrinopurulent exudate in lungs, pleura***.

Collection of material: Nasal swabs, serum and tissue samples

5. Q-fever (*Coxiella burnetii*)

Clinical signs and lesions: No characteristic symptom and lesion.

Collection of material: Nasal swabs, serum, blood and tissue samples

6. Chlamydial infection (*Chlamydia psitttaci*)

Clinical signs and lesions: *Encephalitis:* In young calves fever, hypersalivation, nasal discharge, dyspnoea, serofibrinous peritonitis, enlargement of spleen, lobular pneumonia, edema and congestion of brain and spinal cord, ***meningo-encephalitis***. *Polyarthritis:* Swollen joints, edema of synovial tissues, fibrin flakes in synovial fluid, cellular contents of synovial fluid increases. *Abortions:* No clinical illness in cows, abortion in 7-9th month of gestation, subcutaneous edema, enlargement of lymph nodes, spleenomegaly, petechiae on oral mucous membrane, larynx, trachea, and conjunctiva. Small grey foci on myocardium, granulomatous inflammation in all body organs like liver, meninges, brain, kidneys heart and skin, necrosis of cotyledons and presence of fibrinopurulent exudate in placenta. *Pneumonia:* Bronchopneumonia

Collection of material: Nasal discharge, serum and tissue samples Synovial fluid Fetal stomach contents tissues and serum samples Nasal swabs and lung tissue, samples

7. Leptospirosis (*Leptospira* sp)

Clinical signs and lesions: Fever, ***icterus***, vomiting, dysentry, albuminuria, dehydration, debility, petechiae of pleura, peritoneum, nasal and oral mucosa, liver, retention of bile due to ***pluging of bile canaliculi***, enlargement of spleen and lymphnodes, hemorrhage on myocardium, muscles of urinary bladder, gall bladder, lungs, pancreas. *Cattle:* Icterus, edema of liver, petechiae, hemolytic anemia, ***hemoglobinuria***, ***cholangitis***, grayish white focal necrotic lesion of kidneys.

Collection of material: Paired serum, milk/urine in vials (1 drop of formalin in 20 ml), liver, kidney tissue in 10% formalin.

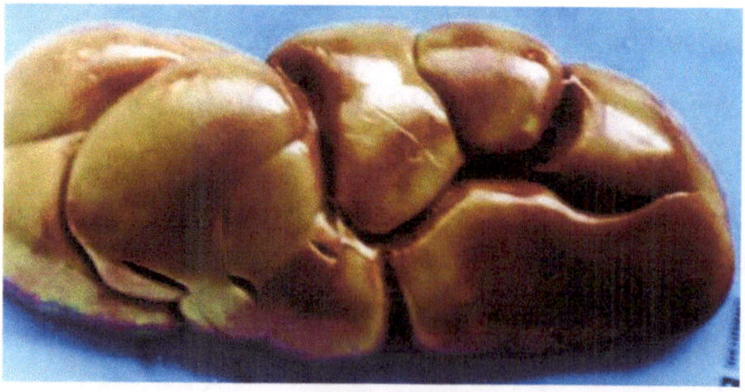

8. Anthrax (*Bacillus anthracis*)

Clinical signs and lesions: Fever, ***bloody discharges from body orifices***, cyanosis, dyspnoea, subcutaneous edema, enlargement of cervical lymph node, ***spleenomegaly***, hemorrhage in intestines, liver, kidneys.

Collection of material: Blood smear from tip of the ear, blood for cultural examination in anticoagulaent, ear tip or Muzzle piece for biological test or Ascoli's test, mark the specimen as "***Anthrax suspect***".

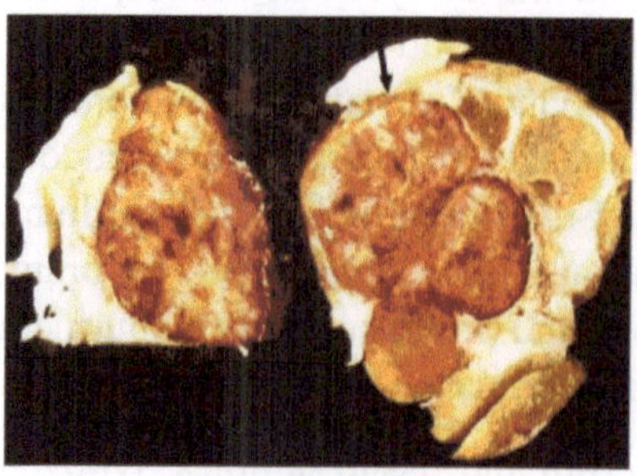

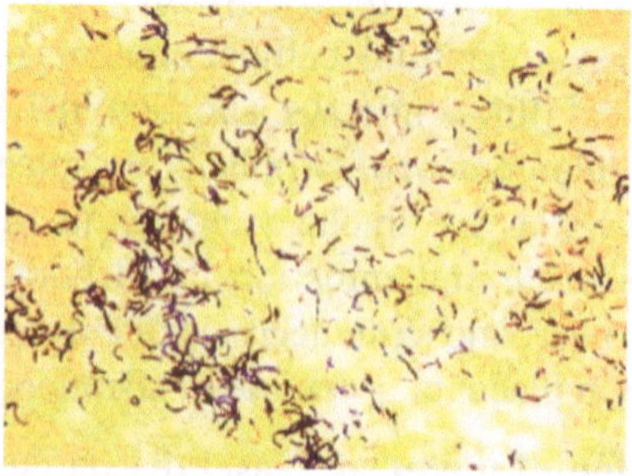

9. Tetanus (*Clostridium tetani*)

Clinical signs and lesions: Prolonged spasmodic contractions of muscles, extension of limbs, ***stiffness***, immobilization of affected parts, lock jaw.

Collection of material: Smear and swabs from lesions.

10. Black leg (*Clostridium chauvoei*)

Clinical signs and lesions: ***Crepitant swelling in muscles*** of affected area particularly at thigh, dark brown or dark red colour of incised muscles, gas mixed exudate, sweatish odour; subcutaneous tissues are gelatinous, blood tinged and yellowish. Empty spaces along the muscle fibers, disease common in growing heifers.

Collection of material: Smear from swelling, affected muscle piece in ice.

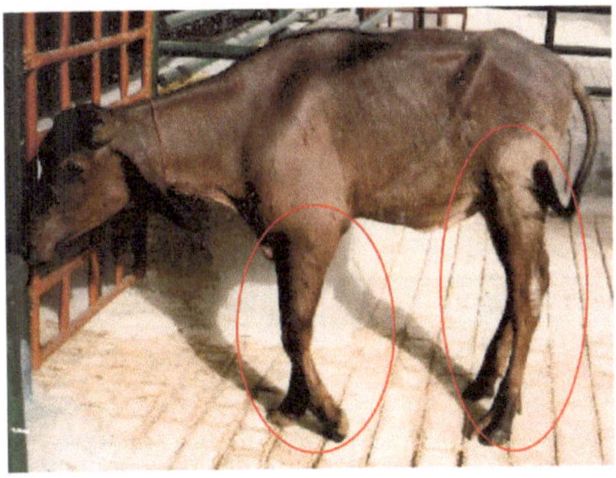

11. Braxy (*Clostridium septicum*)

Clinical signs and lesions: Sudden death, ***edema of abomasal folds***/ wall, hemorrhages in wall of abomasum and small intestines.

Collection of material: Smear from abomasal folds or mucosa; intestinal contents.

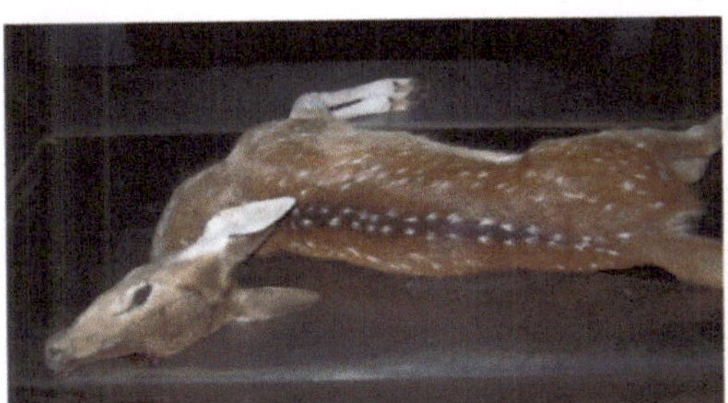

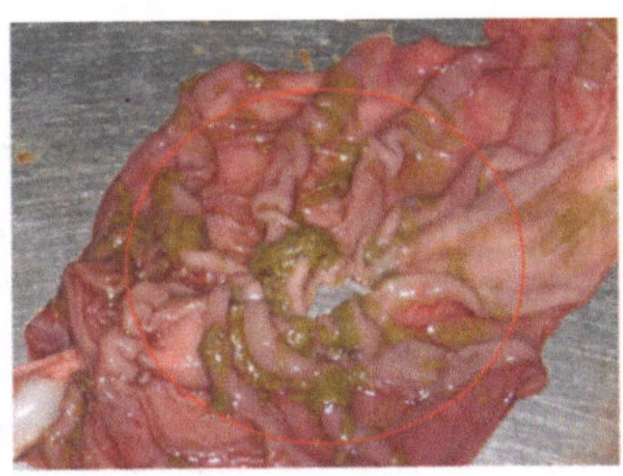

12. Infectious necrotic hepatitis (*Clostridium novyi*)

Clinical signs and lesions: Occurs mainly in sheep, multiple foci of ***necrosis in the liver***, petechiae on epicardium, endocardium, hydropericardium, subcutaneous venous congestion (black disease).

Collection of material: Liver tissue samples

13. Enterotoxemia

	Clinical signs and lesions	**Collection of material**
(*Clostridium* perfringenes type D)	Petechiae and echymotic hemorrhage beneath the epicardial and endocardial surfaces, intestines, abdominal muscles, hydropericardium, mild catarrhal gastroenterities, distention of gall bladder, ***pulpy kidney***.	Intestinal contents
(*Clostridium perfringenes* type A)	Short course, high mortality in lambs, calves, icterus, hemolytic anemia, ***hemoglobinuria***, hydropericardium enlargement of liver, dark and congested kidneys.	Intestinal contents
(*Clostridium perfringenes* type B)	Prostration, pain, diarrhoea, dysentry, death, hemorrhagic enteritis, ulcers in intestines, petechiae on epicardium, endocardium, hydropericardium.	Intestinal contents
(*Clostridium perfringenes* type C)	Hemorrhagic enteritis, ulceration in intestines, peritonitis, hydroperitoneum.	Intestinal contents

14. Strangles (*Streptococcus equi*)

Clinical signs and lesions: Fever, edematous swelling of pharyngeal region, dyspnoea, enlargement of submaxillary lymph nodes, abscess in lymph nodes, catarrhal/ purulent rhinitis, lymphadenitis, ***micro abscess in lungs, liver***, kidneys, spleen, brain, empyema in guttural pouch.

Collection of material: Nasal swab, Serum and tissue samples

15. Campylobacteteriosis (*Campylobacter fetus*)

Clinical signs and lesions: *Cattle:* Mucopurulent endometritis, infertility, prolonged estrus cycle. *Sheep:* ***Abortions***, edema of placenta, death of fetus, vulvitis, vaginitis.

Collection of material: Fetal stomach contents, vaginal mucosa in ice, in pig intestine and liver in 10% formalin, serum, preputial washings from bulls

16. Swine erysipelas (*Erysiplelothrix rhusiopathiae*)

Clinical signs and lesions: Fever, erythema of skin giving it a ***"diamond sking appearance"*** hemorrhage on serous membranes, cutaneous lesions on abdomen in a diamond, rhomboid shape, bright red, purplish or dark bluish in colour, enlargement of joint capsule due to edema, irregular mass of leaves on mitral valve leading to ***vegetative endocarditis***.

Collection of material: Blood smear, swab of pus in ice, skin lesion, kidney, liver and spleen

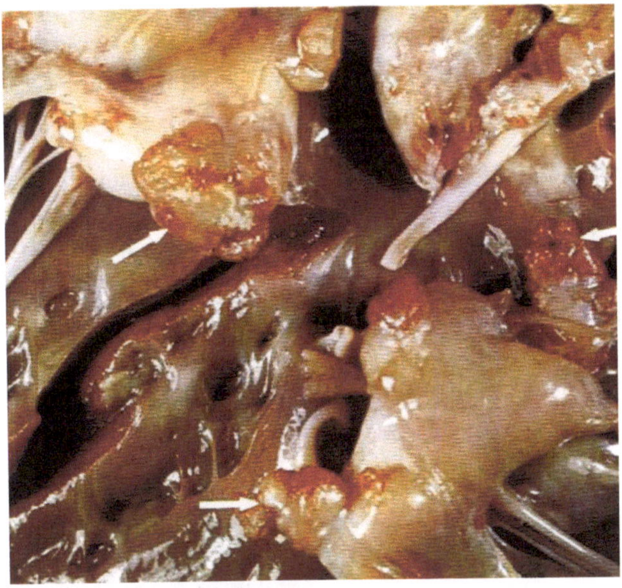

17. Brucellosis (*Brucella sp.*)

Clinical signs and lesions: ***Abortions*** in late gestation, organism localizes in mammary gland/ supra mammary lymph nodes, epididymitis and orchitis in males, sterility in bulls, swelling and induration of scrotum, placenta granular cotyledons, edema of intercotyledonary chorion, yellowish granular necrosis, fetus-edematous, sero-sanguinous fluid in body cavities, bronchopneumonia, granulomatous lesions in mammary gland. In pigs, small nodules in uterus, caseous mass in nodules, the nodule may also occur in spleen, liver kidneys, lymph nodes, epididymis, testicles, seminal vesicles, swelling of joints.

Collection of material: Paired serum one at the time of abortion and 3 weeks thereafter, foetal stomach contents, pieces of lung, spleen, liver, kidney, brain and intestine in separate sterile vials over ice, swabs from uterine discharge and foetal cotyledons, 5 to 10 ml milk in ice.

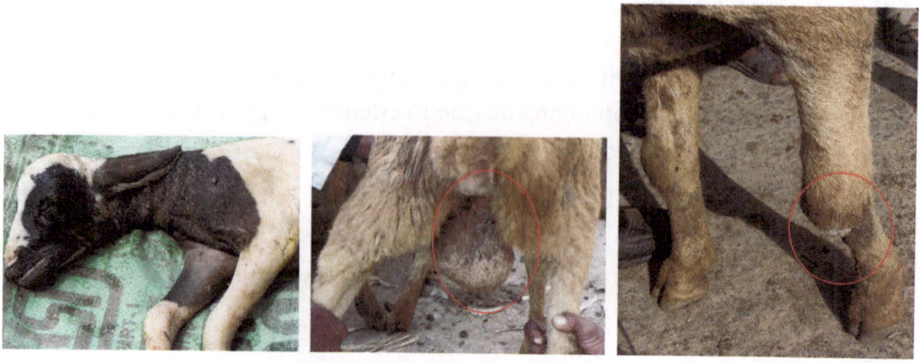

18. Glanders (*Burkholderia mallei*)

Clinical signs and lesions: Copious and persistent catarrhal/ purulent nasal discharge, ***ulcers in nasal mucosa***, chronic cough, ulcers on skin, thickening of superficial lymphatics, abscess in superficial lymph nodes which discharge thick tenacious pus, healed ulcers leaving ***star shaped scars***, granulomatous lesion in lungs, acute purulent bronchopneumonia, granuloma in liver, spleen, Farly.

Collection of material: Smear from discharge, lung, liver and spleen in 10% formalin, paired serum.

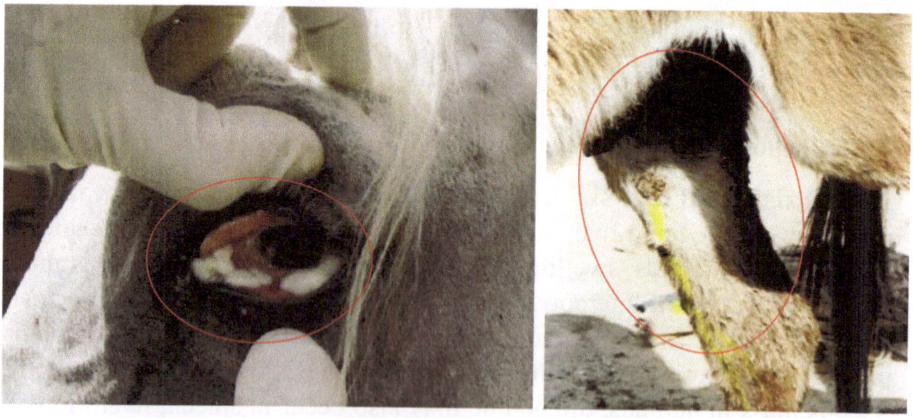

19. Salmonellosis (*Salmonella sp.*)

Clinical signs and lesions: Suppurative polyarthritis in foals, abortions in mare during 6-9th month of gestation, placenta edematous, focal hemorrhage, edema and hemorrhages in fetus, gastroenteritis and septicema in cattle, horse, swine, lesions in ileum and colon, congestion, thickening, red/ yellow/ grey exudate in ulcers, hemorrhage, edema, foci of ***necrosis in liver***, petechiae on pleura, peritoneum endocardium, kidneys, meninges, ulcerative proctitis in pigs.

Collection of material: Liver, spleen, kidney and intestine, faeces, blood, serum, fetal stomach contents and organs pieces over ice and in 10% fromol saline

20. Actinobacillosis (*Actinobacillus lignieresi*)

Clinical signs and lesions: Enlargement of tongue, lymph nodes of head, neck and thorax. Tongue becomes hard due to fibrous tissue proliferation "***wooden tongue***".

Collection of material: Tissues from affected parts in 10% formalin, pus in sterile vial from edge of lesion, slides from pus for sulphur granules.

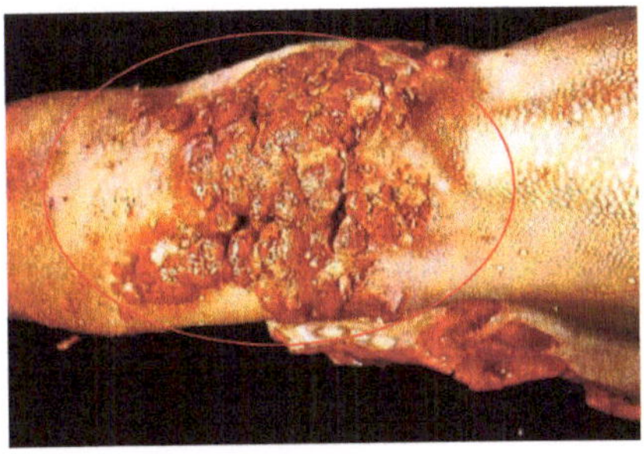

21. Pasteurellosis (*Pasteurella multocida* and *Manhemolytica*)

Clinical signs and lesions: High fever, swelling in neck region extended to the brisket between forelegs, dyspnoea, ***roaring sound***, congestion and consolidation of lungs, abortions in pregnant animals, petechiae on pericardium and other serosal surfaces, congestion of conjunctivae and other mucous membranes, congestion, haemorrhage and oedema in intestines, mesenteric lymphnodes.

Collection of material: Blood smear, nasal swabs and tissue samples

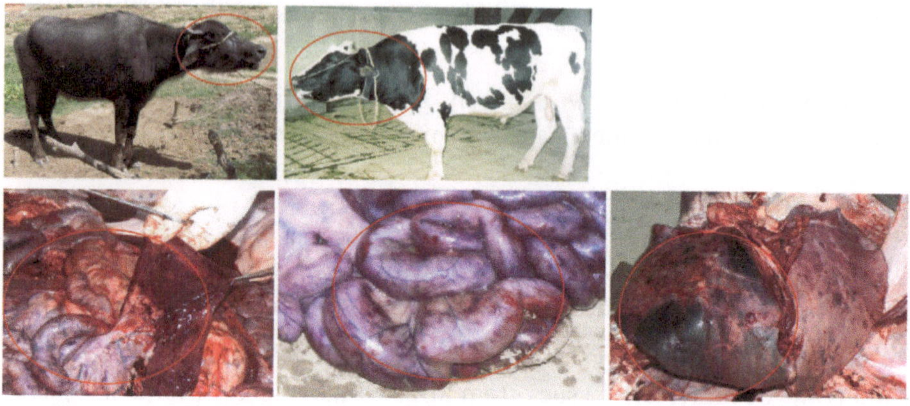

22. Listeriosis (*Listeria monocytogenes*)

Clinical signs and lesions: ***Abortions*** in last quarter of gestation, autolysis of foetus, focal hepatic necrosis, meningitis, encephalitis, abnormal postures, circling movements, presence of ***microabscess in brain***, necrotic foci in liver, spleen, lymph node, myocardium, gastrointestinal tract, and brain.

Collection of material: Half brain in ice, half brain in 10% formalin, fetal stomach contents, blood, CSF and tissue samples

23. Actinomycosis (*Actinomyces bovis*)

Clinical signs and lesions: Large, irregular enlargement of mandible, maxilla "***lumpy jaw***". Cut surface is white, glistening, abscess yellowish pus having sulfur granules.

Collection of material: Tissues from affected parts in 10% formalin, pus in sterile vial from edge of lesion, slides from pus for sulphur granules.

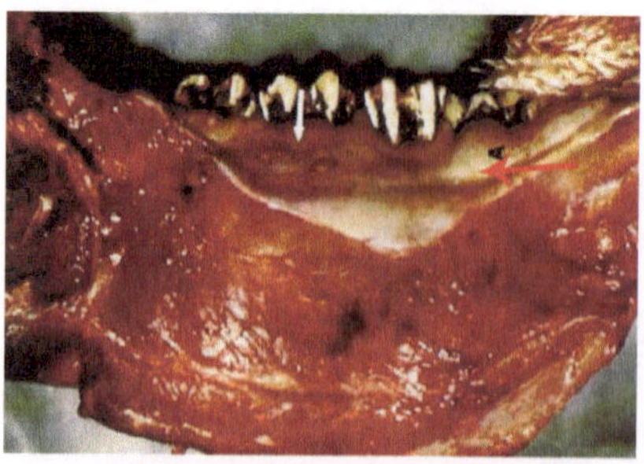

24. Necrobacillosis (*Spherophorus necrophorus*)

Clinical signs and lesions: Necrotic plaques in larynx, pharynx and trachea, "***calf diphtheria***", necrotic foci in spleen, liver, ulceration in rumen, ulcerative necrotizing stomatitis, enteritis in swine, ***foot rot/ pododermatitis*** in cattle, foot rot in sheep, gangrenous dermatitis in foot in horses.

Collection of material: Nasal swabs, swabs from foot lesions and tissue samples

25. Tuberculosis (*Mycobactetrium* sp.)

Clinical signs and lesions: Presence of tubercle in lungs, liver, tubercle looks like necrotic foci bulging from surface, white/ grey/ yellow in colour, oncut-caseous dry and solid, calcification in later stage, size of ***tubercle 1 mm-2 cm***. Chronic wasting disease, emaciation, weakness.

Collection of material: Tuberculin testing; lungs, mediastinal and bronchial lymph nodes in ice and in 10% formalin.

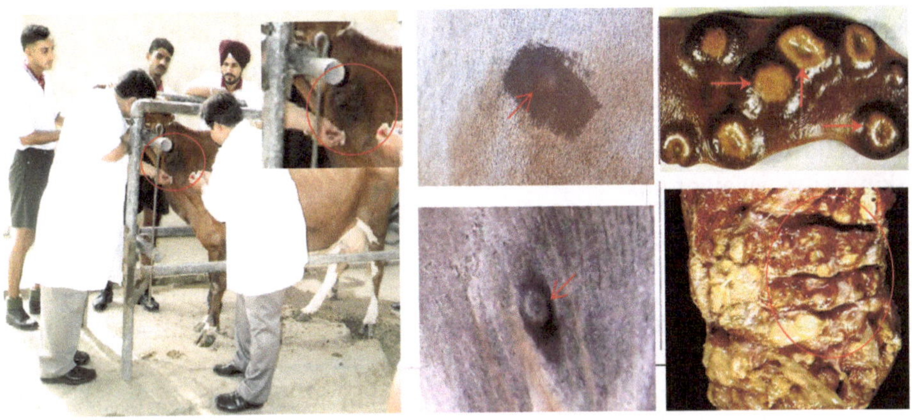

26. Johne's disease (*Mycobacterium paratuberculosis*)

Clinical signs and lesions: ***Chronic diarrhoea***, dehydration, emaciation, hide bound condition, tubercles in mesenteri lymph nodes, small and large intestines and have terminal part of ileum thickened mucosa, transverse ***corrugated folds in mucosa*** of intestines, which remains same on stretching. Granulomatous lesions in liver, spleen, lungs, kidneys, uterus, placenta and lymph nodes.

Collection of material: Smear from rectal mucosa pinch, Johnin testing; Bowel washings in sterile bottle, mesenteric lymph node, part of ileocecal valve and intestine over ice and in 10% formol saline.

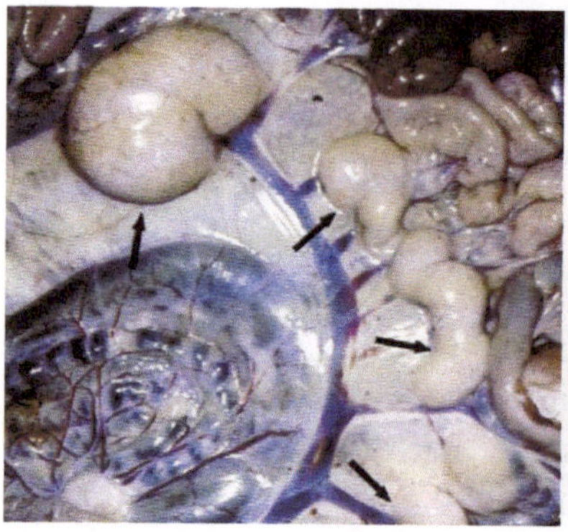

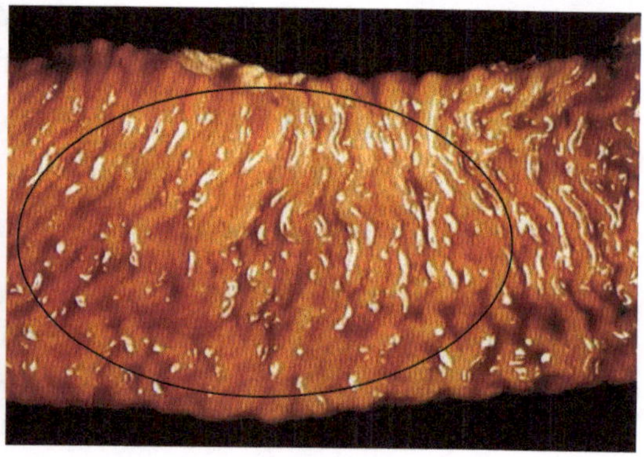

27. Nocardiosis (*Nocardia asteroides* and *Nocardia farcinica*)

Clinical signs and lesions: In dogs, purulent exudate surrounded by granulation tissue in pleura/ peritoneal cavity, brain, visceral organs. In cattle, nocardiosis is known as ***bovine farcy***, chronic suppurative granulomatous lesion on skin, lymphatics and lymph nodes, abortions due to fetal death and placentitis.

Collection of material: Swabs from nasal passage and skin and tissue samples. Skin lesion/ swab of pus.

28. Fowl cholera (*Pasteurella multocida*)

Clinical signs and lesions: *Acute:* Diarrhea, bloody diarrhea, ***cyanotic comb and wattles***, drowsiness, dyspnoea, discharges from beak and nostrils, hemorrhage in intestines, lungs, petechiae on serus membranes, Hemorhage on epicardium, endocardium, and gizzard, enlarged liver. *Chronic:* edema of wattles, rhinitis, sinusitis, swollen joints, torticollis, caseous necrotic foci on lungs, liver, caseous material in peritoneal cavity.

Collection of material: Intestinal contents, nasal swabs and tissue samples

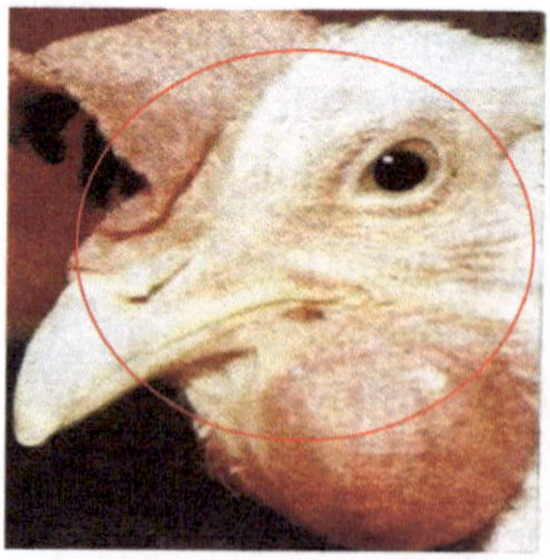

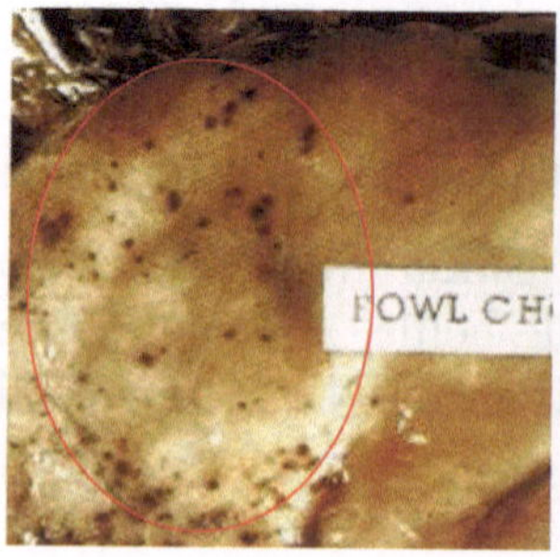

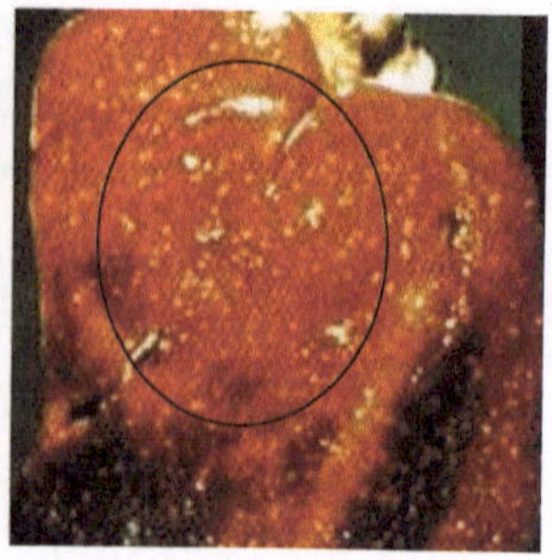

29. Salmonellosis (*Salmonella* Gallinarum)

Clinical signs and lesions: Diarrhoea, solid vent, white/ green colour feces, yellowish necrotic foci on liver, lung, heart; enlargement of liver, catarrhal enteritis,yellowish mass in ceaca, discoloured (ova), ***bronze discoloration of liver, necrotic foci in liver***, enlargement of spleen.

Collection of material: Fecal swabs, heart blood, liver tissue samples

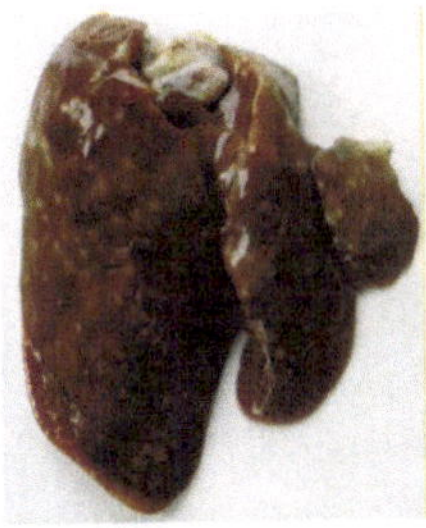
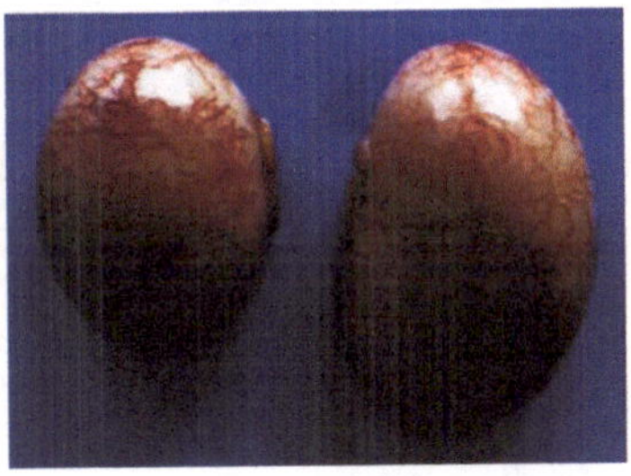
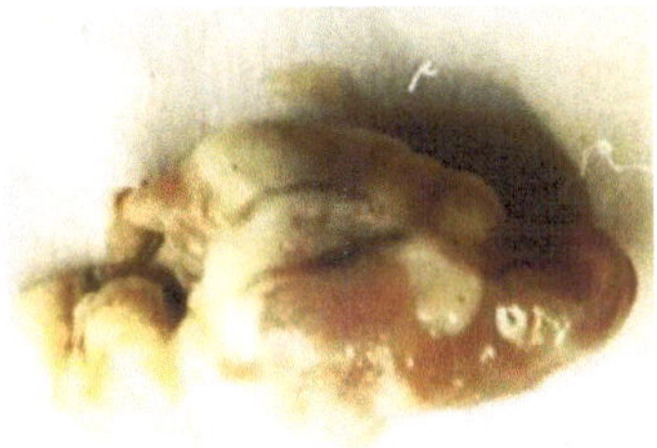

30. Fowl spirochetosis (*Borrelia anserina*)

Clinical signs and lesions: Cynosis of head, ***greenish diarrhoea***, ruffled feathers, organism in blood, one can detect the presence of spirochete in wet smear; anemia, paralysis, ***spleenomegaly***, hemorrhage in spleen, enlarged liver, white necrotic foci on liver, catarrhal enteritis, fibrinous pericarditis.

Collection of material: Blood, serum and tissue samples

31. Chronic respiratory disease (*Mycoplasma gallisepticum* and *E. coli*)

Clinical signs and lesions: Respiratory rales, nasal discharge, cough, decreased egg production, poor weight gain, catarrhal exudate in air sacs, trachea, bronchi, lungs, ***cheesy material in air sacs***, thickened tracheal mucosa, focal pneumonia, fibrinous perihepatitis, pleuritis, edema and petechiae in lungs.

Collection of material: Nasal swabs and tissue samples

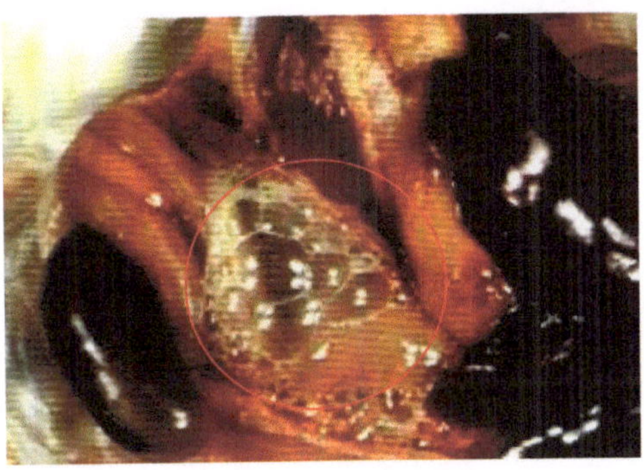

32. Infectious coryza (*Hemophilus gallinarum*)

Clinical signs and lesions: ***Face swollen*** and edematous, foul smelling nasal discharge, lacrimation, sneezing, coughing, dyspnoea, catarrhal rhinitis, sinusitis, air sacculitis, cheesy exudate in sinuses, nasal passage and conjunctival sac.

Collection of material: Nasal swabs and tissue samples

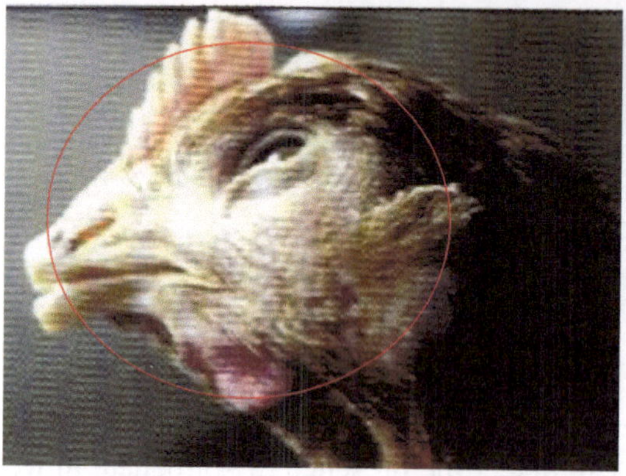

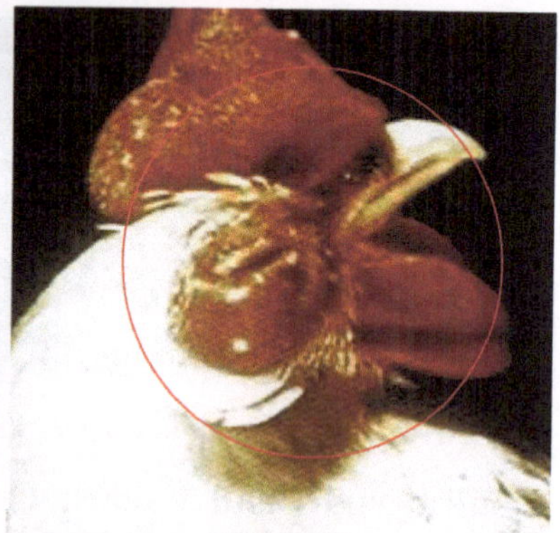

33. Colibacillosis (*E. coli*)

Clinical signs and lesions: *Chicks:* ***Serofibrinous pericarditis***, enlarged liver, bronchopneumonia, tracheitis, distended yolk sac, yolk sac contains foul smelling yellow or curdled/ brown and watery yolk, ***perihepatitis***, adhesions between skin, and abdominal wall/ yolk sac.

Adults: Peritonitis, salpingo-peritonitis, salpingitis, air sacculitis.

Collection of material: Heart blood in sterile vial, tissues from intestine and lymph nodes in 10% formol saline and over ice

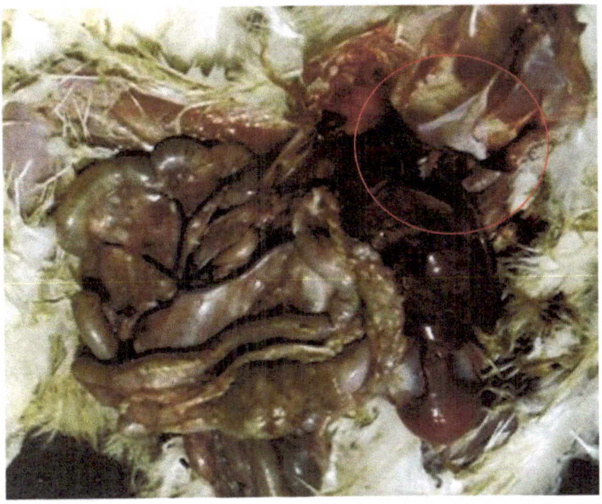 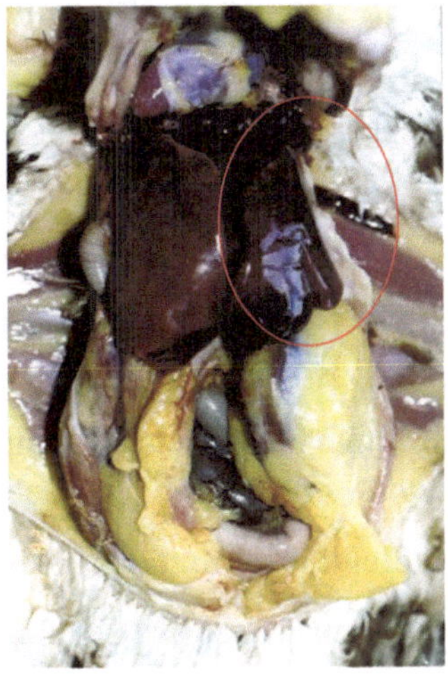

D. Fungul Diseases

1. Aspergillosis (*Aspergillus fumigatus*)

Clinical signs and lesions: *Animals:* Placentitis and abortion in cattle, nodular or diffuse consolidation in lungs, a white mouldy growth. *Poultry*: Dyspnoea, depression, emaciation, accumulation of cheesy material under eyelids, pin head size yellowish nodules in lungs, ***air sacs cloudy*** and thickened with yellowish plaques, necrotic foci in liver, spleen, kidneys, proventriculus. Brooder's pneumonia.

Collection of material: Fetal stomach contents. Air sacs/ lung tissue samples

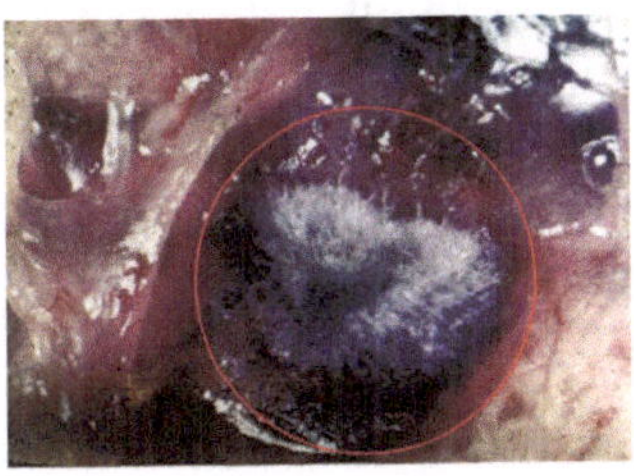 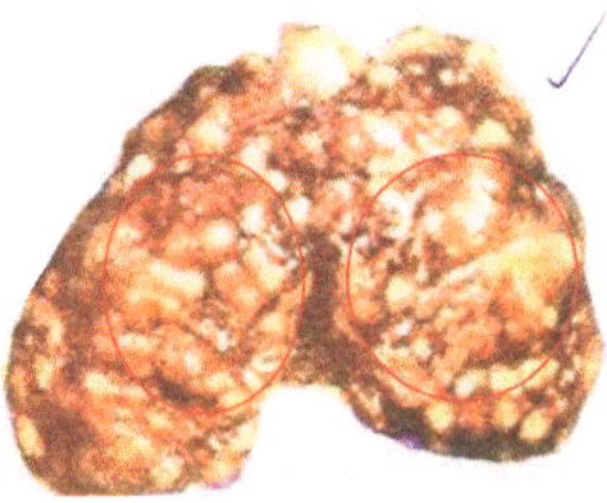 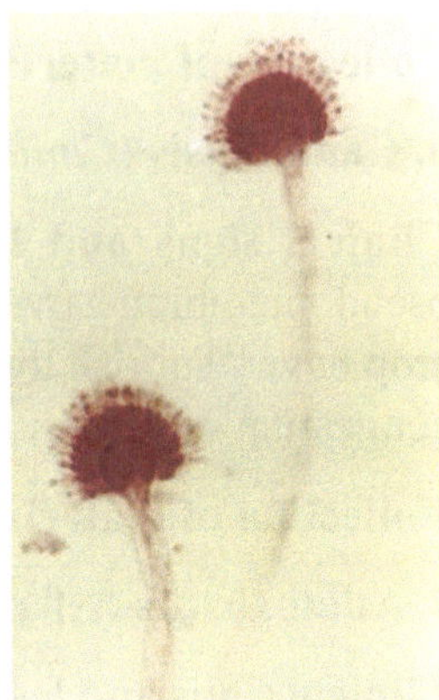

2. Blastomycosis (*Blastomyces dermatidis*)

Clinical signs and lesions: In dogs, grey nodules in lungs, consolidation of lungs, purulent exudate on cut surface. In horse, mammary gland is affected, in cats cutaneous and pulmonary lesions with ***chronic suppurative granulomas***.

Collection of material: Tissue samples

3. Coccidioidomycosis (*Coccidioides immitis*)

Clinical signs and lesions: Low grade fever, cough emaciation, granulomatous lesion in lungs, enlargement of bronchial and mediastinal lymph nodes, ***greyish nodules on lungs***, lymphnodes, liver, spleen meninges, eye and bone marrow.

Collection of material: Tissue samples

4. Cryptococcosis (*Cryptococcus neoformans*)

Clinical signs and lesions: Granulomatous nodules in lungs, peritoneum, nasal mucosa; enlarged lymph nodes, thickened meninges, diffuse and patchy induration of mammary gland.

Collection of material: Tissue samples

5. Histoplasmosis (*Histoplasma capsulatum*)

Clinical signs and lesions: Loss of weight, lymphadenopathy, diarrhoea, weakness, anemia, hepatomegaly, ascites, extensive proliferation of reticuloendothelial cells, lungs-encapsulated nodules of epithelioid cells. Lymphnodes, spleen enlarged due to proliferation of (reticuloendothelial) cells, intestine has nodular mucosal surface.

Collection of material: Tissue samples

6. Candidiasis (*Candida albicans*)

Clinical signs and lesions: Bronchitis, pneumonia, vulvo-vaginitis, white pseudomembrane over skin and mucous membrane. In poultry, mucosa of crop have "Turkish towel appearance", round raised ulcers in crop, esophagus, congestion in proventriculus, abscess formation in proventriculus.

Collection of material: Tissue samples

7. Aflatoxicosis (Aflatoxins; produced by *Aspergillus* sp. *Penicillium* sp.)

Clinical signs and lesions: *Dog:* Anorexia, icterus, prostration, blood in feces, vomition, epistaxis, convulsions, toxic hepatitis, proliferation of small bile duct epithelium, necrosis of hepatic cells, edema of gall bladder. *Poultry:* Hepatitis, hepatomegaly, edema of gall bladder, immunosuppression, diarrhoea, loss of weight, mortality, retarded growth, drop in egg production.

Collection of material: Tissue and feed samples. Poultry feed and tissue samples

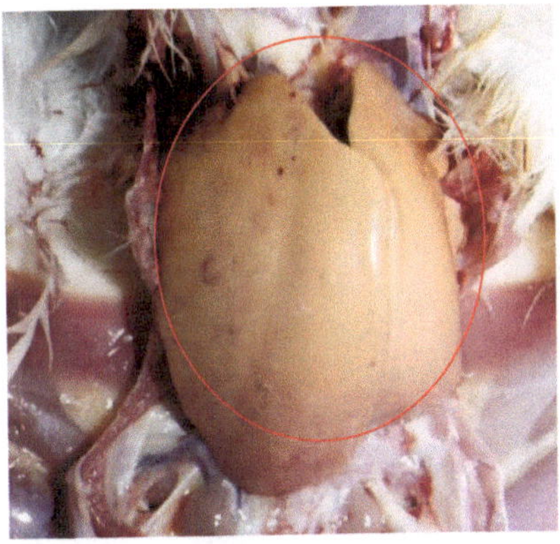
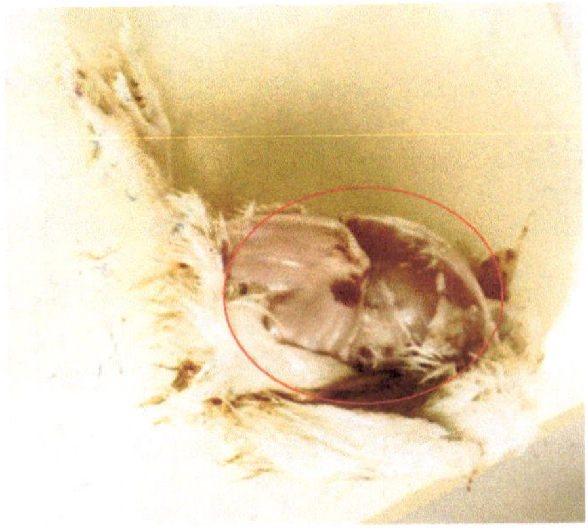

8. Degnala disease (*Fusarium* sp.)

Clinical signs and lesions: Necrosis of tail, ears, extremities, scrotum, gangrene on extremities

Collection of material: Feed (rice straw) samples

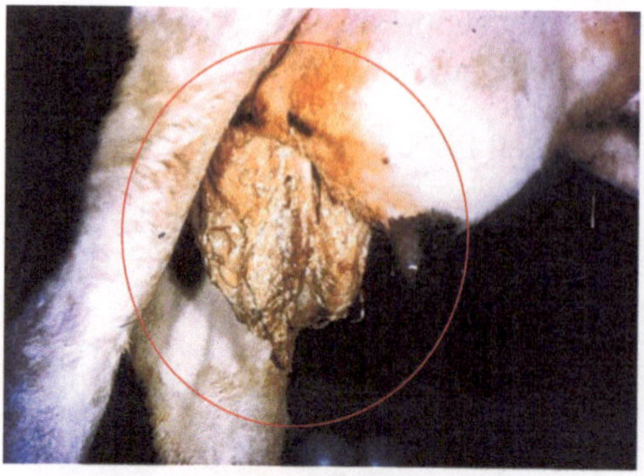

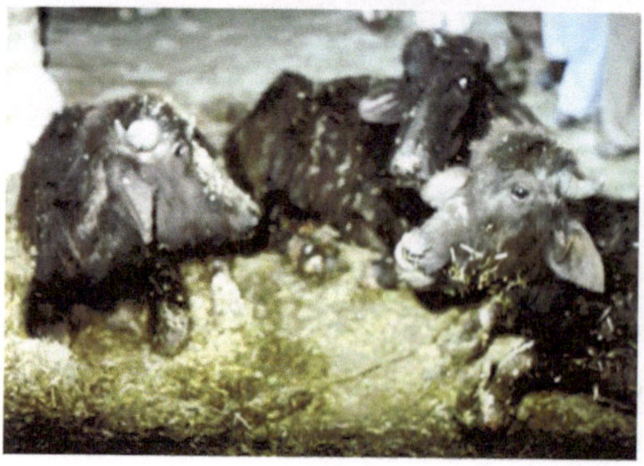

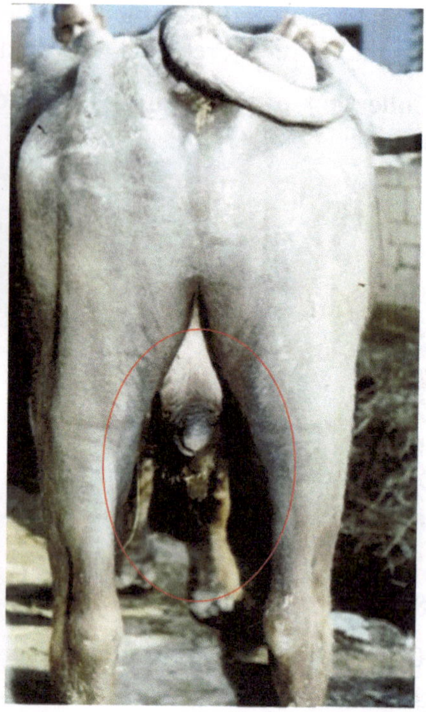

E. Parasitic Diseases

1. Coccidiosis (*Eimeria* sp.)

Clinical signs and lesions: ***Bloody diarrhoea,*** fever, dehydration, emaciation, congestion of intestines, erosions, hemorrhage, ***thickening of the wall of intestines***.

Collection of material: Intestinal contents/ cecal contents

2. Toxoplasmosis (*Toxoplasma gondii*)

Clinical signs and lesions: Lymphadenopathy, myocarditis, pneumonia, ***meningo-encephalitis***, chorioretinitis, lungs resembling pulmonary adenomatosis, enlarged lymphnodes, granulomatous nodules in intestines, focal necrosis in placenta, ***abortion***, granulomatous lesions in fetal brain.

Collection of material: Nasal swabs, cerebrospinal fluid, serum and tissue samples

3. Sarcosporidiosis (*Sarcocystis* sp.)

Clinical signs and lesions: Sarcocysts are found in skeletal muscle or in cardiac muscle, sarcolemma is displaced, no inflammatory reaction, occasionally myositis and muscle necrosis, granulomatous inflammation, in cattle ***eosinophilic myositis***.

Collection of material: Tissue samples

4. Trichomonosis (*Trichnomonas fetus*)

Clinical signs and lesions: Vaginitis in cow, balanitis in bull, endometritis, placentitis, ***early abortions,*** sterility, ***pyometra***.

Collection of material: Fetal stomach contents, vaginal swabs

5. Trypanosomosis/ Surra (*Trypanosoma evansi*)

Clinical signs and lesions: Intermittent fever, gradual emaciation, parasitemia, serous nasal discharge, patchy alopecia, Petechiae on visceral mucosa, incoordination, edema of limbs prostration, ***icterus***, progressive ***anemia***

Collection of material: Blood smear

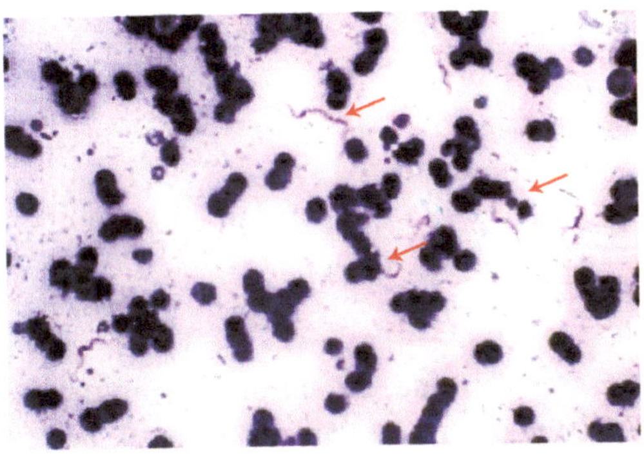

6. Leishmaniasis (*Leismania donovani*)

Clinical signs and lesions: Fever, loss of weight, anemia, cutaneous ulcers, emaciation, enlarged lymph node, spleen, liver, pallor mucous membrane, ulcers in intestines, Leishmania in large macrophages, fibrosis in lymph nodes, In cutaneous forms, nodules on dermis are filled by macrophages, lymphocytes, plasma cells.

Collection of material: Blood smear

7. Babesiosis (*Babesia bigemina*)

Clinical signs and lesions: *Cattle:* Fever, red colour urine, ***hemoglobinuria***, emaciation, thin and watery red tinged plasma, subcutaneous yellow and edematus (swelling), gastroenteritis, icterus, enlarged spleen, hepatomegaly, distended gall bladder, urinary bladder, contain red urine, hemolytic anemia. *Equines:* Fever, anemia, icterus, weakness, hemoglobinuria, subcutaneous edema, ***erythrophagocytosis***, hyperplasia of lymphoid cells in spleen, bone marrow, liver. Hydropericardium, hydrothorax, ascites.

Collection of material: Blood smear

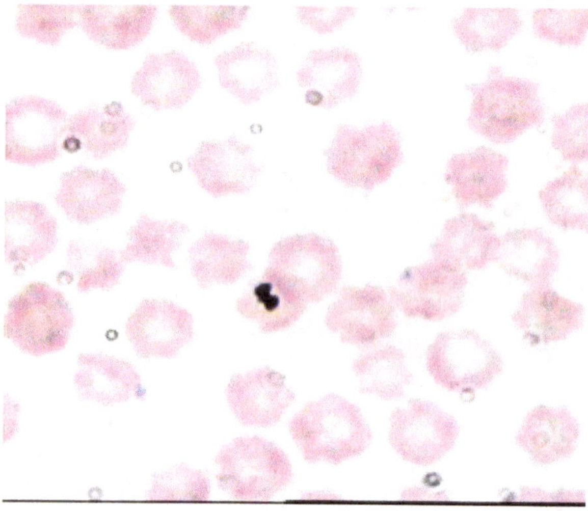

8. Theileriosis (*Theileria annulata*)

Clinical signs and lesions: Fever, loss of appetite, cessation of rumination, reduction in milk production, ***enlargement of superficial lymph nodes***, pulmonary edema, emaciation, coma, anemia leucopenia, emphysema, mottled, yellowish liver, white foci on kidneys, congestion of meninges, focal hemorrhage in brain.

Collection of material: Blood smear

9. Anaplasmosis (*Anaplasma marginale*)

Clinical signs and lesions: ***Anemia***, pallor mucous membrane, icterus, spleen and liver enlarged, gall bladder distended, petechiae on pericardium, catarrhal inflammation of intestines, anaplasma organism in the erythrocytes of peripheral blood.

Collection of material: Blood smear

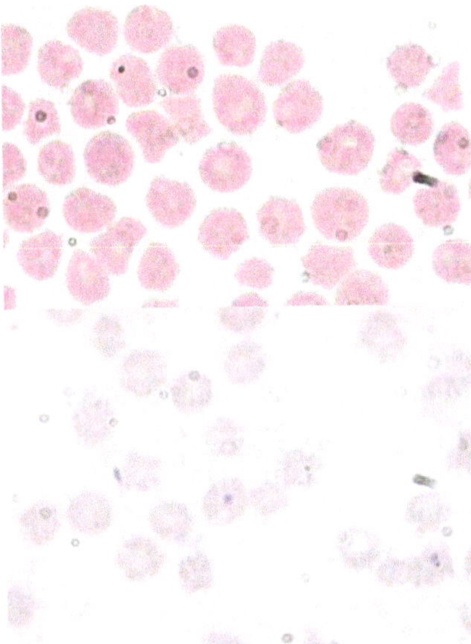

10. Fascioliasis/ Distomiasis (*Fasciola* sp. *Dicrocoelium* sp.)

Clinical signs and lesions: Chronic diarrhoea, debility, anemia, submandibular edema "***bottle jaw***" pot belly (ascites), thickening of wall of bile duct, hydropericardium.

Collection of material: Faecal samples

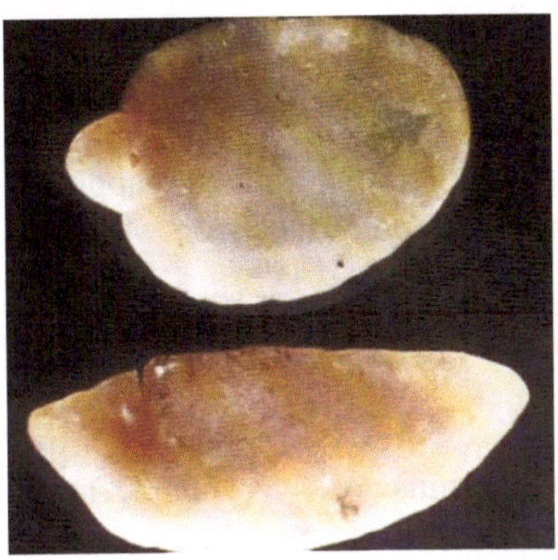

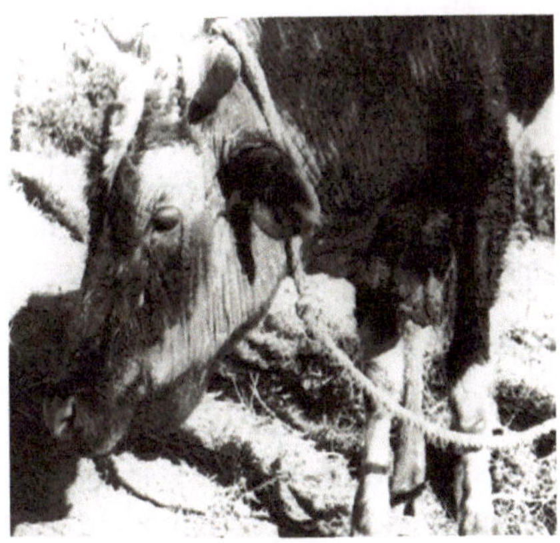

11. Amphistomiasis (*Paramphistomum* sp. *Gigantocotyle* sp *Cotylophoron* sp)

Clinical signs and lesions: Weakness, emaciation, diarrhoea, pale mucous membrane, submaxillary edema, hypoglycemia, flesh coloured flukes "***amphistomes*" *in rumen***, abomasum, duodenum and jejunum, hydropericardium, fat depots are gelatinous, mucosa on intestines becomes thickened, catarhal enteritis.

Collection of material: Fecal samples and rumen contents

12. Schistosomosis (*Schistosoma* sp.)

Clinical signs and lesions: ***Nasal granuloma*** in cattle, minute ulcers in nasal cavity, granulomatous growth in nasal passage causing snoring sound, profuse nasal discharge, pseudotubercles in tissues, parasitic ova in centre and surrounded by macrophages, lymphocytes, giant cells.

Collection of material: Feces and nasal discharge

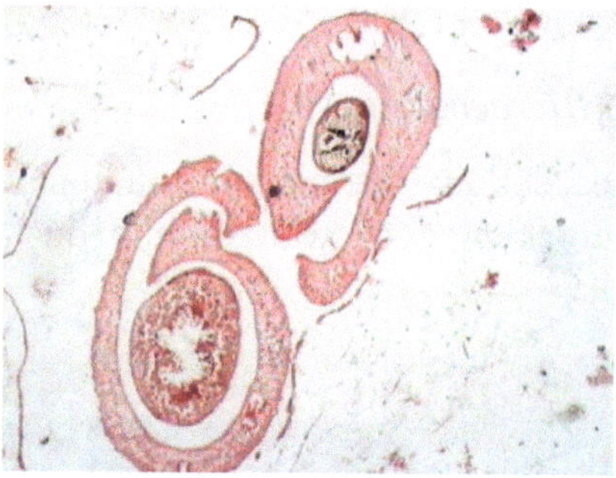

13. Teniasis (Tape worms)

Clinical signs and lesions: Abdominal pain, enteritis, reduced appetite, diarrhoea, emaciation, and irritation, anemia, bloody diarrhoea. Anemia, emaciation and diarrhoea in poultry.

Collection of material: Fecal samples

14. Hydatid disease (*Cysticercus* sp.)

Clinical signs and lesions: Hydatid cysts in muscle, liver, heart, lungs diaphragm in cattle, pigs, sheep and goat

Collection of material: Hydatid cyst

15. Ascariasis (*Neoascaris* sp., *Ascaris* sp., *Parascaris* sp., *Toxocara* sp., *Ascaridia* sp.)

Clinical signs and lesions: Catarrhal enteritis, obstruction in intestines, anemia, emaciation, bloody diarrhoea, ***eosinophilia***, eosinophilic granulomatous lesions in liver, lungs due to migrating larvae.

Collection of material: Fecal samples

16. Strongylosis (*Strongylus* sp.)

Clinical signs and lesions: Diarrhoea, loose foul smelling feces, debility, anemia, edema of lower parts of body, ***thrombosis in anterior mesenteric artery, colic***, petechiae, erosions and thickening of cecal mucosa, catarrhal enteritis, nodules in mucosa and sub-mucosa of cecum.

Collection of material: Fecal samples.

17. Ancylostomiosis (Hook worms)

Clinical signs and lesions: Anemia, weakness, shedding of wool, pallor of mucous membrane, pot belly, diarrhoea, ascites, "***bottle jaw***" condition, enteritis, blood tinged intestinal contents.

Collection of material: Fecal samples

18. Parasitic gastritis (Stomach worms)

Clinical signs and lesions: Anemia, diarrhoea, emaciation, edema of dependent parts, pallor mucous membranes, ***chronic catarrhal gastritis***, hydropericardium, hydrothorax, hyperplastic bone marrow.

Collection of material: Fecal samples

19. Trichinellosis (*Trichinella spiralis*)

Clinical signs and lesions: Catarrhal gastritis, catarrhal enteritis, edema of eyelids, eosinophilia

Collection of material: Fecal samples

20. Trichuriasis (*Trichuris* sp.)

Clinical signs and lesions: Loss of weight, diarrhoea, blood stained feces, anemia-microcytic hypochromic, jaundice.

Collection of material: Fecal samples

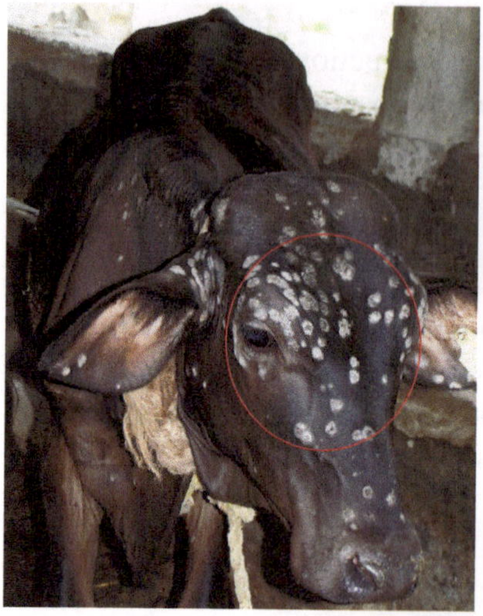

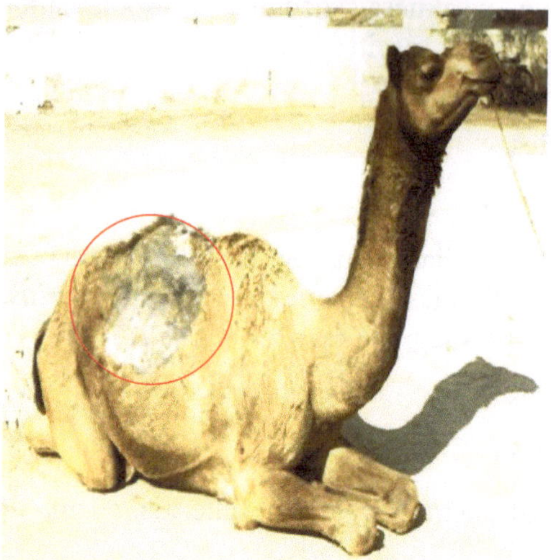

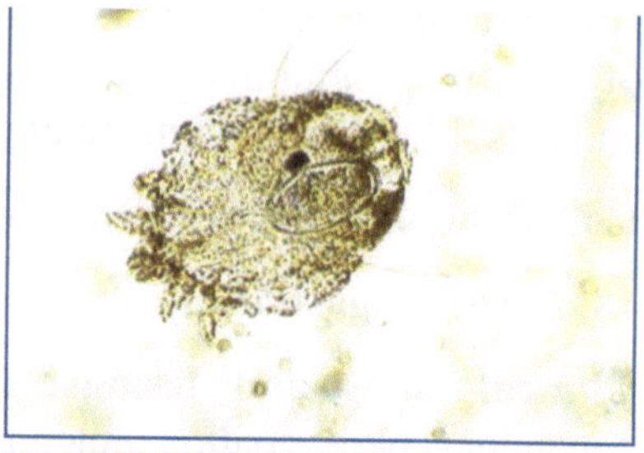

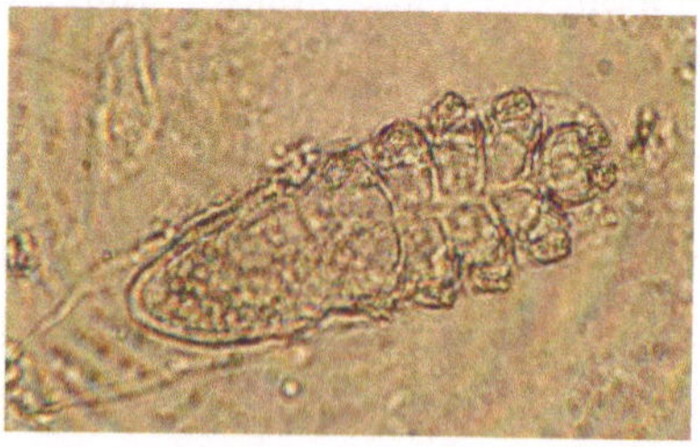

21. Mange

Clinical signs and lesions: Intense itching, Red papular eruptions or abrasion wounds in skin, Loss of hairs, Thickening of skin, Loss of shining of skin and hairs, Hyperkeratosis, Scratch wounds.

Collection of material: Skin scraping

F. Toxic Conditions

1. Cyanide poisoning

Clinical signs and lesions: Convulsions, froth in mouth, gasping, dilated pupils, diarrhoea, micturition, gastroenteritis, focal necrosis in white and grey matter of brain, bright red colour of blood persists for several hours, sub-epicardial and ***sub endocardial hemorrhages***. Prostration, staggering, muscular tremors, paralysis of hind quarters, albuminuria, hematuria, ulcers in abomasum.

Collection of material: Stomach contents, fodder and blood samples

2. Arsenic poisoning

Clinical signs and lesions: Gastritis, enteritis, hemorrhages in intestines, abdominal pain, vomiting, diarrhoea, incoordination, convulsions, ***toxic hepatitis***.

Collection of material: Plants, stomach contents, blood, liver Preserved in 1% solution of mercuric chloride.

3. Mercury poisoning

Clinical signs and lesions: Diarrhoea, hypersalivation, polyuria followed by anuria, muscular tremors, itching on skin, ulcers in stomach, ***cooked appearance of oral mucosa***, nephrosis, hydrothorax, hydropericardium endocardial hemorrhage, perforation in cecum.

Collection of material: Stomach contents

4. Lead toxicity

Clinical signs and lesions: Hypersalivation, grinding of teeth, abdominal pain, diarrhoea, hemorrhage in stomach, intestines, congestion and hemorrhage in kidneys, petechiae on endocardium and epicardium, congestion of meninges. Anemia, ataxia, tremors, blindness, convulsions, laryngeal paralysis leading to roaring respiratory noise.

Collection of material: Blood, urine stomach contents and tissue samples

5. Zinc phosphide toxicity

Clinical signs and lesions: Abdominal pain, animal lethargic with vomiting and convulsions.

Accumulation of gas in stomach, coma, enlargement of heart with dark coloured blood, pulmonary edema, hemorrhage in intestines, congestion of liver, kidneys, endocardial hemorrhage.

Collection of material: Stomach contents

6. Phenol toxicity

Clinical signs and lesions: Depression, shock paralysis, coma, staggering, dilation of pupils, tonic/ clonic muscular spasms, mucous membrane of oral cavity becomes white, coagulative necrosis of the affected tissues, pneumonia, pleuritis, ***cirrhosis*** of liver, gastroenteritis, mucosa of stomach shows coagulative necrosis.

Collection of material: Stomach contents and tissue samples

7. Nitrate/ nitrite

Clinical signs and lesions: Hemolytic anemia, gastroenteritis, depression, cyanosis, dyspnoea, rapid pulse, diarrhoea, convulsions, coma, dark brown colour blood, ***cyanotic mucous membrane***, congestion and hemorrhage in stomach, intestines, serosanguinous pericardial fluid, congestion of liver and kidneys.

Collection of material: Fodder, stomach contents, blood in ice

8. Organochlorine pesticides poisoning

Clinical signs and lesions: Nervous hyperexcitability, muscular twitching convulsions, hypersalivation, abnormal postures, grinding of teeth, cyanosis, congestion of liver, lung and kidneys, blood mixed frothy exudate in trachea and bronchi, congestion of meninges, hemorrhage in endocardium and epicardium. Increased cerebrospinal fluid, enteritis, dehydration, depletion of fat deposits.

Collection of material: Stomach contents, blood and serum samples

9. Organophosphate pesticide poisoning

Clinical signs and lesions: Nausea, abdominal pain, vomiting, diarrhoea, dyspnoea, sweating, muscular twitching, paralysis, convulsions, coma, hemorrhage in heart, lung, gastrointestinal mucosa, pulmonary edema, axonal degeneration, demyelination, degeneration in liver, kidneys, decreased cholinesterase level.

Collection of material: Stomach contents, serum and blood samples

10. Carbamate pesticide poisoning

Clinical signs and lesions: Hypersalivation, increased respiration lacrimation, urination, diarrrhoea, muscular tremors, constriction of pupil, pallor mucous membranes, nausea, vomiting, ataxia. Tachycardia/ Bradycardia, convulsions, incoordination of legs, hepatic necrosis, depletion of lymphocytes in spleen, lymph nodes hemorrhages and congestion in intestines, kidneys, lungs. Lymphocytic infiltration and congestion of meninges. Hyperglycemia, decreased cholinesterase activity.

Collection of material: Stomach content, blood and serum samples

11. Synthetic pyrethroid pesticide poisoning

Clinical signs and lesions: Hyperexcitability, muscular tremors, incoordination, hypersalivation, gastroenteritis, nasal discharge, hyperglycemia, vomiting, convulsions, pallor mucous membrane, abdominal pain, redness of conjunctiva, tongue, lips. Enlargement of liver, axonal edema, degeneration of nerve fibers, depletion of lymphoid tissue in spleen. Immunosuppressive effect.

Collection of material: Fat tissue, liver, stomach contents, blood in ice, blood and serum samples

12. Phenothiazine toxicity

Clinical signs and lesions: ***Photosensitization***, hemolytic anemia, jaundice, ***hemoglobinuria***, diarrhoea, colic, corneal ulceration, abortion, prostration, coma, hepatomegaly, spleenomegaly, edema of kidneys, dark coloured urine in urinary bladder, dermatitis.

Collection of material: Stomach content and urine samples

13. Thalium toxicity

Clinical signs and lesions: Vomiting, diarrhoea, respiratory distress, conjunctivitis, paralysis of esophagus, erythema, adominal pain, ***ulcers in stomach*** and intestines, lymphopenia, eosinopenia, neutrophilia, shift to left, acanthosis and parakeratosis, intraepithelial abscess, congestion of dermal capillaries, purulent brounchopneumonia, ulceration in esophagus, carrdiac hypertrophy, subendocardial hemorrhage, enlargement of spleen.

Collection of material: Stomach contents and skin tissue samples

14. Lantana poisoning (*Lantana camera* plant)

Clinical signs and lesions: Edema of face, ear, redness of muzzle, bloody diarrhoea, ***icterus, hemorrhagic gastroenteritis***, subcutaneous edema, epicardial hemorrhage, swollen liver, distended gall bladder, enlarged hepatocytes, vacuolar degeneration in kidney tubular epithelium, hylaine casts, ***bilirubinuria***, uremia.

Collection of material: Stomach contents plants and urine samples

15. Ratti poisoning

Clinical signs and lesions: Needle can be seen in skin, ***profuse swelling and congestion at the site of needle prick***, hypersalivation, nasal discharge, clonic convulsions, incoordination of legs, congestion and edema, subcutaneously, Enlargement and edematous lymph nodes, petechiae on endocardium.

Collection of material: Serum and blood samples

16. Ergot poisoning

Clinical signs and lesions: Incoordination of legs, staggering, hyperexcitability, convulsions, diarrhoea, paralysis, coma, blindness, lameness, gangrene on extremities, ***ulceration on oral mucosa***, stomach, intestine, degeneration of neurons in brain.

Collection of material: Stomach contents

17. Warfarin poisoning

Clinical signs and lesions: Diarrhoea, vomiting, hematoma at joints, stiffness of legs, lameness, ***cyanosis of mucous membrane***, prostration, hemorrhage in intestines, liver, lungs, large quantity of unclotted blood in intestines, pallor of liver, viscera.

Collection of material: Stomach contents

18. Strychnine poisoning

Clinical signs and lesions: Stomach contents, intestinal contents, urine, liver, kidney in ice.

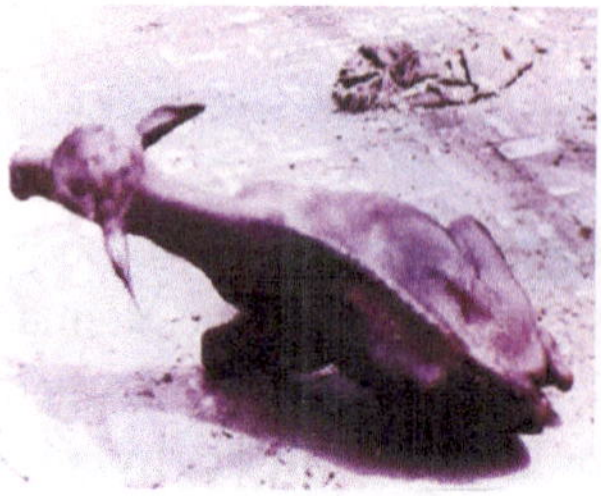
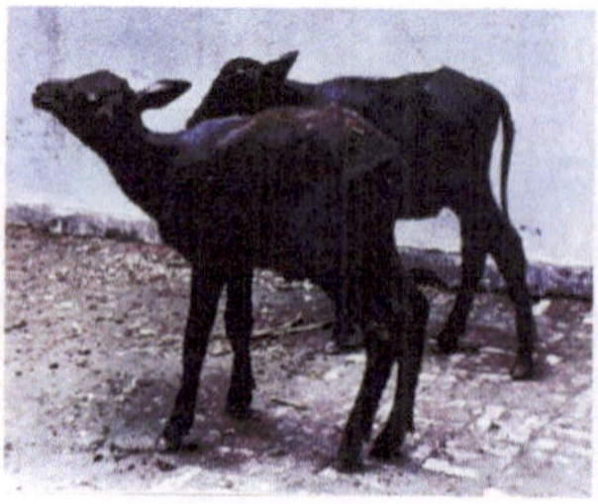
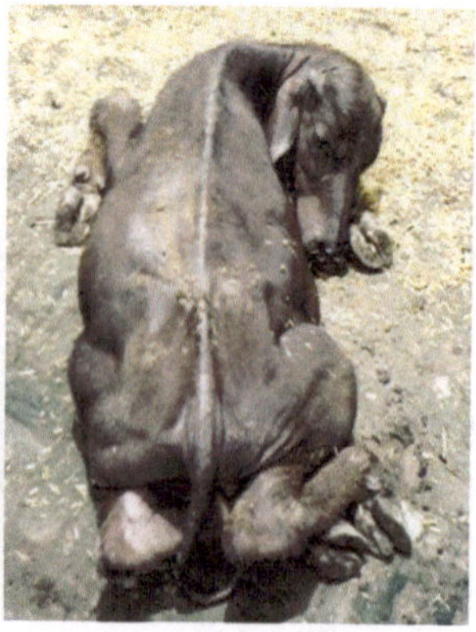

19. Bracken Fern poisoning

Clinical signs and lesions: Hematuria, Cancer in urinary bladder.

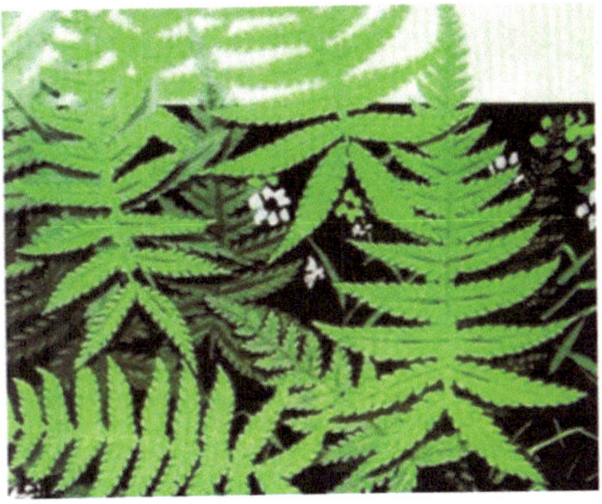

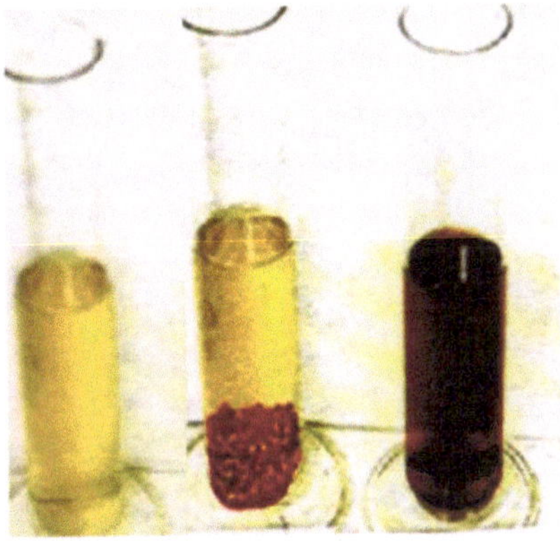

G. Miscellaneous conditions (materials for diagnosis)

	Collection of material
Encephalitis	Cerebrospinal fluid in heparinized vials, half of brain tissue in 10% formol saline, brain tissue in 50% glycerol.
Alkaloids	Liver, stomach contents and brain tissue in ice.
Diarrhoea/ Enteritis	Faecal sample in sterile vial, serum, tissues of intestine, mesenteric lymph nodes in 10% formol saline.
Abortion/ Metritis	Faetal stomach content tide off or in sterile vials, serum of dam after 21 days of abortion, vaginal discharges in sterile conditions, tissues of placenta, foetal liver, stomach, kidney in 10% formol saline.
Mastitis	Milk in sterile test tubes from all quarters separately for microbiology and California mastitis test
Pneumonia	Nasal discharge/nasal swabs, lung tissue/pieces in sterile vials, lung tissue and mediastinal lymph node in 10% formol saline.
Dermatitis	Skin scrapings in 10% KOH, skin tissue in 10% formol saline.
Nephritis	Urine sample in sterile vial, kidney tissue in 10% formol saline.

28

Miscellaneous Information for Diagnosis and Prevention of Diseases

- Epidemiological definitions
- List of tests for international trade
- OIE listed diseases
- Solutions and reagents
- Age and body weight of animals
- Rectal temperature of animals
- Normal values of blood vascular system
- Vaccination schedule

Epidemiological Definitions

Incidence: The proportion of sampled animals that develop a condition of interest over a defined period of time. It is the measure of the occurrence of disease over time in a defined group of susceptible animals. Incidence can also be applied to measuring the occurrence of new cases of disease in an ever-changing population over time.

Prevalence: The proportion of sampled animals that display a condition of interest at a given point in time. It is a single measurement of each animal in a group. It is usually a static measure in which the time is short (1-7 days).

Morbidity and Morbidity rate: *Morbidity-* The state of being diseased. The ratio of the number of sick individuals to the total susceptible population. *Morbidity rate-* Morbidity rate is the percentage/ proportions of affected animals out of total population in a particular disease outbreak. e.g. Out of 100 animals, 20 are suffering from diarrhea. The morbidity rate of diarrhea will be 20%.

Mortality and Mortality rate: *Mortality-* Death, Death rate. *Mortality rate-* Mortality rate is the percentage/ proportions of animals out of total population died due to disease outbreak. e.g. In a population of 100 animals, 20 falls sick and 5 died. The mortality rate will be 5%.

Case fatality rate: Case fatality rate is the percentage/ proportions of animals died among the affected animals. In a population of 100 animals, 20 falls sick and 5 died. The case fatality rate will be 25%.

Epidemic (Epizootic): Rapidly spreading (as a disease) so that many animals or people have it concurrently.

Pandemic: Prevalent (as a disease) throughout an entire country or continent or the world.

Panzootic: A disease, which affects all animals in an area.

Enzootic: Occurring endemically among animals, i.e., continuously prevalent among animals in a certain region.

Ecology: The study of the relation of organisms to their environment, habits, and modes of life.

Ecosystem: The complex of a living community and its environment, functioning as an ecological unit in nature.

Climate: The prevailing weather conditions that affect life.

List of Tests for International trade

Sl.No	Disease Name	Prescribed tests	Alternative tests
1.	Foot and mouth disease	ELISA*, VN	CF
2.	Vesicular stomatitis	CF, ELISA, VN	-
3.	Swine vesicular disease	VN	ELISA
4.	Rinderpest	ELISA	VN
5.	Peste des petits ruminants	VN	ELISA
6.	Contagious bovine pleuropneumonia	CF, ELISA	-
7.	Lumpy skin disease	-	VN
8.	Rift Valley fever	VN	HI, ELISA
9.	Bluetongue	Agent id., AGID, ELISA, PCR	VN
10.	Sheep pox and goat pox	-	VN
11.	African horse sickness	CF, ELISA	VN
12.	African swine fever	ELISA	IFA
13.	Classical swine fever (hog cholera)	NPLA, FAVN, ELISA	-
14.	Highly pathogenic avian influenza	-	AGID, HI
15.	Newcastle disease	-	HI

Sl.No	Disease Name	Prescribed tests	Alternative tests
16.	Anthrax	-	-
17.	Aujeszky's disease	ELISA, VN	-
18.	Echinococcosis/Hydatidosis	-	-
19.	Leptospirosis	-	MAT
20.	Rabies	VN	ELISA
21.	Paratuberculosis (Johne's disease)	-	DTH, ELISA
22.	Heartwater	-	ELISA, IFA
23.	New World screwworm (*Cochliomyia hominivorax* and Old World screwworm *Chrysomya bezziana*)	-	Agent id.
24.	Trichinellosis	Agent id.	ELISA
25.	Q fever	-	CF
26.	Leishmaniosis	-	Agent id.
27.	Bovine brucellosis	BBAT, CF, ELISA, FPA	-
28.	Bovine genital campylobacteriosis	Agent id.	-
29.	Bovine tuberculosis	Tuberculin test	-
30.	Enzootic bovine leukosis	AGID, ELISA	PCR
31.	Infectious bovine rhinotracheitis/ infectious pustular vulvovaginitis	VN, ELISA, Agent id. (semen only)	-
32.	Trichomonosis	Agent id.	Mucus agg.
33.	Bovine anaplasmosis	-	CF, Agg. Card
34.	Bovine babesiosis	-	ELISA, IFA
35.	Bovine cysticercosis	-	Agent id.
36.	Dermatophilosis	-	-
37.	Theileriosis	Agent id., IFA	-
38.	Haemorrhagic septicaemia	-	Agent id.
39.	Bovine spongiform encephalopathy	-	-
40.	Malignant catarrhal fever	-	VN, IFA, PCR
41.	Trypanosomosis (Tsetse-transmitted)	-	IFA
42.	Ovine epididymitis (*Brucella ovis*)	CF	ELISA
43.	Caprine and ovine brucellosis (excluding *Brucella ovis* infection)	BBAT, CF	Brucellin test, FPA
44.	Contagious agalactia	-	-
45.	Caprine arthritis/encephalitis & Maedi-visna	AGID, ELISA	-
46.	Contagious caprine pleuropneumonia	CF	-
47.	Enzootic abortion of ewes (ovine chlamydiosis)k	-	CF
48.	Scrapie	-	-

Sl.No	Disease Name	Prescribed tests	Alternative tests
49.	Ovine pulmonary adenomatosis (adenocarcinoma)	-	-
50.	Nairobi sheep disease	-	-
51.	Salmonellosis (*S.* abortusovis)	-	Agent id.
52.	Contagious equine metritis	Agent id.	-
53.	Dourine	CF	IFA, ELISA
54.	Equine encephalomyelitis (Eastern and Western)	-	HI, CF, PRN
55.	Equine infectious anaemia	AGID	ELISA
56.	Equine influenza	-	HI
57.	Equine piroplasmosis	ELISA, IFA	CF
58.	Equine rhinopneumonitis	-	VN
59.	Glanders	Mallein test, CF	-
60.	Equine viral arteritis	VN, Agent id. (semen only)	-
61.	Horse mange	-	Agent id.
62.	Venezuelan equine encephalomyelitis	-	HI, CF, PRN
63.	Epizootic lymphangitis	-	-
64.	Japanese encephalitis	-	-
65.	Surra (*Trypansoma evansi*)	-	-
66.	Atrophic rhinitis of swine	-	-
67.	Porcine brucellosis	ELISA	BBAT, FPA
68.	Enterovirus encephalomyelitis (previously Teschen/Talfan diseases)	-	VN
69.	Transmissible gastroenteritis	-	VN, ELISA
70.	Porcine reproductive and respiratory syndrome	-	ELISA, IFA, IPMA
71.	Porcine cysticercosis	-	Agent id.
72.	Infectious bursal disease (Gumboro disease)	-	AGID, ELISA
73.	Marek's disease	-	AGID
74.	Avian mycoplasmosis (*Mycoplasma gallisepticum*)	-	Agg., HI
75.	Avian chlamydiosis	-	-
76.	Fowl typhoid and Pullorum disease	-	Agg., Agent id.
77.	Avian infectious bronchitis	-	VN, HI, ELISA
78.	Avian infectious laryngotracheitis	-	AGID, VN, ELISA
79.	Avian tuberculosis	-	Tuberculin test, Agent id.,

Sl.No	Disease Name	Prescribed tests	Alternative tests
80.	Duck virus hepatitis	-	-
81.	Duck virus enteritis	-	-
82.	Fowl cholera (avian pasteurellosis)	-	-
83.	Fowl pox	-	-
84.	Myxomatosis	-	AGID, CF, IFA
85.	Tularemia	-	Agent id.
86.	Rabbit haemorrhagic disease	-	HI
87.	Acariosis of bees	-	-
88.	American foulbrood	-	-
89.	European foulbrood	-	-
90.	Nosemosis of bees	-	-
91.	Varroosis	-	-
92.	*Tropilaelaps* infestation of honey bees (*Tropilaelaps clareae, T. koenigerum*)	-	-
93.	Cysticercosis	-	Agent id.
94.	Bunyaviral diseases of animals (excluding Rift Valley fever)	-	-
95.	Salmonellosis	-	Agent id.
96.	Mange	-	Agent id.
97.	Border disease	Agent id.	-
98.	Bovine viral diarrhea	Agent id.	-
99.	West Nile encephalitis	-	-
100.	*Campylobacter jejuni* and *C. coli*	-	-
101.	Cryptosporidiosis	-	-
102.	Hendra and Nipah virus diseases	-	-
103.	Swine influenza	-	-
104.	Toxoplasmosis	-	-
105.	Verocytotoxigenic *Escherichia coli*	-	-
106.	*Listeria monocytogenes*	-	-

*Please refer to *Terrestrial Manual* chapters to verify which method is prescribed

Note: The tests prescribed by the *Terrestrial Animal Health Code* for the purposes of international trade are printed in blue in this *Terrestrial Manual.*

Abbreviations

Agent id.	Agent identification	HI	Haemagglutination inhibition
Agg.	Agglutination test	IFA	Indirect fluorescent antibody
AGID	Agar gel immunodiffusion	IPMA	Immunoperoxidase monolayer assay
BBAT	Buffered *Brucella* antigen test	MAT	Microscopic agglutination test
CF	Complement fixation	NPLA	Neutralizing peroxidase-linked assay
DTH	Delayed-type hypersensitivity	PCR	Polymerase chain reaction

Agent id.	Agent identification	HI	Haemagglutination inhibition
ELISA	Enzyme-linked immunosorbent assay	PRN	Plaque reduction neutralization
FAVN	Fluorescent antibody virus neutralization	VN	Virus neutralization

OIE Listed Diseases

Earlier, the member countries made use of lists of diseases notifiable to the OIE. There were previously 2 lists, List A and List B. The list A diseases were accorded higher priority being of nature with chances of quicker spread and heavy losses.

Whether a disease, which was earlier included in List "A" and "B" is to remain in the new single list or it has to be deleted or a new disease has to be added in this new list has been decided (and would be decided on a continuous basis) on the basis of a decision-making model based upon 4 basic criteria: a) International spread, b) Significant spread within naive populations, c) Zoonotic potential, and d) Emerging diseases.

The decision-making model and the decision tree application are described in the Terrestrial Animal Health Code available on OIE website. Each disease of list was evaluated on its potential of international spread, than its zoonotic potential.

The revision which has been made in previous list(s) on the basis of the laid out criteria has resulted in deletion some diseases from the list. Several new emerging diseases have been added. There has been a change in name of some ailments and a change also in the species category of others. The single list finally approved by the International Committee is included in Article 2.1.1.3 of the code.

The new list is given below:

1) Category of multiple species diseases

- Anthrax
- Aujeszky's disease
- Bluetongue
- Brucellosis *(Brucella abortus)*
- Brucellosis *(Brucella melitensis)*
- Brucellosis *(Brucella suis)*

- Crimean Congo haemorrhagic fever
- Echinococcosis/ hydatidosis
- Foot and mouth disease
- Heartwater
- Japanese encephalitis
- Leptospirosis
- New world screwworm *(Cochliomyia hominivorax)*
- Old world screwworm *(Chrysomya bezziana)*
- Paratuberculosis
- Q-fever
- Rabies
- Rinderpest
- Rift Valley fever
- Trichinellosis
- Tularemia
- Vesicular stomatitis
- West Nile fever

2) Category of cattle diseases

- Bovine anaplasmosis
- Bovine babesiosis
- Bovine genital campylobacteriosis
- Bovine spongiform encephalopathy
- Bovine viral diarrhoea
- Bovine tuberculosis
- Contagious bovine pleuropneumonia
- Enzootic bovine leukosis
- Haemorrhagic septicaemia
- Infectious bovine rhinotracheitis/infectious pustular vulvovaginitis

- Lumpy skin disease
- Malignant catarrhal fever
- Theileriosis
- Trichomonosis
- Trypanosomosis (Tsetse-transmitted)

3) Category of sheep and goat diseases

- Caprine arthritis/encephalitis
- Contagious agalactia
- Contagious caprine pleuropneumonia
- Enzootic abortion of ewes (Ovine chlamydiosis)
- Nairobi sheep disease
- Maedi-visna
- Ovine epididymitis *(Brucella ovis)*
- Peste des petits ruminants
- Salmonellosis *(S. abortusovis)*
- Scrapie
- Sheep pox and goat pox

4) Category of equine diseases

- African horse sickness
- Contagious equine metritis
- Dourine
- Equine encephalomyelitis (Eastern)
- Equine encephalomyelitis (Western)
- Equine infectious anaemia
- Equine influenza
- Equine piroplasmosis
- Equine rhinopneumonitis
- Equine viral arteritis

- Glanders
- Surra *(Trypanosoma evansi)*
- Venezuelan equine encephalomyelitis

5) Category of swine diseases

- African swine fever
- Classical swine fever
- Nipah virus encephalitis
- Porcine cysticercosis
- Porcine reproductive and respiratory syndrome
- Swine vesicular disease
- Transmissible gastroenteritis

6) Category of avian diseases

- Avian chlamydiosis
- Avian infectious bronchitis
- Avian infectious laryngotracheitis
- Avian mycoplasmosis (M. *gallisepticum*)
- Avian mycoplasmosis (M. *synoviae*)
- Duck virus hepatitis
- Fowl cholera
- Fowl typhoid
- Highly pathogenic avian influenza
- Infectious bursal disease (Gumboro disease)
- Marek's disease
- Newcastle disease
- Pullorum disease
- Turkey rhinotracheitis

There are three more categories of diseases, diseases of Bees, of lagomorphs (rabbits and hares) and camel. Six diseases have been included in the list of

Bee diseases whereas Camel pox and Leishmaniosis have been included in camel category. Two viral diseases Myxomatosis and Rabbit haemorrhagic disease have been included in the category of lagomorphs.

The Report of OlE Terrestrial Animal Health Standards Commission/January 2005 with the report of the OlE Ad-hoc Group on Diseases/ Pathogenic agents, notification on a new list of terrestrial Animal diseases is surely a culmination of insights of renowned international experts on the animal diseases. It is hoped that new method and technology used in notification will serve to better disease management across continents.

OIE List of Disease

Sl. No.	OIE list of Diseases	Sl. No.	OIE list of Diseases
	List A Diseases		
1.	Foot and mouth disease **(NB: version adopted May 2006)**	25	Leishmaniosis
2.	Vesicular stomatitis	**Bovine Diseases in List B**	
3.	Swine vesicular disease	27	Bovine brucellosis
4.	Rinderpest	28.	Bovine genital campylobacteriosis
5.	Peste des petits ruminants	29.	Bovine tuberculosis
6.	Contagious bovine pleuropneumonia	30.	Enzootic bovine leukosis
7.	Lumpy skin disease	31.	Infectious bovine rhinotracheitis / Infectious pustular vulvovaginitis
8.	Rift valley fever	32.	Trichomonosis
9.	Bluetongue	33.	Bovine anaplasmosis
10.	Sheep pox and goat pox	34.	Bovine babesiosis
11.	African horse sickness	35.	Bovine cysticercosis
12.	African swine fever	36.	Dermatophilosis
13.	Classical swine fever (hog cholera)	37.	Theileriosis
14.	Avian influenza (**NB: version adopted May 2005**)	38.	Haemorrhagic septiaemia (**NB: version adopted May 2005**)
15.	Newcastle disease	39.	Bovine spongiform encephalopathy
16.	**Multispecies Diseases in List B**	40.	Malignant catarrhal fever
17.	Anthrax	41.	Trypanosomosis (tsetse-transmitted)
18.	Aujeszky's disease		**Sheep and Goat Diseases in List B**
19.	Echinococcosis/hydatidosis	42.	Ovine epididymitis (*Brucella ovis*)
20.	Leptospirosis	43.	Caprine and ovine brucellosis (excluding *Brucella ovis*)
21.	Rabies	44.	Contagious agalactia
	Paratuberculosis (Johne's disease)	45.	Caprine arthritis/encephalitis & Maedi-visna
23	Heartwater	46.	Contagious caprine pleuropneumonia

Sl. No.	OIE list of Diseases List A Diseases	Sl. No.	OIE list of Diseases
24	New World screwworm *(Cochliomyia hominivorax)* and Old World screwworm *(Chrysomya bezziana)*	47.	Enzootic abortion of ewes (ovine chlamydiosis)
48.	Trichinellosis	73.	Scrapie
49.	Q fever	74.	Ovine pulmonary adenomatosis (adenocarcinoma)
50.	Nairobi sheep disease	75.	Avian infectious bronchitis
51.	Salmonellosis (S. abortusovis)	76.	Avian infectious laryngotracheitis
Equine Diseases in List B		77.	Avian tuberculosis
52.	Contagious equine metritis **(NB version adopted May 2005)**	78.	Duck virus hepatitis
53.	Dourine	79.	Duck virus enteritis
54.	Equine encephalomyelitis (Eastern and Western)	80.	Fowl cholera (avian pasteurellosis)
55.	Equine infectious anaemia	81.	Fowl pox
56.	Equine influenza		**Lagomorph Diseases in List B**
57.	Equine piroplasmosis	82.	Myxomatosis
58.	Equine rhinopneumonitis	84.	Tularemia
59.	Glanders	85.	Rabbit haemorrhagic disease
60.	Horse pox	86.	BEE Diseases in List B
61.	Equine viral arteritis	87.	Introductory note on bee diseases
62.	Horse mange	88.	Acariosis of bees
63.	Venezuelan equine encephalomyelitis	89.	American foulbrood
64.	Epizootic lymphangitis	90.	European foulbrood
65.	Japanese encephalitis	91.	Nosemosis of bees
66.	Surra (*Trypanosoma evansi*)	92.	Varroosis
Swine Diseases in List B		93.	Tropilaelaps infestation of honey bees (*Tropilaelaps clareae, T. koenigerum*)
67.	Atrophic rhinitis of swine	94.	Fowl typhoid and Pullorum disease
68.	Porcine brucellosis	95.	Swine influenza
69.	Enterovirus encephalomyelitis (previously Teschen/Talfan diseases)	96.	Toxoplasmosis
70.	Transmissible gastroenteritis	97.	Verocytotoxigenic *Escherichia coli*
71.	Porcine reproductive and respiratory syndrome	98.	*Listeria monocytogenes*
72.	Porcine cysticercosis		
Diseases Not Covered by List A and B			
99.	Infectious bursal disease (Gumboro disease)	106.	Mange
100.	Marek's disease	107.	Border disease
101.	Avian mycoplasmosis *(Mycoplasma gallisepticum)*	108.	Bovine viral diarrhoea

Sl. No.	OIE list of Diseases List A Diseases	Sl. No.	OIE list of Diseases
102.	Avian chlamydiosis	109.	West Nile encephalitis
103.	Cysticercosis	110.	*Campylobacter jejuni* and *Campylobacter coli*
104.	Bunyaviral diseases of animals (excluding Rift Valley fever)	111.	Crytosporidiosis
105.	Salmonellosis	112.	Hendra and Nipah virus diseases

Solutions and Reagents

1. Normal Saline Solution (NSS)

Sodium chloride : 0.85gm

Distilled Water : 100ml

2. Phosphate buffered saline (PBS)

Sodium Chloride : 8gm

Potassium Chloride : 0.2gm

Disodium hydrogen Phosphate (Na_2HPO_4) : 1.44gm

Potassium di hydrogen Orthophosphate (KH_2PO_4) : 0.24

Distilled water : 1000ml

Dissolve in 100ml of distilled water and adjust the pH to 7.4, if required. Make the final volume to 1000ml. Dispense the solution into aliquots and sterilize them by autoclaving for 20 minutes at 15lb psi. store at room temperature

3. 50% Buffered Glycerine saline

PBS (pH – 7.4) : 50 parts

Glycerin : 50 parts

4. 25% Buffered glycerine saline:

PBS (pH – 7.4) : 75 parts

Glycerine : 25 parts

5. 10% Formal Saline

Formaldehyde (40%) : 100ml

Sodium chloride : 8.5gm

Distilled water : 900ml

Duration of fixation is 24 to 48 hours. Keeping quality of the solution is poor. This is not used as a routine fixative because of poor nuclear chromatin staining.

6. 10% Buffered neutral formalin

Formaldehyde	: 100ml
Distilled water	: 900ml
Sodium dihydrogen phosphate	: 4gm
Disodium hydrogen phosphate	: 6.5gm

Duration of fixation is 24 to 48 hrs. It is best overall fixative and recommended for routine use.

7. Zenker's fluid:

Potassium dichromate	: 25gm
Mercuric chloride	: 50gm
Sodium sulphate	: 10gm
Distilled water	: 1000ml
Glacial acetic acid	: 50ml (Added just before use)

Potassium dichromate and mercuric chloride are dissolved in the distilled water by heating. After cooling the solution it is filtered and stored as a stock solution without adding glacial acetic acid.

Duration of fixation is 3 to 18 hours. Used for hard tissues.

8. Boun's fluid

Saturated aquous picric acid	: 750ml
Formaldehyde	: 250ml
Glacial acetic acid	: 50ml

Duration of fixation is 6 to 24 hours or longer. Best fixative for nuclear details, spleen, lymph nodes and other glandular structures.

Hank's Medium

Hank's Solution –I

NaCl	:	80 g
KCl	:	4 g
$MgSO_4$, $7H_2O$	:	2 g
$CaCl_2$, $2H_2O$	:	1.85 g or $CaCl_2$ - 0.7 g
Distilled water up to	:	1000 ml

Hank's Solution –II

Na_2HPO_4, $2H_2O$	:	0.75 g
or		
Na_2HPO_4, $12H_2O$	:	1.5 g
KH_2PO_4	:	0.65 g
Dextrose	:	20 g
Phenol red (0.4%)	:	50 ml
or		
Phenol red (1%)	:	20 ml

Hank's Solution –III

$NaHCO_3$	:	1.4 g
Distilled water	:	100 ml

Hanks I and II are autoclaved separately at 15 lbs pressure for 30 min and kept at 4°C till use. Hanks III is to be prepared fresh before adding it to the Hanks medium.

Hank's maintenance medium

Lactalbumin hydrolysate	:	5 g
Yeast extract	:	0.5 g
Hanks I	:	100 ml
Hanks II	:	100 ml
Hanks III	:	25 ml

Penicillin : 1 lakh units

Streptomycin : 0.2 g

Distilled water up to : 1000 ml

The medium is sterilized by passing through EKS filter pads.

Hank's growth medium

Lactalbumin hydrolysate : 5 g

Yeast extract : 0.5 g

Hanks I : 100 ml

Hanks II : 100 ml

Hanks III : 25 ml

Serum : 120 ml

Penicillin : 1 lakh units

Streptomycin : 0.2 g

Distilled water upto : 1000 ml

The medium is sterilized by passing through EKS filter pads.

Preparation of Phenol red

10 g of phenol red powder dissolved in 300 ml of 0.1 N NaOH. Solution is filtered and stored in the refrigerator.

Glycine buffer, pH 9.5-10.5

Sodium hydroxide : 5.1 g

Sodium chloride : 104 g

Glycine : 156 g

Distilled water up to : 1000 ml

Alsever's solution

Dextrose : 29.50 g

Sodium chloride : 4.20 g

Sodium citrate : 8.00 g

Citric acid : 0.55 g

Distilled water up to : 1000 ml

Phosphate buffer saline

PBS (Solution A)

NaCl	: 64 g
KCl	: 1.6 g
$Na_2HPO_{4,}$ $7H_2O$	: 17.36 g
KH_2PO_4	: 1.6 g
Distilled water	: 6400 ml

PBS (Solution B)

Calcium chloride	: 0.8 g
Distilled water	: 800 ml

PBS (Solution C)

Magnesium chloride ($MgCl_2$, 6 H_2O)	: 1.7 g
Distilled water	: 800 ml

All the solutions (A, B and C) are sterilized separately at 20 lbs at 115°C for 30 minutes in an autoclave.

Final preparation of Phosphate Buffer Solution (PBS)

After cooling, add solution B to A and then C to BA. 1 lakh I.U. of crystalline penicillin 100 mg of dihydro-streptomycin per litre of PBS are added with sterile precautions. This is finally distributed in smaller flasks of 100, 250 and 500 ml capacities and stored in refrigerator.

Trypsin-versene solution

NaCl	: 10 g
KCl	: 0.250 g
Na_2HPO_4	: 1.90g
KH_2PO_4	: 0.25g
Trypsin	: 1.7g
EDTA	: 1.4 g
0.4% Pheno red	: 1 ml
Distilled water	: 1000 ml

Mix the contents by putting it on a magnetic stirrer and filer it through disposable filter (0.22 μ) and dispensed in sterilized container and keep at –20°C until further use.

Virus transport medium

The two common virus transport media used are (1) 50% glycerine phosphate buffer saline, and (2) Hank's balanced salt solution (HBSS) containing 0.5% bovine serum albumin or 1% FCS and antibiotics.

BSA (fraction V)	: 5 g
or	
FCS	: 10 ml
Penicillin	: 10 lakhs units
Streptomycin	: 1 g
Mycostatin	: 25,000 units
HBSS	: 1000 ml

Adjust the pH 7.0 and sterilize by membrane filtration and aliquot into screw capped glass vials. As soon as the specimen is collected, it should be maintained at an optimum pH (7.2 – 7.4) and should be transported on ice to the laboratory.

Serum

Serum from foetal or adult origin is available from commercial companies. The serum should be heat inactivated at 56°C for ½ hr in a water bath and then kept frozen at -20°C until further use.

10% sodium bicarbonate solution

$NaHCO_3$	: 100 g
Distilled water	: 1000 ml

Dissolve the sodium bicarbonate in 1000 ml of distilled water. Filter sterilize and dispense in sterile bottles. Store at 4°C until further use.

Trypan blue (0.4%) for viable counts

Trypan blue stain	: 0.2 g
Normal saline solution	: 50 ml

Dissolve the trypan blue in 50 ml NSS. Filter and aliquot in 5-10 ml quantity. Store at room temperature. It is also available as a 0.4% trypan blue solution.

Age and Body Weight of Animals

Animal	Body weight at maturity (kg)	Age at maturity	Life span (yrs)	Weight at birth (kg)
Cattle (*Bos taurus/indicus*)	464-653	5 yrs	20-25	25-45
Horse (*Equus caballus*)	450	3-5 yrs	20-25	45-55
Sheep (*Ovies aries*)	34-80	2 yrs	10-18	2.0-4.0
Goat (*Capra hircus*)	26-102	2 yrs	10-15	2.5-3.5
Swine (*Sus scrofa*)	70-128	-	16-18	1.0-2.0
Chicken (*Gallus domesticus*)	1.5-3.3	20-30 wks	2-5	0.049-0.065
Rabbit (*Oryctolagus cuniculus*)	3.0-4.9	1 yr	5-8	0.04-0.08
Turkey (*Meleagris gallapavo*)	5.0-14.8	28-35 wks	-	0.52-0.56

Rectal Temperature of Animals

Animal	°C	°F
Beef cow	38.3 (36.7-39.1)	101 (98.0-102.4)
Camel	37.5 (34.2-40.7)	99.5 (93.6-105.3)
Cat	38.6 (38.1-39.2)	101.5 (100.6-102.5)
Chicken	41.7 (40.6-43.0)	107.1 (105.0-109.4)
Dairy cow	38.6 (38.0-39.3)	101.5 (100.4-102.8)
Dog	38.9 (37.9-39.9)	102 (100.2-103.8)
Donkey	37.4 (36.4-38.4)	99.3 (97.5-101.1)
Goat	39.1 (38.5-39.7)	102.3 (101.3-103.5)
Mare	37.8 (37.3-38.2)	100 (99.1-100.8)
Pig	39.2 (38.7-39.8)	102.5 (101.6-103.6)
Rabbit	39.5 (38.1-40.1)	103.1 (101.5-104.2)
Sheep	39.1 (38.3-39.9)	102.3 (100.9-103.8)
Stallion	37.6 (37.2-38.1)	99.7 (99.0-100.6)

Normal Values of Blood Vascular System

Parameters	Cow	Horse	Sheep	Dog	Pig
RBC Count (million/µl)	7	7	11	7	7
White cell count (10^3/µl)	9	9	8	12	15
Hemoglobin (gm/dl)	12	12.5	11	13.5	12
Hematocrit (Volume % of red cells)	40	42	32	45	42
Sedimentation rate	0/30 0/60	2 to 12/10 15 to 20/30	0/30 0/60	1 to 6/30 5 to 25/60	0 to 6/30 1 to 40/60

Parameters	Cow	Horse	Sheep	Dog	Pig
Coagulation time (min)	6.5	11.5	2.5	25	3.5
Blood pH	7.3 (7.20-7.55)	7.4 (7.35-7.43)	-	7.5 (7.32-7.68)	7.4
Specific gravity	1.043	1.060	1.042	1.059	1.060
Heart rate/ min average & range	60-70	32-44	70-80	70-120	60-80
Blood pressure (mm Hg, syst/ diast)	134/88	80/50	114/68	148/100	169/108
Carotid pressure mm Hg	125-166	169 (159-194)	114 (90-140)	155 (120-176)	169 (144-185)
Blood volume (% of body wt.)	7.7	9.7	8.0	7.2	8.0
Diameter of red cells (µm)	5.6	5.6	5.0	7.3	6.2
DLC					
Neutrophils (%)	30	55	40	60	40
Lymphocytes (%)	60	30	50	25	50
Monocytes (%)	5	10	6	8	8
Eosinophils (%)	5	4	4	5	2
Basophils (%)	1	1	1	1	1

Vaccination Schedule

Disease	Vaccination period
A. Vaccination in cattle and buffalo	
FMD (Oil)	• 1st vaccination on 3rd week • 2nd vaccination on 3 – 3½ month • 3rd vaccination on 6th month • Then every year
FMD	• 1st vaccination in the age of 4 – 6 month • Then after every 6 month
Brucellosis	• In the age of 4 – 8 month
Black quarter	• In the age of 6 month • Then after every year
H.S.	• In the age of 6 month • Then after every year before rainy season
B. Vaccination in sheep and goat	
In pregnant sheep	• 2 months of pregnancy period • 4 months of pregnancy period
C. Vaccination in pig	

Disease	Vaccination period
Vaccine of swine fever	• 1st vaccination in the age of 6 weeks • Then after every year
D. Vaccination in dog	
Rabies	• 1st vaccination in the age of 3 months • Then after every year
Distemper	• 1st vaccination in the age of 12 weeks
Liver Infection Parvovirus infection Leptospirosis	• There is one vaccine for these 3 diseases • Vaccination in the age of 6-12 weeks
E. Vaccination in chicken	
Marek disease	• Immediately after birth in chicks
Ranikhet disease (RDF)	• 1st vaccination within 1-7 days • 2nd vaccination in between 4-5 weeks
Ranikhet disease (R2B)	• Vaccination in between 8-10 weeks
Ranikhet disease (oil emulsion and neutral)	• Vaccination in between 16-18 weeks
Chicken pox	• Vaccination in between 6-8 weeks
Gambaro disease (neutral)	• Vaccination in the age of 15-20 days • Then after 16-18 weeks
Infectious bronchitis	• Vaccination in the age of 4-16 weeks (i/v) • Then after 16-18 weeks
Infectious respiratory disease	• Vaccination in the age of 8 weeks (ILT)
Diarrhoea	• Vaccination in the age of 6 weeks

Clinical Pathology and Disease diagnosis

S.no.	Clinical Pathology Test	Name of Disease /Agent
1.	Blood smear examination	Trypanosomosis, Theileriosis, Babesiosis, Anaplasmosis, Leishmaniosis, Ehrlichiosis, Hepatozoonosis, Schistosomosis, Microfilariasis. Anthrax, Canine Distemper (inclusions in neutrophils), TRP (shift to left), Fowl spirochetosis, *Haemoproteus columbiae* (Pigeon malaria), Leukemia.
2.	Bone marrow examination	Leukemia, Chicken anaemia
3.	Serum examination for biochemical	
(i)	Hyperglycemia	Diabetes
(ii)	Hypophosphatemia	Post Parturient Haemoglobinuria, Pica, Rheumatism like syndrome
(iii)	Hypocalcimia	Osteomalacia, Rickets, Milk fever, Eclampsia in bitch, Lactation tetany in mare

4.	Urine examination	
(i)	Ketoneuria (Ketone bodies in urine)	Ketosis
(ii)	Glycosuria	Diabetes
(iii)	Haematuria	Bracken fern poisoning
(iv)	Spirochete	Leptospirosis
5.	Faecal examination	Tapeworm infestation, Liver fluke infestation, Roundworm infestation, Coccidiosis, Cryptosporidiosis, Amoebiosis, Giardiosis, Histomoniasis
6.	Milk examination	Mastitis, Brucellosis (MRT)
7.	Skin scraping examination	Mange(*Sarcoptes, Psoroptes, Chorioptes, Demodectic*), Lice infestation, Ringworm infection, Favus, Tick paralysis, Fowl spirochetosis
8.	Synovial fluid examination	Rheumatism - Presence of Ragocytes (immune complex in neutrophils)
9.	Semen examination	TB, IBR, Brucella (by PCR)
10.	Cytopathology	Cancer, Rabies (by corneal smear examination), Lymph node biopsy for Theileriosis, Rotavirus, Coronavirus, Parvovirus infection
11.	Cerebrospinal fluid examination	Trypanosomosis, Brain tumours, Listeriosis
12.	Microbiological examination	Anthrax, Hemorrhagic septicaemia, Pox

Index

D

Q

R

S

W

X

Y

Z